A MANUAL OF
MEDICAL LABORATORY TECHNOLOGY

ARVIND H. PATEL

Adjunct Professor of Microbiology

Division of Biology, Chemistry, and Physics

Essex County College

Newark, New Jersey

authorHOUSE

AuthorHouse™
1663 Liberty Drive
Bloomington, IN 47403
www.authorhouse.com
Phone: 833-262-8899

Published by AuthorHouse 05/11/2021

ISBN: 978-1-7283-0767-1 (sc)
ISBN: 978-1-7283-0766-4 (e)

Library of Congress Control Number: 2019904201

Print information available on the last page.

Table of Contents

Section I: Hematology

Section II: Clinical Chemistry

Section III: Immunology/Serology

Section IV: Clinical Microbiology

Section V: Blood Banking/Immunohematology

Section VI: Body Fluids

PREFACE TO THE SECOND EDITION

The overwhelming response to the first edition served as an impetus to work harder for the preparation of the second edition. The author has spent enough time preparing quality content to fulfill the needs of medical laboratory students and related professionals.

The author has added chapters on automation in hematology, immunohematology, and microbiology disciplines. There are over 100 neat diagrams throughout the book to facilitate the understanding of the concepts.

In chemistry, chemical reactions have been included to ease the understanding of the underlying principles. Since most chemical determinations use enzymes as reagents, a detailed description of enzymes has been included too.

To learn more about the author, please visit the website, www.mltahpatel.us.

May I assure my readers that everything possible has been done to make this title worth its name.

I earnestly request the readers of this book to feel free to make any constructive suggestions they might be inclined to do.

Arvind H. Patel, M.Sc.; MT (ASCP)

ACKNOWLEDGMENTS

I would like to thank Dr. Rakesh Panchal and Dr. Paresh Soni for their key suggestions in upgrading the quality of the material. Additionally, I am grateful to Dr. Bhairavsinh Raol, Dr. Arti Raval, Dr. Shweta Agrawal, Dr. Rachana Shukla, Dr. Harsha Soni, and Dr. Sneha Trivedi for their unlimited technical help.

Importantly, I wish to thank to Minaxi Patel for encouraging me during the preparation of this project.

Finally, I am thankful to Mahbube Akar and Jose Bautista for making images for this title.

ACKNOWLEDGMENTS

DEDICATION

This book is dedicated to my talented son, **Ravi Patel** (M.D. candidate at School of Medicine, Boston University).

Chapter 1

Scope of Medical Laboratory Technology

Definition

Medical Laboratory Technology (MLT) is a branch of medicine concerned with the performance of the laboratory determinations and analysis used in the diagnosis and treatment of diseases and the maintenance of health.

Nature of work

There are five major areas in most clinical laboratories:

A. Hematology
B. Clinical Chemistry
C. Immunology
D. Microbiology
E. Blood Banking

In a small laboratory, a medical technologist might do some work each day in each area. In a medium-sized laboratory, a technologist may rotate from one area to another, perhaps, changing every week or every month. In a large laboratory, a technologist will usually work in only one area.

A. Hematology: The technologist studies the blood cells: (i) the white cells (leukocytes) to help in the diagnosis of infections, leukemia, and other conditions (ii) the red cells (erythrocytes) to help in the diagnosis of anemia to determine the type of anemia.

B. Clinical Chemistry: The technologist does quantitative determinations of chemical constituents of blood, cerebrospinal fluid, urine, and other fluids.

C. Immunology: The technologist detects antigen-antibody reactions in disease states.

D. Microbiology: The technologist isolates and identifies bacteria, fungi, and animal parasites that cause diseases.

E. Blood Banking: The technologist does pretransfusion testing (collection of donor's blood, separation of blood components, identification, and cross-matching of red cells) to ensure safe transfusions.

Careers

Laboratory professionals are the detectives of the healthcare world. They search for clues to help in the diagnosis and treatment of a disease or injury and to help patients stay healthy.

Clues to solving the mystery of diseases are found in our bodies. Laboratory tests check the makeup of our blood, urine, body fluids, and tissues for early warning signs of diseases. To perform these tests, laboratory professionals work in various capacities in a clinical laboratory:

1. Administration
2. Education
3. Bench Technologist
4. Chief Technologist
5. Research and Development

Areas of work

1. Hospital laboratories
2. Private laboratories
3. Public health laboratories
4. Laboratory supply companies (sales and technical consultation)
5. Computer industry
6. Commercial and industrial laboratories
7. University settings (education and research)
8. Veterinary medicine
9. Military

The employment outlook in the USA

Healthcare is one of the fastest-growing industries in the United States. More than one-quarter million people work in medical laboratory services alone. As the population grows older and medical knowledge expands, there is an increasing need for highly skilled and educated professionals. Today, there are more jobs for medical laboratory professionals than educated people to fill those jobs. For educated professionals, the future long-term employment looks very bright into the next century. The need is great everywhere throughout the country.

About 4-5 billion laboratory tests are performed each year because 70% of medical decisions of a physician on any one patient depend on laboratory test results. According to the infographics prepared by Pearson Education and the University of Cincinnati Medical Laboratory Service Program, the projected growth of laboratory professionals from 2012 to 2022 is 22%. In other words, more job opportunities will be created. There are mainly three contributing factors for the shortage of laboratory professionals:

1. About 83.7 million population aged 65 and over in 2050
2. About 50% decline in educational programs since the 1970s National Accrediting Agency for Clinical Laboratory Sciences (NAACLS) report
3. Inclusion of newly developed laboratory tests (e.g., molecular diagnostics) all the time to improve early detection and diagnosis of diseases and better prognosis

The highest employment for CLS and MLT professionals by State (May 2015) is listed in Table 1.1 (a) and (b), respectively.

Table 1.1: Highest employment for (a) CLS and (b) MLT professionals by State (May 2015)

(a) *CLS professionals*

State	Employment
Texas	12,560
California	10,790
Florida	10,380
New York	9,640
Pennsylvania	7,890

(b) *MLT professionals*

State	Employment
California	17,670
Texas	11,890
Pennsylvania	8,140
New York	7,440
Ohio	7,000

Interestingly, clinical microbiology laboratories are making rapid changes to meet daunting challenges. Currently, a vacancy rate in U.S. microbiology laboratories is >10% with an additional 17.4% of the medical technologists awaiting to retire in the next 5 years.

Conclusion

The practice of modern medicine would be impossible without the tests performed in the clinical laboratory. The medical technologist performs a full range of laboratory tests from simple premarital blood tests to more complex tests to complete the laboratory diagnosis of diseases such as AIDS, diabetes, Covid-19, and cancer. The medical technologist is also responsible for confirming the accuracy of test results and reporting laboratory findings to the pathologist and other doctors. Thus, they hold life and death in their hands because the information they give to the doctor influences the medical treatment a patient will get.

Chapter 2

Safety Measures and First Aid

Introduction

Every pathological specimen received for laboratory examination is considered to be potentially infectious. Therefore, medical laboratory personnel should strictly follow the rules and regulations of a medical laboratory while working in the laboratory. This practice avoids minor as well as major accidents. But, accidents are apt to occur in some cases even by a systematic and experienced medical personnel. Therefore, first aid is of great value to prevent any major damage to the laboratory worker.

The ten commandments for clinical laboratory personnel are:

1. Treat all biological materials as potentially infective
2. Do not attempt to recap, break, or bend needles
3. Wear disposable gloves
4. Wash hands using a disinfectant
5. Prohibit mouth pipetting, eating, smoking, or chewing gum in the laboratory. Leave pens/pencils in the laboratory. Do not chew your pen/pencil, bite your fingernails, rub, or pick your nose
6. Always wear a laboratory coat or gown
7. Use a biological safety cabinet
8. Decontaminate laboratory work surfaces at least daily with freshly prepared chemical germicide (e.g., 1-10% sodium hypochlorite)
9. Routinely decontaminate equipment
10. Immediately decontaminate large and small blood and body fluid spills. Dispose the biological waste only in a designated container that is labeled with a biohazard sign as shown in Fig. 2.1.

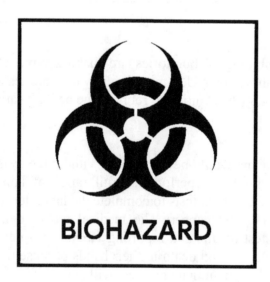

Fig. 2.1: The biohazard sign to be affixed to the biological waste container.

Furthermore, it is also advisable to take the following three general precautionary measures:

1. Keep poisonous and dangerous chemicals in a separate locked cupboard.
2. Care should be taken to ensure that all gas taps work efficiently and that no gas leaks after turning the taps off. Do not attempt to find gas leaks with the help of a lighted match.
3. Keep fire extinguishers at readily accessible places.

First aid in accidents and poisoning

It is required to keep an up-to-date first aid box. In addition to this, laboratory personnel should undergo a first aid training program. Thus, the combination of first aid facility and trained personnel could help in the elementary treatment of laboratory personnel met with an accident. The discussion is restricted to burn cases and chemical poisoning cases.

Burns

There are two types of burns, namely small burns, and extensive burns. So, first aid depends upon the severity of burns.

(i) Small burns

Immerse small burns in cold water or an ice bag or apply a cold wet pack on the trunk or face.

1. Cooling must be constant until the pain disappears
2. Use non-adhesive dressings, e.g., plastic films
3. Consult a physician
4. Do not break the blisters

(ii) Extensive burns

1. Keep patient in a flat position
2. Remove clothing from the burned area
3. Cover with a clean cloth
4. Keep patient warm
5. Hospitalize the patient immediately

Note: Do not use ointments, greases, powders, etc. Electric burns with shock may require artificial respiration. Use non-conductive material to pull the victim.

Chemical poisoning

The general procedure to be followed in chemical poisoning is as under:

1. Remove the noxious agent that is in contact with the patient
2. Place the unconscious patient in a prone position (i.e., lying on the abdomen) with head turned to one side and tongue pulled forward
3. Keep patient warm and recumbent
4. Be prepared to administer mouth to mouth artificial respiration if the patient experiences difficulty in breathing

5. Do not leave the patient without an attendant
6. Do not administer alcohol without medical advice because it accelerates the absorption of some poisons
7. Summon and obtain medical attention as soon as possible without interrupting this general procedure

Also, the nature of first aid treatment varies according to the site of the body damaged by the poison. The mode of first aid treatment for some common parts of the body is briefly discussed below:

Mouth

1. Induce vomiting immediately
2. Give 2-4 glasses of water or milk
3. Place the victim in a position of comfort
4. Identify the poison
5. Administer an appropriate antidote

Skin and eyes

1. Remove poison from contact with skin/eyes
2. Flood affected area with water for at least 15 minutes
3. Remove clothing, including all contaminated articles on the patient
4. Arrange to identify the poison and consult a physician

First aid in the case of acids and corrosive chemicals (e.g., HCl, HNO_3, H_2SO_4):
External
Use the general procedure as outlined earlier under chemical poisoning.

Internal

1. Do not induce vomiting
2. Do not give carbonates or sodium bicarbonate
3. Administer aluminum hydroxide gel or milk of magnesia in large amounts followed by milk or egg white beaten with water

First aid in the case of alkalis and caustic chemicals (e.g., $NH_3 + H_2O \longleftrightarrow NH_4OH_{aq.}$)

External
Use the general procedure as outlined earlier under chemical poisoning.

Internal
All steps in the case of acids except step (3). Administer large amounts of diluted acetic acid (1%), vinegar (1:4), citric acid (1%), or lemon juice followed by milk or egg white beaten with water.

A safety data sheet (SDS), originally called material safety data sheet (MSDS), is a document that provides information about the hazardous chemicals. It is prepared in alignment with the UN's globally harmonized system of classification and labeling of chemical (GHS) that the manufacturer, importer, or distributor of a chemical compound is required to provide downstream users. The occupational safety and health administration (OSHA) regulates SDSs in the US. Nowadays, SDSs are electronically available. The contact information is:

Occupational Safety and Health Administration
200 Constitution Ave NW
Washington, DC 20210
Phone: 1-800-321-6742
www.OSHA.gov

Caution

1. Do not give syrup of ipecac or do anything to induce vomiting. It can do more harm than good.
2. Do not wait for signs and symptoms to develop, call the poison control center for guidance. The U.S. National Poison Control Center at 1-800-222-1222 if you have any questions about a possible poisoning. This toll-free number is routed to the poison control center that serves your area.

Chapter 3

Laboratory Instruments

Introduction

Every medical laboratory student should understand the principle, working, proper use, and care to be taken while handling the following laboratory instruments:

1. Microscope
2. Centrifuge
3. Analytical balance
4. Colorimeter and spectrophotometer
5. Water bath
6. pH meter
7. Paper electrophoresis
8. Thin-layer chromatography
9. Gas chromatography

1. The compound light microscope (see Fig. 3.1)

The compound microscope is the primary tool in the medical laboratory. Laboratory diagnosis of certain diseases (e.g., malaria, amoebic dysentery, and leukemia) is not possible without a microscope. It enlarges the image of objects that otherwise cannot be seen at all. This enlargement of objects is called magnification. It is measured in micrometer (μm) and nanometer (nm), equaling 0.000001 m and 0.000000001 m, respectively. However, the smallest metric unit of length called angstrom (0.0000000001 m) is not in use.

Many different types of compound microscopes are available. The principle underlying all these microscopes remains the same. It consists of an optical system and an illumination system. Therefore, a medical laboratory student has to understand the principles and the relationship between magnification, resolving power, and illumination.

Magnification
There are two lens-systems in a compound microscope:

a. Objective (produces a real image)
b. Ocular (produces a virtual image)

Usually, there are three types of objectives:

1. A low power objective
2. A high power objective
3. An oil-immersion objective

The total magnification is the magnification of its objective multiplied by that of its ocular. Therefore, the total magnification of the microscope with a 10x objective and 10x ocular would be 100x. In the case of 100x objective and 10x ocular, the total magnification through the microscope is 1,000x. A compound light microscope is limited to about 2000x magnification. Beyond this limit, neither eyes nor the brain would be able to recognize the image. Except for viruses, one can view bacteria, fungi, algae, protozoa, and blood cells. Viruses can be studied with the help of electron microscopes. The electron microscopes could magnify objects up to 500,000x with a resolving power of < 1 nm. Unlike light microscopes, they use a beam of electrons and electro-magnets for focusing instead.

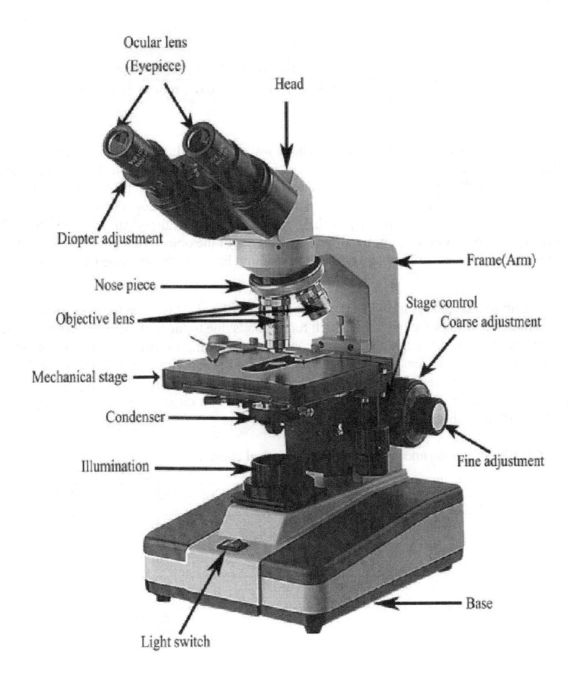

Fig. 3.1: The binocular microscope.

Resolving power

The ability of a lens to show two closely adjacent points as distinct and separate is called its resolving power:

Naked eye = 0.1 mm
Light microscope = 0.2 µm
Electron microscope = 2.5 nm

$$\text{Resolving power} = \frac{\text{Wavelength of the light in nm } (\lambda)}{2 \times \text{Numerical aperture of an objective lens}}$$

It is obvious from this relationship that the shorter wavelength of light should be used to visualize smaller structures. For example, blue light gives greater resolution than red. But, it is of limited value to increase the resolution by decreasing the wavelength of the visible light. This is just because of a relatively narrow spectrum of visible light. Therefore, a considerable increase in the resolution of a light microscope is possible by increasing the numerical aperture (NA). The numerical aperture is a function of the effective diameter of the objective with its focal length and the light-bending power (refractive index) of the medium between the specimen and the objective.

When a beam of light passes from a microscope slide into the air, it is refracted at so great an angle that it completely misses the objective. Such refraction is due to the high refractive index of glass compared to air. This difficulty can be overcome by interposing immersion oil (e.g., cedarwood oil) between the objective lens and the specimen slide as shown in Fig. 3.2. This can be understood from the similarity of the refractive index of glass and immersion oil, decreasing the refraction. This results in greater resolution, leading to the formation of a clear image. The usual figures for the NA of different objectives are given in Table 3.1.

Table 3.1: Magnification and corresponding numerical aperture

Magnification	Numerical Aperture (NA)
10x	About 0.25
20x	About 0.45
40x	About 0.65
100x	About 1.30

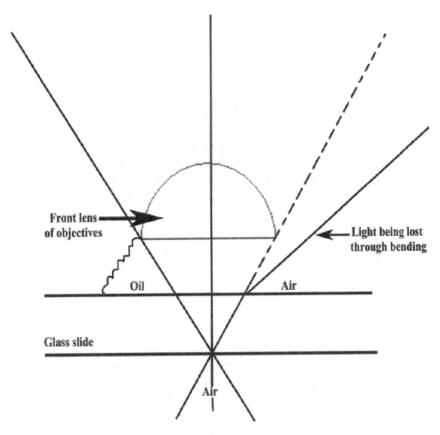

Fig. 3.2: The working of an oil-immersion lens.

Illumination

It is necessary to have uniform illumination that can form the perfect image. The main difficulty in proper illumination is with a glare. There are many glare-developing sources. For example, stray light from windows reaching the eye interferes with the formation of a perfect image. Great variation in the intensity of ordinary daylight restricts its use as a source of illumination. Therefore, artificial light (e.g., a tungsten lamp) sources are usually used to control the intensity, color, and size of the light rays.

The size of the cone of light entering the objective depends upon the type of objective being used. The size of the cone of light is adjusted by the iris diaphragm. The requirement of the size of the cone of light for low-power, high-power, and oil-immersion objectives is in the order given below: low-power, high-power, oil-immersion.

Thus, an increase in the magnification of the objective lens needs a larger cone of light to enter it. Furthermore, the working distance decreases, and the angle of aperture of the objective lens increases while increasing the magnification of the objective lens as shown in Fig. 3.3. This explains why the iris-diaphragm is opened almost fully when an oil-immersion lens is in use.

Use of a microscope

One who wants to work with a microscope should understand the principles, the systematic use, and care to be taken while handling the microscope. Important steps for using a microscope are given below:

1. Place a specimen slide on the stage and center the area to be examined over the hole of the stage
2. Adjust the light source in such a way that the maximum amount of light can pass through the specimen
3. Examine with the low-power objective and shift it to the high-power objective
4. Focus the objective by racking the objective slowly upwards with the coarse adjustment until the specimen comes into approximate focus followed by fine adjustment
5. Adjust the mirror and the iris-diaphragm to give a well-illuminated image with fine details.
6. Examine the different fields of the specimen slide by moving it with the help of the mechanical stage
7. Use oil-immersion objective (100x) for the maximum magnification opening the iris fully

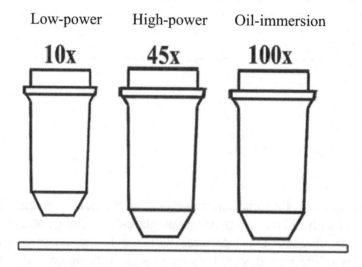

Fig. 3.3: The working distances of three objectives.

Precautions
1. Do not touch the lenses of the objectives
2. Wipe the lenses of the objectives and the condenser with a lens paper. Clean the mirror and the upper surface of the upper lens with a soft cloth
3. Use very little xylol to remove oil dried on a lens. Do not use too much xylol or alcohol as these may dissolve the cement holding the lens
4. Keep the fixed stage clean and dry
5. Use machine oil to lubricate controlling mechanical parts
6. Cover the microscope by a light plastic cover when it is not in use
7. Consult a proper scientific instrument repairer or the maker if the microscope is damaged optically or mechanically

2. Centrifuge

When a suspension of a solid in liquid is allowed to stand for some hours without disturbance, solid matter sediments at the bottom slowly. The force that works here is the gravitational force. The rate of sedimentation can be made faster by applying centrifugal force. The gravitational force can be developed by spinning tubes. The centrifuge is used for this purpose. The factors affecting the settlement of particles include:

1. Shape and size of the particles
2. Viscosity and the specific gravity of the liquid
3. The speed of centrifugation (i.e., revolutions per minute)
4. Time of centrifugation
5. Length of radius

Thus, the centrifuge is a piece of basic equipment for a clinical laboratory. Usually, a motor-driven centrifuge is operated from a mains electricity supply. It is available in various capacities. Thus, the number of buckets may be four, six or more. Also, there may be an auto-stop switch.

Precautions
1. Place the centrifuge on a firm base
2. Use centrifuge tubes made of strong glass of the correct length
3. Balance the opposite tubes of a pair carefully
4. Place the cover in its place before turning it on
5. Increase the speed of the centrifuge gradually
6. Do not try to stop the centrifuge by holding the shaft
7. Keep the centrifuge clean and dry

Uses
1. Clinical biochemistry (e.g., separation of serum or plasma)
2. Blood banking (e.g., washing of erythrocytes with normal saline)
3. Hematology (e.g., determination of a packed cell volume)
4. Urinalysis (e.g., recovery of urine sediment)

3. Analytical balance

An analytical balance is a common instrument of any analytical laboratory. It should be used carefully because of its high price and delicacy. Basically, it consists of two hanging pans at two ends of a beam. This assembly is inside the glass cabin to protect it from dust and wind friction.

Precautions
1. Place the analytical balance on a firm bench
2. Level the analytical balance by adjusting the leveling screws (a spirit level or a plumb-line is used as an indicator during leveling)
3. Release the beam by gentle turning of the knob and see that the beam is resting on its knife-edge with the pointer swinging within the scale using the screw nuts at both the ends of the beam
4. Place the weights with the help of forceps in the right pan and the object (e.g., chemical) to be weighed in the left pan

5. Always have the balance at rest before adding or removing the weights or objects
6. Close the glass windows of the balance before taking the final reading
7. Keep the balance clean, using a small camel hairbrush

An expensive single pan electronic balance is used in research laboratories for accurate weighing.

4. Colorimeter and spectrophotometer {see Fig. 3.4 (a), (b)}

A photoelectric colorimeter is an indispensable instrument for biochemical assay techniques in a clinical laboratory. Essentially, it consists of a source of light, a simple lens, a filter system (prisms or gratings in case of photometers), a photocell, and a galvanometer. It should be used very carefully because it is a very expensive and sensitive instrument.

The knowledge of Beer's law is essential to understand the working mechanism of photoelectric colorimeters. The law states that 'the concentration of a substance is directly proportional to the amount of light absorbed or inversely proportional to the logarithm of transmitted light.' Mathematically,

$$A = abc = \frac{100}{\%T}$$

$$= 2 - \log (\%T)$$

Where A = Absorbance
a = proportionality constant
b = the length of the column of solution through which light passes
c = concentration of the substance in question

(a) Filter photometer

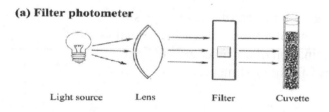

Light source   Lens   Filter   Cuvette

(b) Spectrophotometer

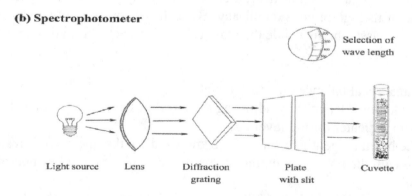

Selection of wave length

Light source   Lens   Diffraction grating   Plate with slit   Cuvette

Fig. 3.4 (a), (b): Types of photoelectric colorimeters.

Graphically, a linear curve is obtained when one plots a graph between the absorbance of light and percent transmittance of light. This linearity is lost at a very high concentration of a chemical substance to be assayed.

In other words, Beer's law is not followed after a certain concentration of the substance in a colored solution. Therefore, the specimen is diluted before the estimation and the final result is multiplied by the dilution factor to obtain the actual concentration of the substance in the undiluted specimen.

A specific colored waveband can be selected from the mixture of white light and passed into the cuvette. It is necessary to know which wavelength is to be used for measuring the optical density (OD) of a specific color. The use of a desired wavelength of light is possible either by using different filters in a filter photometer or by adjusting the desired wavelength in a spectrophotometer (Fig. 3.4(b)).

A key component of photoelectric colorimeters is a photocell. The light-emitting through the cuvette filled with a colored solution strikes the photocell. Thus, a photocell is an agency which converts light energy into electricity. The galvanometer measures the electricity. Thus, the higher the color intensity of a colored solution, the greater is the absorbance (optical density) of light. Furthermore, percentage transmission (% T) decreases in this case.

There are two types of spectrophotometers available, namely analog and digital. Also, the number of beams may be one or two depending upon the model.

Precautions
1. Keep the photoelectric instrument, including cuvettes clean
2. Warm the instrument for 10 minutes before measurement of OD of a colored solution
3. Select the wavelength of light to be used (e.g., using a filter in a filter photometer)
4. Calibrate the instrument using distilled water as a blank, adjusting at 100% transmittance
5. Put the cuvette filled with a colored solution after cleaning the outer surface using a tissue paper
6. Measure the OD of a solution with low intensity first followed by a solution of high intensity of a similar color, thus avoiding washing of a cuvette in between
7. Switch off the power by using a power switch in the photocolorimeter instrument
8. Take the filter out in case of a filter photometer and replace it in the protective box
9. Keep the instrument covered with a plastic cover when it is not in use

Note: It is advisable to use a stabilizer to minimize the effect of voltage fluctuations

5. Water bath

A water bath is a simple laboratory apparatus. It controls the desired temperature of test tubes for a given time limit. It is preferable to incubators because of the uniformity of its temperature.

The water bath is equipped with an electrical thermostat. Thus, it is possible to set at a required temperature with the help of an adjustable temperature knob. Thereafter, the temperature is maintained accurately for a given time of incubation. The adjustable temperature range is from room temperature to 100°C. Nowadays, dry heating blocks replace water baths in clinical laboratories.

Precautions
1. Use distilled or deionized water. Renew it regularly
2. Check the actual temperature of the water with the help of a thermometer
3. Keep the level of water in a water-bath just above the height of the column of the contents in test tubes
4. Use an aluminum-made rack to hold test tubes

Uses
1. Serological tests {e.g., Widal (tube) test}
2. Assay of enzymes (e.g., alanine transaminase)

6. pH meter

The term, pH, was introduced by the Danish biochemist SPL Sørensen in 1909. It is a sensitive and costly apparatus. It is used for an accurate measurement of the pH of a test solution. pH meter is a potentiometer that measures the potential of an indicator electrode in contact with the test solution. The potential of the electrode, in turn, is measured concerning a calomel reference electrode whose potential is already known.

Principle
When a pair of electrodes, namely a pH-sensitive glass electrode and a reference electrode, are dipped in a given solution, generating electromotive force (emf). Electromotive force, sometimes called voltage, is not truly a force rather it is a measurement of energy per unit charge. In other words, it is the potential difference in charge between the two points in a circuit. According to the Nernst equation, the emf of the complete cell (E_{cell}) is equal to the potential developed by the glass electrode (E_{glass}) minus that of the calomel electrode ($E_{cal.}$):

$$E_{cell} = E_{cal.} - E_{glass}$$

The potential of the calomel electrode is determined by the standard H^+ electrode and it has a potential of 0.246 at 25°C. On the other hand, the potential of the glass electrode depends on the temperature and pH of the test solution.

Precautions
1. Soak the new glass electrode in 0.1 M HCl for several hours before use to activate it
2. Stir the test solution for thorough mixing, using the magnetic stirrer
3. Bring the temperature of the test solution to room temperature
4. Keep buffers in the refrigerator
5. Wash the electrode before and after use with the help of distilled water
6. Warm the pH meter before use by turning the switch on for 15 minutes
7. Standardize the pH meter before using standard buffers
8. Keep the electrode immersed in distilled water when it is not in use

16

9. Use heparinized plasma to measure blood pH

7. Paper electrophoresis

Recent advances in analytical techniques have effectively been used in obtaining and identifying substances in the state of high purity. Physical methods like fractional precipitation, distillation, and crystallization have been used in the separation and purification of chemical compounds. These methods work quite successfully in many cases but some difficulties arise where the individual components of the compounds have similar physical and chemical properties. For example, fractional distillation methods could be safely used in case of a mixture of liquids which have a good range of boiling point differences. However, this method could be used in the case of liquid air as well as rare gases where the boiling points of individual components are very close to each other. Likewise, after treating the biological materials by the usual classical methods, one is usually left with many compounds such as a mixture of amino acids which are similar in properties to each other. In such cases, the extremes of temperature, pH, organic solvents, and the use of oxidizing and reducing agents are avoided as these may irreversibly change the structure of the molecule and destroy their biological activity.

Such complicated separations were achieved successfully by the techniques of chromatography and paper electrophoresis. These methods resolve the individual components under relatively mild conditions and utilize differences in the basic physical properties of the individual molecules such as their mass, size, shape, charge, and adsorption properties. The paper electrophoresis method has an edge over the paper chromatographic method, as in the latter, substances with low distribution coefficients are not properly separated. Such difficulties are not faced with the technique of paper electrophoresis which involves the migration of charged substances under the influence of electric current. Paper electrophoresis is an incomplete form of electrolysis that is widely used in the separation of biological materials and many other rare and costly substances. In compounds or a mixture of compounds where some ionize and others do not, the degree of separation can be effectively made by the use of paper electrophoresis.

This method owes its development to the painstaking research of Arne Wilhelm Kaurin Tiselius of Sweden who was awarded the Nobel Prize in 1948.

Technique
The paper to be used for electrophoresis is first wetted with an electrolytic solution which is normally a buffer solution (e.g., barbitone buffer at pH 8.6). The wet paper is placed in a vessel made up of anodic and cathodic compartments in such a manner that the two ends dip inside the solution. Test solutions are put on the middle portion of the paper and are dried. A current of the order of 2-10 V/cm is then passed through the solution. Buffer solutions serve the purpose of conductors and the wet paper as a conducting bridge between the two compartments. The substances move either to the cathode or anode, depending on the nature of the charge which they possess as shown in Fig. 3.5.

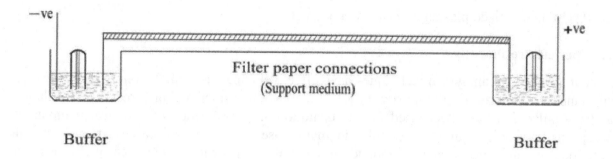

Fig. 3.5: Paper electrophoresis.

The movement of the substances is expressed by electrophoretic mobility (μ) which is defined as:

$$\mu = \frac{\text{distance moved/unit time}}{\text{electrical field strength}}$$

$$\mu = \frac{\text{cm/sec}}{\text{volt /cm}}$$

$$= cm^2 \, volt \, sec^{-1}$$

The movement of the substances depends on many factors which are listed below:

(i) Size and nature of the charge
The bigger the charge the faster will be the movement, and the smaller the size the slower the movement.

(ii) Environmental factors
The concentration of electrolyte, ionic strength, dielectric properties, chemical properties, temperature, viscosity, and the presence of non-polar molecules have their individual and independent role to play.

(iii) pH effect
The direction of the movement of the substances will depend on the pH of the solution, especially with those substances which have both positive and negative charges like amino acids.

$$
\begin{array}{c}
COO^- \\
| \\
H_3N\!-\!\!-\!C\!-\!\!-H \\
| \\
R
\end{array}
$$

We see that the addition of HCl will cause the following reaction:

$$
\begin{array}{c}
COO^- \\
| \\
H_3N\!-\!\!-\!C\!-\!\!-H \\
| \\
R
\end{array}
+ H^+ \longrightarrow
\begin{array}{c}
COOH \\
| \\
H_3N\!-\!\!-\!C\!-\!\!-H \\
| \\
R
\end{array}
$$

Whereas addition of NaOH results in:

$$
\begin{array}{c}
COO^- \\
| \\
H_3N\!-\!\!-\!C\!-\!\!-H \\
| \\
R
\end{array}
+ OH^- \longrightarrow
\begin{array}{c}
COO^- \\
| \\
H_2N\!-\!\!-\!C\!-\!\!-H \\
| \\
R
\end{array}
+ H_2O
$$

When the pH is low enough, the amino acid will be positively charged and will migrate towards the cathode, and at a sufficiently higher pH value, it will be negatively charged and will migrate towards the anode. At some intermediate pH value, the isoelectric point (IEP), no migration in an electrical field will occur in either direction. Different amino acids have different R groups. Their net charges at a given pH value will differ, offering the possibility of separation by electrophoresis.

Paper moistened with a buffer solution has a resistance which depends on the nature and the amount of buffer solution on paper. The resistance is constant in the beginning and by Ohm's law, $I = V/R$.

Thus, it is evident that the passage of current generates heat on the paper. The heat so produced causes evaporation of the water of buffer solution. As the solvent evaporates, salt is left behind on the paper. The increase of voltage increases the amount of salt on the paper which affects the electrophoretic mobility of substances. It has been seen that the usual maximum amount of heat that can be tolerated is 0.15 watts/cm^3.

(iv) Diffusion

When the samples are put on the paper they tend to diffuse along with the paper. The diffusion depends on the molecular size. It has been observed that diffusion occurs even when no potential is applied to the system.

(v) Electro-osmosis

When a buffer solution is placed in the compartment, it moves towards the cathode which means that the water is positively charged. In the test substance, the positive and negative charges move towards the cathode, and anode, respectively. Thus, the speed of the anions and cations would be affected. However, in general, this effect is ignored in electrophoresis experiments.

Applications

Paper electrophoresis has been widely used in the field of large molecules such as proteins, enzymes, and nucleic acids. Now, it is also used in the separation of peptides, nucleotides, amino acids, and abnormal hemoglobin (see Fig. 3.6). Outside the biological science, electrophoresis has played a little part in the problems of ion separation, possibly because quantitative analysis is more important and because good ion-exchange procedures are available. Much work has been done on the best methods of separation of serum proteins. This method is considered to be one of the most standard hospital biochemical procedures. Various diseases are shown to exhibit specific patterns following electrophoresis. The diseases affecting the liver, kidneys, malignancies, etc., show a change in the number of different bands and occasionally a band in a different position which is of diagnostic significance. The proteins of the other components of blood, e.g., the red cell could be separated by similar procedures.

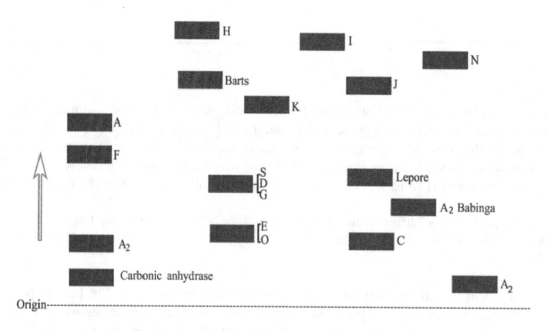

Fig. 3.6: Relative mobilities of some abnormal hemoglobins
on cellulose acetate (Tris buffer, pH 8.9).

20

8. Thin-layer chromatography

Thin-layer chromatography is one of the comparatively recent analytical methods added to the list that includes adsorption chromatography, partition chromatography, paper chromatography, gas-liquid chromatography (GLC), gas-solid chromatography (GSC), electrochromatography, ion-exchange chromatography, etc. It has found wide applicability in the separation and identification of both organic and inorganic substances. The main advantage of thin-layer chromatography (TLC) lies in the fact that the technique can carry out separation and identification of unknown substances in very small amounts and in a very short time. None of the other methods can match it in this regard. Even paper chromatography which has earned the reputation of carrying out the separation in very small amounts has been exceeded by this method. For example, TLC can carry out separation or identification in still smaller amounts and in much less time than is taken by paper chromatography.

Like paper chromatography, thin-layer chromatography is a micro chromatographic technique in which glass plates are coated with thin layers of adsorbents like alumina, silica gel, cellulose powder, etc. These adsorbents adhere to the glass plates firmly due to the presence of binding materials added to the adsorbent slurry. The adsorption plates are sometimes called chromatostrips or chromatoplates and are similar to paper strips in paper chromatography, but they are much easier to handle.

The credit for discovering this new technique goes to two Russian workers, N.A. Izmailov and M.S. Schraiber, who in the year 1938 attempted the separation of plant extracts on alumina-coated glass plates and got a satisfactory separation. This discovery did not attract the attention of other workers until 1949. In that year, J.E. Meinhard and N.F. Hall showed some satisfactory separation with the new method. They were also the first to describe an apparatus for coating glass plates with adsorbents. But the technique could not gain popularity because of the difficulties involved in the preparation of suitable adsorbents and applying them in uniform layers on glass plates.

The method which was practically given up was reinvented by the untiring efforts of Egon Stahl, a German worker, who not only found practical equipment for coating glass plates with adsorbents but also demonstrated the usefulness of this technique on a wide range of materials. Since 1958, the use of TLC has been so widespread that it has entered almost every phase of analysis. This is because the technique has been developed to such an extent that good and reproducible results are obtained readily and in comparatively less time. Since Thin-layer chromatography is based fundamentally on adsorption and separation chromatography, the same theoretical principles are involved in it.

TLC has been used in the separation and identification of a large variety of organic compounds: alkaloids, terpenes, vitamins, hormones, dyes, drugs, sugars, alcohols, aldehydes, acids, and many others. TLC has also found useful application in the analysis and identification of inorganic compounds.

Materials and technique

Adsorbents and applicators are the two essential items of the TLC technique, although other accessories like glass plates, aligning tray, activating oven, developing chamber, etc., play their roles. The efficiency of the former two plays a very important part in the success of the technique.

Applicator

There are various types of applicators for spreading the adsorbent in the form of slurry over the glass plates. Adjustable applicators are available for spreading layers of various degrees of thickness ranging from 250µ to 2 mm over glass plates.

Adsorbent

The character of the adsorbent is of the greatest importance in this technique. Silica gel and alumina are mostly used and have proved to be quite suitable. They are used along with some binding materials like plaster of Paris to fix the thin and porous layer on the glass plates. Besides, Kieselgel has also been used for making thin layers. Cellulose powders with and without binding materials are also in use. Various types of cellulose powders, including ion-exchange cellulose powder, are much in use.

Preparation of thin-layers

The adsorbents are mixed thoroughly with requisite quantities of water or mixtures of water and alcohol with the help of a mechanical stirrer for about two minutes to form a homogeneous slurry. Then, it is immediately spread over well-cleaned glass plates of standard size (20x20 cm or 20 x 5 cm) arranged in a row on an aligning tray with the help of the applicator. The applicator is first adjusted according to the thickness of the layer, after which the slurry is put inside the applicator and the latter is drawn by hand over the glass plates arranged on the aligning tray. The coated glass plates are then allowed to dry at room temperature for 10 minutes to 2 hours during which the binder present in the adsorbent sets the adsorbent firmly over the glass plates.

After air drying, the coated glass plates are activated by drying in an oven at a suitable temperature depending on the adsorbent. Similarly, the heating period varies. After activation, the plates are stored in a vacuum desiccator until they are used. If the plates are not stored in a desiccator and exposed to air or kept for a long time without being used, the efficiency of the plates decreases.

The samples to be analyzed are applied in the same way as in paper chromatography. Usually, a small amount, e.g., 4 microliters of the solution of the substance or a mixture in a micropipette is applied to the starting point near one of the edges (narrow edge) of the chromatoplates in such a manner that the drop becomes as small as practicable and then dries up. The smaller the diameter of the spot, the better is the resolution, 5-10 micrograms are sufficient for one operation. Substances are usually applied about 2 cm away from the edge of the plate.

The plates are then put in the chromatography chamber, usually much smaller than the paper chromatography chamber. The chamber should be saturated with the solvent vapor sufficiently ahead of the actual operation. Its walls should be lined up with filter paper soaked with the solvent to maintain steady saturation inside the chamber. The solvent is put inside the chamber to a thickness of 1cm. The spotted chromatoplates are developed by the ascending technique. The plates are held vertically inside the chamber. They can also be developed by the descending technique with certain modifications of the chamber. The development takes much less time than in the case of paper chromatography. When the development is complete, the plates are taken out and allowed to dry in the air inside a clean, dust-free chamber at room temperature. Then, developed plates are activated by keeping them in an oven adjusted at a specified temperature (100°-250°C).

Detection of the movement of spots and determination of Rf values are similar to those in paper chromatography. Detection of spots can be made by spraying the chromatogram with visualizing reagents (e.g., ninhydrin), or in some cases, it may be done by seeing the chromatogram in UV light.

Partition and ion-exchange TLC can be performed in the same way. Two-dimensional thin-layer chromatography has also been achieved with success by developing the single plate in two directions at right angles to each other, utilizing two different solvent systems. Thin-layer chromatography has shown good success in the separation of mixtures of various types of compounds.

9. Gas chromatography: (see Fig. 3.7)

Gas chromatography (GC), also sometimes called vapor-phase chromatography (VPC) or gas-liquid partition chromatography (GLPC), is a very sensitive and versatile analytical technique for volatile organic mixtures.

The separation of mixture components occurs based on their affinity for the stationary phase (GC column). The carrier gas (mobile phase) carries mixture components down the column depending upon the components' relative mobilities. Gas chromatography can best be summarized in the following five areas.

(i) Carrier gas
The carrier gas serves as a mobile phase. Additionally, the type of carrier gas usage directly affects the column efficiency and resolution. Helium and argon gases are commonly used in the GC technique. Sometimes, nitrogen (packed columns) finds its application as a carrier gas. The choice of carrier gas in the GC method depends on the type of a column as well as the type of a detector being used. The choice of carrier gas is as under:

$$He > Ar > N_2 > H_2$$

All carrier gases are available in pressurized tanks equipped with pressure regulators, gauges, and flow meters. It is of utmost importance that a carrier gas meets the 99.9995% specification (UHP grade). Significant damage occurs to the column if heated above 70°C in the presence of trace amounts of O_2 in the column. This explains why a gas clean filter is used to trap O_2 and moisture.

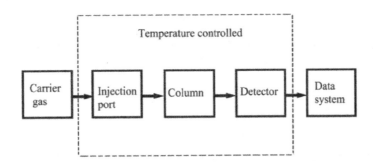

Fig. 3.7: Block diagram of gas chromatography.

(ii) Injection port

Manually, a glass microsyringe is used to introduce a sample mixture into a chromatograph. GC equipped with packed columns need 1-10µL of the sample. The needle of the syringe is carefully inserted through the septum to go all the way to the heated block. The heated block has a temperature of 50°C higher than the column oven to vaporize the sample being introduced into the chromatograph. GC with capillary (tubular) columns makes use of either split or splitless injection techniques because capillary columns usually have a much smaller cross-section area than that of packed columns. This feature enables to handle low sample volumes and low flow rates of the carrier gas. In the case of a split injection device, samples contain the target analyte(s) in relatively high concentrations. Autosamplers are now available to inject a sample mixture automatically into the inlets. Autosampler provides better reproducibility and time optimization.

(iii) Column

The column is considered to be the heart of a GC technique. Glass is widely used as a material in constructing columns. Some columns are also made up of stainless steel. There are two types of columns used in the gas chromatography:

   a. Tubular (capillary) columns
   b. Packed columns

a. Tubular (capillary) columns: Tubular columns have many applications. They are fragile because they make use of fused silica (pure form of glass) in the inner wall with a coating of a thin film of liquid called a stationary phase ("wall-coated open tubular columns"). These columns are strengthened by covering capillary tubes with a thin outside coating of polyamide. Capillary columns measure 5-100m in length and 0.1-0.5mm in the inside diameter. These columns have a very small sample capacity.

b. Packed columns: Packed columns have limited applications (e.g., fixed gas analysis) because they have lower column efficiency and poor resolution than that of capillary columns. They range from 0.5-10m in length and 2-4mm in the inside diameter. These columns have a larger sample capacity due to increased column diameter.

Many compounds (polar and non-polar) are used as the stationary phase in gas-liquid chromatography (GLC). Key attributes for such compounds include low volatility, thermostability, chemical inertness, and solvent characteristics. It should be kept in mind that high temperatures and high flow rates decrease the retention time but deteriorate the quality of separation.

(iv) Detector

There are many types of detectors available. An ideal detector should have the following characteristics:

   ● adequate sensitivity
   ● reproducibility
   ● good stability
   ● a wide temperature range
   ● ease of operation

- reliability
- a short response time irrespective of the flow rate
- non-destructive

Different types of GC detectors are listed below:

- Thermal conductivity detector (TCD)
- Flame ionization detector (FID)
- Electron capture detector (ECD)
- Mass spectrometer detector (MSD)
- Flame photometric detector (FPD)
- Hall detector (electrolytic conductivity)
- Photoionization detector (PID)
- Fourier transform infrared (FTIR)

The selection of a particular detector depends on some important factors, namely the nature of compounds being analyzed, the sensitivity of the detector being considered, a linear and dynamic range of the detector being debated, and so on. It needs to be emphasized here that thermal conductivity detector (TCD) and flame ionization detector (FID) are *universal detectors*.

(v) Data recorder and analysis

Gas chromatography instrument and a recorder are integrated in order to draw a chart with peaks, corresponding to the relative amounts of the different components in the sample mixture. The identification of analytes of a sample mixture relies on the order in which they exit from the column and their retention times in the column. A chart (chromatogram) is prepared using a detector response (y-axis) against retention time (x-axis). Quantification of an analyte is made by calculating the area of the peak in the chromatogram, using a mathematical function of integration because the area under a peak is proportional to the concentration of an analyte present in the original sample. In most modems (GC-MS systems), the use of a computer software helps in drawing and integrating peaks, and matching MS spectra to library spectra.

Uses
- Pharmaceutical
- Food
- Environmental
- Industrial
- Research
- Forensic science

Section I: Hematology

Chapter 4

Hemopoiesis

Introduction

The formation of mature blood cells involves intermediate stages with different characteristics. This phenomenon is termed as hemopoiesis. There is a cellular hierarchy of progenitor cells that proliferate and differentiate via distinct lineages. Young blood cells are constantly produced to replace the short-lived mature blood cells, e.g., $1\text{-}2 \times 10^{11}/L$ erythrocytes and platelets/day and $7 \times 10^{10}/L$ granulocytes/day. The production rates of blood cells can increase tenfold if needed.

Organs engaged in the production and destruction of blood cells include bone marrow, spleen, liver, thymus, lymph node, and the reticuloendothelial system. Bone marrow serves as the primary organ in hematopoiesis. It is 100% hemopoietic tissue at birth followed by fat displacement at the age of four years. In adults, both hemopoietic tissue and fat cells are in equal amounts. Spleen and liver are primary sites for extramedullary hemopoiesis if activated in adults. Lymphocytes (B and T) are produced by the spleen, lymph node, lymphatic nodules, and thymus.

The reader will find a short description of the intermediate stages of this chapter. Factors affecting the formation of blood cells. These factors fall into two broad classes:

a. Humoral factors
- Erythropoietin (from the kidney) stimulates the formation of erythrocytes
- Crude bacterial and tissue extracts stimulate increased formation of neutrophils

b. Nutrient factors
These are important factors governing hemopoiesis. Some of them are vitamin B12, folic acid, and iron.

1. Erythropoiesis: (see Fig. 4.1)

In the early embryo, the formation of red cells takes place first in the mesoderm of the yolk sac. The next phase of the formation of red cells is chiefly in the liver and to some extent in the spleen. Formation of red cells occurs in a fetus's bone marrow at about the fifth month and decreases in the liver as it increases in the red bone marrow. At birth, all bones are filled with red marrow and later on with yellow marrow (i.e., fatty tissue). This process takes place first in the distal then intermediate and lastly in the proximal bones. Fetal marrow is very cellular (stromal stem cells). But, marrow normally contains 50% marrow cells and 50% fat in adults. Red cells are destroyed in the reticuloendothelial system.

Stages of development
Proerythroblast (pronormoblast)
1. It is approximately 12-20 μm in diameter.
2. The cytoplasm (agranular) stains deep blue.
3. The round-shaped nucleus stains a reddish-purple and contains several darker staining nucleoli.
4. It is devoid of hemoglobin.

5. High nuclear: cytoplasmic ratio.

Basophilic erythroblast
1. It shows a very close resemblance to the pronormoblast.
2. It shows active mitosis.
3. It is approximately 10-16 μm in diameter.
4. The nucleus is relatively large with clumped chromatin and stains deeply without nucleoli.
5. The cytoplasm is basophilic due to cytoplasmic ribosomes.

Polychromatic erythroblast
1. It is approximately 8-14 μm in diameter.
2. It shows active mitosis.
3. The cytoplasm shows a polychromatic staining reaction (a gray-green cytoplasm).
4. The nucleus decreases in size and stains deeply due to the clumping of the chromatin.
5. The synthesis of hemoglobin just begins from this stage.

Orthochromatic erythroblast (normoblast)
1. It varies from 8-10 μm in diameter.
2. Mitosis ceases.
3. The cytoplasm is acidophilic due to an increase in hemoglobin.
4. The nucleus is eccentric, small with condensed chromatin, and becomes pyknotic[1].
5. A bluish shade due to cytoplasmic ribosomes is a characteristic of the cell.

Polychromatic erythrocyte (reticulocyte)
1. It is a flat and disc-shaped cell.
2. It has a fine basophilic network of reticulum in the cytoplasm.
3. Its relative proportion in normal blood is 0.02 to 2%.
4. It has no nucleus.

Erythrocyte (red blood cell) see chapter 12.

2. Leukopoiesis: (see Fig. 4.1)

The development of leukocytes is conveniently discussed in three major groups:

   a. granulocytic (myeloid) series
   b. lymphocytic series
   c. monocytic series

a. Granulocytic (myeloid) series

It is a characteristic of these cells to contain either a neutrophilic, eosinophilic, or basophilic granules in the cytoplasm. Furthermore, mature cells of the series have lobulated (segmented) polymorphic nuclei. This is the reason why these cells are called polymorphonuclear leukocytes (polymorphs).

---

[1] Pyknosis is a stage in the degeneration of the nucleus which breaks up and finally disappears due to lysis or extrusion.

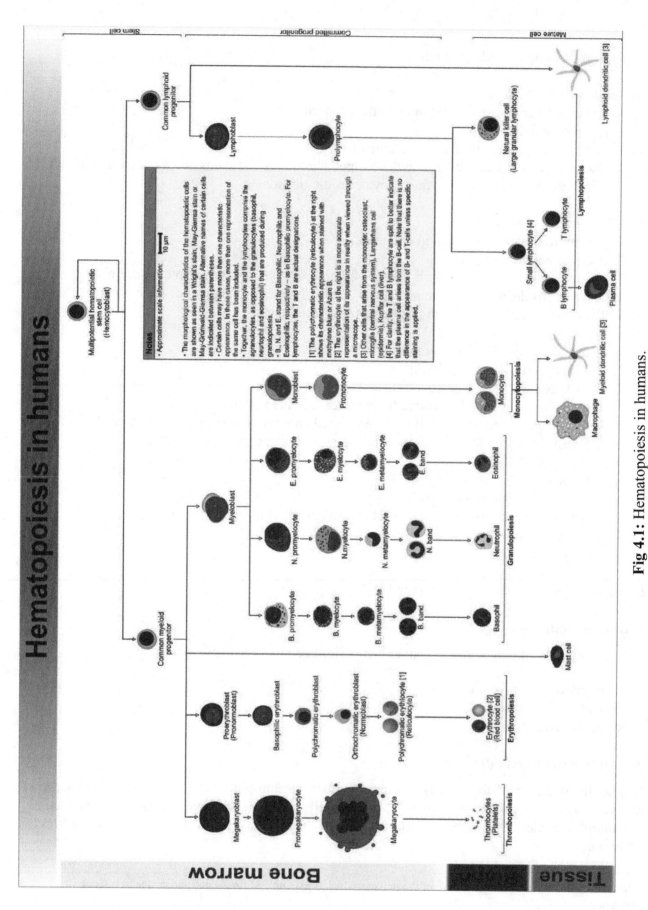

Fig 4.1: Hematopoiesis in humans.

Myeloblast
1. It is 15-20 μm in diameter.
2. The cytoplasm may be non-granular or may show a few azurophilic granules. It stains moderately deep blue.
3. The nucleus is spherical or oval and occupies about four-fifths of the total cell area. It stains reddish-purple, giving an even and reticular appearance.
4. Usually, 2-5 nucleoli of medium size are present.

Promyelocyte
1. It resembles the myeloblast except that the basophilic cytoplasm contains eye-catching azurophilic granules.
2. Its diameter is in the range of 22-25 μm.
3. The oval-shaped nucleus may still contain identifiable nucleoli and diffuse chromatin.

Myelocyte
1. It is 10-18 μm in diameter (It may be as large as 25 μm at the very early stage).
2. Usually, the cytoplasm is pale blue but it becomes pink in the late myelocyte. Moreover, there is clear granulation.
3. The nucleus is round or oval and the thick nuclear chromatin strands stain more unevenly and deeper than in the promyelocyte.
4. Nucleoli are not seen.

Metamyelocyte
1. It is from 14-20 μm in diameter.
2. The cytoplasm is pink with fine neutrophil granules.
3. The nucleus is kidney- or U-shaped with clumped chromatin.
4. Both protein biosynthesis and cell-division have ceased.

Band (stab) cell
1. It measures 12-15 μm in diameter (smaller than metamyelocytes).
2. The nucleus is indented like a thin crescent, appearing 'S'-like in shape.
3. The cytoplasm is acidophilic and contains fine reddish granulation.
4. Chromatin is coarse and clumped.

Mature cells of the myeloid series:
see chapter 11.

b. Lymphocytic series

The precursor cell is called a lymphoblast. The transition from lymphoblast to lymphocyte is brief. The intermediate cell is known as promyelocyte.

Lymphoblast
1. It measures 15-20 μm in diameter.
2. Non-granular cytoplasm stains deep blue at the periphery and lighter at the center.
3. Nucleus is large, round, and contains moderately fine chromatin and a well-defined nuclear membrane..

4. One or two nucleoli are present.
5. Uncontrolled growth and division leads to a form of cancer called acute lymphoblastic leukemia (ALL).

Prolymphocyte[2]
   1. It measures 10-18 μm in diameter (smaller than lymphoblast)
   2. The cytoplasm is in the form of broadband and stains blue.
   3. Nuclear chromatin tends to be clumped without a definite nucleolus.

Large lymphocyte and small lymphocyte
see chapter 11.

c. Monocytic series

There are two intermediate cells during the development of a mature monocyte. The precursor cell is called the monoblast.

Monoblast
   1. It measures 18-22 μm in diameter.
   2. The cytoplasm stains deep blue and the clear unstained area surrounding the nucleus called the perinuclear zone.
   3. The smooth nuclear chromatin is less definite and stains mauve.
   4. Several nucleoli may be present but are not so prominent as in the lymphoblast.

Promonocyte
   1. It is approximately 20 μm in diameter.
   2. The cytoplasm stains gray-blue and may contain fine azurophilic granules.
   3. A large and convoluted nucleus present that has a folded appearance.
   4. Loose chromatin appears as a network and no definite nucleoli are visible.

Monocyte
see chapter 11.

Plasma cell series

It is believed that the plasma cell is formed from the stem cell (hemohistioblast). The precursor cell (plasmablast) and intermediate cell (pro-plasma cell) are characterized below:

Plasmablast
   1. The shape, size, and staining reaction of plasmablast are very similar to the lymphoblast.
   2. Its average size is 18 μm.
   3. Cytoplasmic granules are not seen.
   4. It is not easy to resolve nucleoli even if their presence up to six.

---

[2] Hairy cells with prominent central nucleoli mimick prolymphocytes.

Pro-plasma cell
1. It varies from 15-25 μm in size.
2. Non-granular cytoplasm stains dark blue showing a pale perinuclear halo.
3. Usually, the nucleus is eccentric but may be present at the center.
4. The nuclear chromatin looks like a loose mesh.
5. Several obvious nucleoli may be seen.

Plasma cell
1. It is usually oval and varies from 14-20 μm in its size.
2. Non-granular cytoplasm stains deep blue with a clear perinuclear halo and may contain one or more vacuoles even in the normal condition.
3. The nucleus lies to one side of the cell with a wheel-like pattern of chromatin arrangement.

3. Megakaryocyte series and formation of platelets: (see Fig. 4.1)

Like the erythrocytes and most of the leukocytes, platelets are formed in the bone marrow. There are three precursor cells in the order given below before mature platelets are formed. They are briefly characterized as under:

Megakaryoblast
1. It varies from 50-100 μm in diameter.
2. The cytoplasm stains intensely blue and forms an irregular rim around the nucleus.
3. The nucleus is large and oval or kidney-shaped with poorly defined chromatin and several dark blue staining nucleoli.
4. It comprises less than 1% of all the megakaryocyte series in the normal bone marrow.
5. It may show 2, 3, or 4 nuclei due to mitotic division as a normal finding.

Promegakaryocyte (basophilic megakaryocyte)
1. This cell is much larger than the megakaryoblast.
2. Basophilic cytoplasm with a finely granular appearance.
3. The nucleus is large and indented.

Megakaryocyte (granular megakaryocyte)
1. It is the largest cell seen in the marrow and may measure up to 100 μm in diameter.
2. Bulky cytoplasm contains many azurophilic granules.
3. The multilobed or indented nucleus is small as compared to the volume of cytoplasm and chromatin is arranged in coarse, deeply staining strands.
4. The late stages of maturation (budding megakaryocyte) are differentiated into granular platelets in pseudopodia-like structures.

Platelets (thrombocytes)
1. They are small cytoplasmic fragments formed after detachment from the irregular margin of the megakaryocyte. Over 1,000 platelets are produced by one megakaryocyte.
2. They are without a cell nucleus.
3. They vary from 2-3 μm in diameter and occasionally from 1-4 μm.
4. The cytoplasm stains light blue with an azurophil staining material at the center.
5. They live for 8-10 days.

Chapter 5

Collection and Care of Blood Specimens

It is of utmost importance to keep the blood specimens unchanged after their collection. This is one of the factors influencing the test results. Therefore, blood specimens are to be transported and stored carefully after they are collected.

1. Anticoagulants

Those chemical agents which prevent blood clotting are called "anticoagulants". The choice of an anticoagulant depends upon the nature of the test to be performed. Furthermore, it is also required to add the appropriate quantity of an anticoagulant to the blood specimen. Some important anticoagulants are summarized in Table 5.1.

Table 5.1: Anticoagulants

Anticoagulant	Concentration, mg/mL	Mode of Action	Use(s)
Ethylenediamine tetraacetate (EDTA)	1.5 ± 0.25	Chelates calcium ions	Complete blood count
Trisodium citrate ($Na_3 C_6 H_5 O_7$, $2H_2O$)	3.2	Converts the calcium into a non-ionized form	ESR, coagulation tests, blood transfusion, PT, PTT
Potassium oxalate	2	Precipitates calcium ions	Blood pH, estimation of lactate, pyruvate, and urea
Heller and Paul mixture: Ammonium oxalate (3 parts) and Potassium oxalate (2 parts)	2	Precipitates calcium ions	Hematocrit, Sedimentation, and specific gravity determinations
Fluoride oxalate: Sodium fluoride (1 part) and Potassium oxalate (5 parts)	4	-Inhibits the glycolytic decomposition of glucose -Precipitates calcium ions	Blood sugar and C.S.F. sugar determinations
Lithium heparin	0.2	Neutralizes thrombin	Osmotic fragility tests, electrolytes, NH_3, and other biochemical determinations

Note: Aqueous solution of an anticoagulant is pipetted into clean and dry containers. Then, they are dried.

2. Collection

Some patients resist puncturing. Therefore, the phlebotomist has to persuade the patient gently. Analysis of blood is performed, using either venous or capillary blood. In some tests (e.g., platelet count), venous blood is the only satisfactory blood specimen, giving satisfactory results.

a. Venous blood

It is most frequently obtained by venipuncture. Before a phlebotomist begins the blood collection, it is required to do positive identification of the patient, explain the procedure, and get the consent. The procedure is as under:

1. Ask the patient to sit or lie down with the forearm resting on a suitable support.
2. Warm the arm for better circulation, distending the veins.
3. Locate the site of the venipuncture (The veins on the front of the elbow called antecubital veins are usually preferred because they are easily visible and not slippery). Select a vein on the dorsum of the hand in obese patients.
4. Tie a tourniquet a few cm above the elbow without obliterating the arterial pulse at the wrist and smack the skin over the site of the vein.
5. Ask the patient to clench the fist to make the vein prominent (If the veins are seen blurry, instruct the patient to exercise the forearm by flexion and extension for a few times).
6. Sterilize the skin over the vein with a small pad of cotton moistened with 70% alcohol.
7. Insert a sterile disposable needle (facing the bevel uppermost) fitted onto a disposable syringe of suitable capacity. Care is to be taken to avoid a semi- or counter-puncturing.
8. Loosen a tourniquet once the blood appears in the syringe to avoid hemoconcentration due to congestion.
9. Pull the piston slowly until the barrel of the syringe is filled up to the desired mark, holding the syringe firmly by the thumb of the other hand.
10. Place a small pad of cotton soaked with 70% alcohol at the site of venipuncture and withdraw the needle quickly. Ask the patient to press the cotton pad till the bleeding stops.
11. Detach the needle and deliver the blood from the syringe into a suitable container and mix with anticoagulant thoroughly by gentle shaking (4-5 times) of the container. Prepare blood films directly from the blood in the syringe.

Note: Arterial blood is less frequently used, e.g., blood gas determination. It is similar in composition to capillary blood.

Vacutainer glass or plastic tubes are also used in the blood collection procedure. According to the nature of additive (s) present in each Vacutainer tube, they are named differently based on the stopper color as shown in Table 5.2.

Table 5.2: Some routinely used Vacutainer tubes with different stopper colors

Stopper color	Additive(s)
Lavender (Purple)	Potassium EDTA
Green	Lithium heparin
Grey	Sodium fluoride and Potassium oxalate
Light blue	Sodium citrate
Light yellow	Sodium polyanethol sulfonate (SPS)*

*Used for blood culture specimens.

Vacutainer tubes are more expensive than disposable plastic syringes, thus limiting their use only in developed countries, e.g., the USA. Therefore, disposable plastic syringes are still used in developing countries.

b. Capillary blood

As capillary (peripheral) blood specimens may give discrepant results, they should be used only when venous blood is not possible. A free flow of blood gives satisfactory blood specimens for some tests. The steps of the procedure are given below:

1. Select the site for skin puncture.
2. Rub the selected sites with lint to promote blood circulation. (In infants, the heel is bathed in hot water).
3. Sterilize the site with a small pad of cotton soaked with 70% alcohol and allow it to dry before pricking.
4. Grasp the part firmly and make a bold puncture smartly to a depth of 2-3 mm with the help of a sterile disposable lancet.
5. Wipe off the first drop that contains tissue juices and foreign matters, causing inaccurate results.
6. Fill the pipette quickly to the calibrated mark after the formation of a compact drop. Do not exert undue pressure. If necessary, gentle pressure may be applied.
7. Press a small pad of cotton moistened with 70% alcohol till bleeding stops.

Ideally, blood films (e.g., thin and thick smears in malarial parasite test) are made immediately after the withdrawal of blood. Either heparinized or plain capillary tubes are used to collect blood for ultramicro techniques in pediatrics.

3. Transportation and storage

In some cases, blood specimens are to be transported from one place to another. For example, blood specimens from patients' residences are to be carried to a clinical laboratory. Sometimes, they are also to be sent from a small laboratory to a large laboratory for a test that is not performed in a small laboratory. Blood specimens should be labeled and arranged in a specially designed ice-box (4°C) for transportation. Mail service can be used in carrying these samples to a distantly situated laboratory. Here, blood specimens should be carefully packed and should carry a paper label, 'potentially infective specimen'.

In hematological tests, the nature of the component under test decides the storage limit. Except for leukocyte and platelet counts, blood may safely be stored overnight at 2°-8°C. It is advisable to count leukocytes and platelets within 2 hours.

Certain changes occur if blood is stored at room temperature (18°-25°C), e.g., swelling of erythrocytes, an increase of osmotic fragility, prothrombin time, and a decrease of ESR. Blood films are prepared immediately and protected from dust, flies, and other foreign contaminants. If collected in EDTA, smears may safely be prepared for up to two hours. Hemoglobin remains unchanged for several days if blood is collected under aseptic conditions in a sterile container.

If a biochemical determination is to be delayed, serum or plasma specimens should be stored at 2°-8°C (refrigerator). The time limit for storage depends on the nature of the component to be assayed. For tests listed below, serum specimens can satisfactorily be stored at 2°-8°C for 5 days:

1. lactate dehydrogenase (LDH)
2. alanine transaminase (ALT)
3. aspartate transaminase (AST)

Serum for bilirubin determination can be stored for one week if kept in the dark under refrigeration. Furthermore, the stability of some blood components can be increased by the addition of thymol, e.g., the storage of uric acid for several days. But, in some determinations, e.g., ammonia, lactate, pyruvate, and pH, whole blood is used immediately where very rapid changes keep on occurring.

Chapter 6

Normal Hematological Values

Introduction

Blood is a red fluid filling the heart and blood vessels. It is kept in continuous circulation by the pumping action of the heart. It flows through arteries (oxygenated blood) and veins (deoxygenated blood). It consists of an opaque and pale-yellow fluid called plasma that contains minute solid corpuscles. These corpuscles are:

1. Red blood cells (erythrocytes)
2. White blood cells (leukocytes)
3. Platelets (thrombocytes)

In normal human blood, erythrocytes outnumber the leukocytes by 500 to 1. Plasma contains 91-92% of water and solids from 8-9%. The solids consist of proteins, glucose, cholesterol, nitrogenous compounds, electrolytes, hormones, enzymes, gases, complement, and antibodies. Blood has the following specific physical properties:

a. Viscosity is four to six times that of water
b. Specific gravity varies between 1.041-1.067
c. pH value of approximately 7.35-7.45
d. Characteristic odor and a salty taste

The total blood volume in an adult is about six liters. In other words, it is about one-thirteenth of body weight and plasma volume about one-twentieth of body weight. The amount of blood varies with age, sex, the quantity of fat and muscle in the body, activity, state of hydration, condition of the heart and blood vessels, and so on. The volume of cells and plasma is approximately equal.

Functions

1. To carry O_2 from the air in the lungs to the tissues, and CO_2 from the tissues to the lungs
2. To carry digested food materials (e.g., glucose, amino acids, and fats) absorbed from the intestine and transport them to the body cells for utilization
3. To transport hormones from the glands to the tissues, requiring them to act as regulators
4. To carry the waste products of metabolism (e.g., urea and creatinine) to the excretory organs, namely the kidneys, the lungs, the intestine, and the skin
5. To help maintain the fluid balance between blood and body cells
6. To help maintain the body temperature at a normal value. Regulation of body temperature is attributed to water possessing the following properties:

   a. high specific heat
   b. high conductivity
   c. high latent heat of evaporation

7. To help maintain the normal acid-alkali balance of the tissues owing to the presence of the plasma electrolytes (e.g., K^+, Na^+, Cl^-, and HCO_3^-)

8. To constitute a defense mechanism of the body against the invasion of harmful organisms due to the presence of phagocytes and lymphocytes
9. To undergo clotting to prevent loss of blood after an injury

Normal hematological values

It is impossible to state 'normal values' or the 'normal range' for laboratory results of hematological tests performed on healthy individuals. The following governing factors are responsible for this difficulty:

1. The sex, age, physique, and occupation
2. Genetic and ethnic background
3. Geographical distribution, particularly altitude
4. The physiological and environmental conditions under which the samples are collected (e.g., diet, emotional stress, and hospitalization)
5. The method and timing of sample collection, conveyance, and preservation
6. Variation in the testing technique used

Also, the overlapping of hematological values from completely healthy and unhealthy individuals occurs because the borderline between them is indefinite. Therefore, the concept of 'normal values' and 'normal range' is being replaced by 'reference values' and 'reference limits'. Here, the variable factors are well described while establishing the 'reference values' for the population under survey in a specific test. It includes a relatively small number of individuals, assuming them to be representatives of the population as a whole. At present, 'reference values' have been established for only a limited number of hematological tests (e.g., red cell indices).

Normal hematological values are determined by a compilation of data from a 'normal' population in each laboratory. Table 6.1 provides data to serve as a rough guide to the 'normal range' that applies to many but not to all healthy persons.

Ethylenediaminetetraacetic acid (EDTA) is the anticoagulant of choice for most hematological test procedures, e.g., CBC with the automated or manual differential count. It is recommended that a full EDTA tube is filled and mixed promptly (by inverting the tube gently at least 6 times). Thus, whole blood is used in most hematological test methods. Heparin (green top tube) and citrate (blue top tube) are not suitable anticoagulants for hematological analysis.

Table 6.1: Hematological reference values

Test	SI unit*	Traditional unit
Red blood cell count	$\times 10^{12}$ cells /L	$\times 10^6$ cells /µL
Men	5.5 ± 1.0	5.5 ± 1.0
Women	4.8 ± 1.0	4.8 ± 1.0
Infants (full-term, cord blood)	5.0 ± 1.0	5.0 ± 1.0
Children, 3 months	4.0 ± 0.8	4.0 ± 0.8
Children, 1 year	4.4 ± 0.8	4.4 ± 0.8

* SI (Systeme International) unit is the recommended method of reporting clinical laboratory results.

Table 6.1 (cont.): Hematological reference values

Test	SI unit*	Traditional unit
Children, 3-6 years	4.8 ± 0.7	4.8 ± 0.7
Children, 10-12 years	4.7 ± 0.7	4.7 ± 0.7
Hemoglobin	**g/L**	**g/dL**
Men	155 ± 25	15.5 ± 2.5
Women	140 ± 25	14.0 ± 2.5
Infants (full-term, cord blood)	165 ± 30	16.5 ± 3.0
Children, 3 months	115 ± 20	11.5 ± 2.0
Children, 1 year	120 ± 15	12.0 ± 1.5
Children, 3-6 years	130 ± 10	13.0 ± 1.0
Children, 10-12 years	130 ± 15	13.0 ± 1.5
Hematocrit/Packed cell volume	**L/L**	**%**
Men	0.47 ± 0.07	47 ± 7
Women	0.42 ± 0.05	42 ± 5
Infants (full-term, cord blood)	0.54 ± 0.10	54 ± 10
Children, 3 months	0.38 ± 0.06	38 ± 6
Children, 3-6 years	0.40 ± 0.04	40 ± 4
Children, 10-12 years	0.41 ± 0.04	41 ± 4
Mean corpuscular volume (MCV)	**fL**	**μm^3**
Adults	86 ± 10	86 ± 10
Infants (full-term, cord blood)	106	106
Children, 3 months	95	95
Children, 1 year	78 ± 8	78 ± 8
Children, 3-6 years	81 ± 8	81 ± 8
Children, 10-12 years	84 ± 7	84 ± 7
Mean corpuscular hemoglobin (MCH)	**pg/cell**	**pg/cell**
Adults	29.5 ± 2.5	29.5 ± 2.5

* SI (Systeme International) unit is the recommended method of reporting clinical laboratory results.

Table 6.1 (cont.)**:** Hematological reference values

Test	SI unit*	Traditional unit
Children, 3 months	29.0 ± 5.0	29.0 ± 5.0
Children, 1 year	27.0 ± 4.0	27.0 ± 4.0
Children, 3-6 years	27.0 ± 3.0	27.0 ± 3.0
Children, 10-12 years	27.0 ± 3.0	27.0 ± 3.0
Mean corpuscular hemoglobin concentration (MCHC)	**g/L**	**g/dL**
Adults	325 ± 25	32.5 ± 2.5
Children	325 ± 25	32.5 ± 2.5
Red cell distribution width (RDW)	$11.0 - 15.0\ \%$	$11.0 - 15.0\ \%$
Reticulocytes *(relative)*	**%**	**%**
Adults and children	0.2 - 2	0.2 - 2
Infants (full-term, cord blood)	2 - 6	2 - 6
Reticulocytes *(absolute)*	**x10⁹ cells/L**	**x10³ cells/μL**
Adults and children	25 - 85	25 - 85
Infants (full-term, cord blood)	150	150
Red-cell volume	**mL/kg**	
Men	30 ± 5	-
Women	25 ± 5	-
Plasma volume	45 ± 5	-
Total blood volume	70 ± 10	-
Red cell life span	120 ± 30 days	-
Leukocyte count *(total)*	**x10⁹ cells /L**	**x10³ cells / μL**
Adults	7.5 ± 3.5	7.5 ± 3.5
Infants (full-term, first day)	18 ± 8.0	18 ± 8.0
Infants, 1 year	12 ± 6.0	12 ± 6.0
Children, 4-7 years	10 ± 5.0	10 ± 5.0
Children, 8-12 years	9.0 ± 4.5	9.0 ± 4.5
Differential leukocyte count *(absolute)*	**x10⁹ cells /L**	**x10³ cells / μL**

* SI (Systeme International) unit is the recommended method of reporting clinical laboratory results.

Table 6.1 (cont.)**:** Hematological reference values

Test	SI unit*	Traditional unit
Adults		
Neutrophils	2.0 - 7.5	2.0 -7.5
Lymphocytes	1.5 - 4.0	1.5 - 4.0
Monocytes	0.2 - 0.8	0.2 - 0.8
Eosinophils	0.04 - 0.4	0.04 - 0.4
Basophils	<0.01- 0.1	<0.01 - 0.1
Infants (first day)		
Neutrophils	5.0 - 13	5.0 - 13
Lymphocytes	3.5 - 8.5	3.5 - 8.5
Monocytes	0.5 - 1.5	0.5 - 1.5
Eosinophils	0.1 - 2.5	0.1 - 2.5
Basophils	<0.01 - 0.1	<0.01 - 0.1
Infants (three days)		
Neutrophils	1.5 - 7.0	1.5 - 7.0
Lymphocytes	2.0 - 5.0	2.0 - 5.0
Monocytes	0.3 - 1.1	0.3 - 1.1
Eosinophils	0.2 - 2.0	0.2 - 2.0
Basophils	<0.01 - 0.1	<0.01 - 0.1
Children (six years)		
Neutrophils	2.0 - 6.0	2.0 - 6.0
Lymphocytes	5.5 - 8.5	5.5 - 8.5
Monocytes	0.7 - 1.5	0.7 - 1.5
Eosinophils	0.3 - 0.8	0.3 - 0.8
Basophils	<0.01 - 0.1	<0.01 - 0.1
Differential leukocyte count (*relative*)	%	%
Neutrophils	38 - 80	38 - 80

* SI (Systeme International) unit is the recommended method of reporting clinical laboratory results.

Table 6.1 (cont.): Hematological reference values

Test	SI unit*	Traditional unit
Lymphocytes	15 - 49	15 - 49
Monocytes	0 - 13	0 - 13
Eosinophils	0 - 8	0 - 8
Basophils	0 - 2	0 – 2
Platelet count	$x10^9$ cells /L	$x10^3$ cells / μL
Adults	150 - 400	150 - 400
Mean platelet volume (MPV)	7.5 - 12.5 fL	7.5 - 12.5 μ³
Bleeding time (Duke's method)	1 - 3 min	1 - 3 min
Prothrombin time (PT)	11 - 13.5 secs	11 - 13.5 secs
INR	0.9 - 1.1	0.9 - 1.1
Activated partial thromboplastin time (APTT)	27 - 35 secs	27 - 35 secs
Thrombin Time (TT)	11 - 15 secs	11 - 15 secs
Prothrombin - consumption index	0 - 30 %	-
	g/L	mg/dL
Plasma fibrinogen	2 - 4	200 - 400
Fibrinogen antigen	1.49 - 3.53	149 - 353
D - Dimer	< 0.005	< 0.5
Iron (serum):	**μmol/L**	**μg/dL**
Adult males	13 - 31	75 - 175
Adult females	5 – 29	28 -162
Total iron-binding capacity (TIBC) (serum)	45 - 73	250 - 410
Iron (transferrin) saturation	**%**	**%**
Adult males	20 - 50	20 - 50
Adult females	15 - 50	15 - 50
Serum ferritin	**μg/L**	**ng/mL**
Adult males	12 - 300	12 - 300
Adult females	12 - 150	12 - 150

* SI (Systeme International) unit is the recommended method of reporting clinical laboratory results.

Sedimentation rate (Westergren's method at $20° \pm 3°C$)

Table 6.1 (cont.)**:** Hematological reference values

Test	SI unit*	Traditional unit
	mm/h	mm/h
Men 17-50 years	1 - 7	1 - 7
>50 years	2 - 10	2 - 10
Women 17-50 years	3 - 9	3 - 9
>50 years	5 - 15	5 - 15

* SI (Systeme International) unit is the recommended method of reporting clinical laboratory results.

Chapter 7

Hemoglobins and their Determinations

Introduction

Most of the cells in the blood are erythrocytes. Millions of erythrocytes circulate in the bloodstream. The erythrocytes contain a conjugated protein called hemoglobin. Hemoglobin is a pigment (coloring matter) containing iron. The color of blood is red owing to the presence of hemoglobin combined with oxygen. It is estimated that there are about 750 g of hemoglobin in the circulating blood of a 70 kg man. About 6.25 g of hemoglobin is produced and destroyed daily. Furthermore, one erythrocyte contains about 600 million molecules of hemoglobin.

Hemoglobin has a more important function than just giving color to the blood. It can combine loosely with oxygen. It is this ability that makes it possible for the erythrocytes to deliver oxygen to the cells of the body.

Oxygen is a part of the air breathed into the lungs. The erythrocytes in the bloodstream pass through the lungs where the hemoglobin picks up oxygen. The erythrocytes, traveling through the bloodstream, release oxygen to the body cells.

When the oxygen is released, hemoglobin takes up carbon dioxide from the cells. This gas is a waste product that is formed when the cells burn food. The erythrocytes combined with carbon dioxide return to the lungs. Thus, an exchange of oxygen and carbon dioxide occurs during respiratory activity.

Normal Hemoglobins

Hemoglobin consists of iron-containing heme molecules, linked to globin chains (see Fig. 7.1). The heme is formed from succinyl coenzyme A and glycine, involving a key enzyme called δ-aminolevulinic acid synthetase (ALA synthetase). Hemoglobin synthesis involves the following steps:

1. 2 succinyl-CoA + 2 glycine $\longrightarrow$ pyrrole

2. 4 pyrrole $\longrightarrow$ protoporphyrin IX

3. protoporphyrin IX + Fe^{++} $\longrightarrow$ heme

4. heme + polypeptide $\longrightarrow$ hemoglobin chain (alpha or beta)

5. 2 alpha chains + 2 beta chains $\longrightarrow$ hemoglobin A

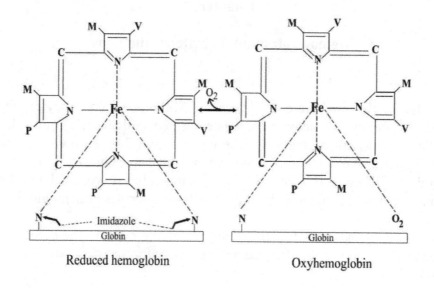

Reduced hemoglobin   Oxyhemoglobin

Fig. 7.1: Imidazole conjugation in hemoglobin.

There are two pairs of globin chains. Each globin moiety has a molecular weight of about 64,000 daltons. Based on the total number and sequence of amino acids forming a globin chain, they are classified into four groups:

1. Alpha chains (α): composed of 141 amino acids
2. Beta chains (β): composed of 146 amino acids
3. Gamma chains (γ): composed of 146 amino acids
4. Delta chains (δ): composed of 146 amino acids

Alpha chains are present in all normal hemoglobins, namely Hb F, Hb A, and Hb A2. The formation of all forms of globin is under genetic control.

Hemoglobin F
It is present in newborn children. It consists of two alpha chains and two gamma chains ($\alpha2\ \gamma2$). Normally, it is replaced by hemoglobin A by the end of the first year.

Hemoglobin A
It is present in adults. It consists of two alpha chains and two beta chains ($\alpha2\ \beta2$). It persists throughout life.

Hemoglobin A2
It is also present in a small quantity in adults. It consists of two alpha chains and two delta chains ($\alpha2\ \delta2$).

Approximate percentages of these normal hemoglobins in healthy neonates and adults are given in Table 7.1.

Table 7.1: Distribution (%) of normal hemoglobin in neonates and adults

Hb type	Neonate (%)	Adult (%)
F	75	<1
A	25	>97
A2	<1	<3

Hemoglobin abnormalities (hemoglobinopathy, hemoglobin variants)

Hemoglobins with abnormal globin chains are called abnormal hemoglobins. The phenomenon of occurrence of abnormal hemoglobins in the circulating blood is termed as 'hemoglobinopathy'. Hemoglobinopathy may develop in either of the following two ways:

a. Abnormal hemoglobins may result from minor changes in the globin residues. These changes take place from mutations of the α chains (e.g., hemoglobin, namely I, P, Q, and D) or of the β chains (e.g., hemoglobin, namely S, C, D, E, G, J, L, and N) of hemoglobin A. For example, both Hb S and Hb C are formed due to the replacement by amino acids valine and lysine, respectively at position 6 in the beta chain of Hb A. Out of these abnormal, only a few (i.e., hemoglobin, namely S, C, D, and E) are of clinical significance.

b. Abnormal hemoglobins are the result of suppression of α- or β- chain biosynthesis of Hb A. This is well exemplified by thalassemia. Several forms of thalassemia are grouped below:

1. Alpha thalassemia (an alpha chain deficiency): e.g., Hb Barts (γ4) and Hb H (β4).
2. Beta thalassemia (a beta chain deficiency): e.g., Cooley's anemia.
3. Thalassemia major (the thalassemia gene is homologous): It can cause serious disease.
4. Thalassemia minor (the thalassemia gene is heterozygous): It is called a trait form. Usually, the effects are mild and may not require any treatment.

Estimation of hemoglobin

Hemoglobin can be determined by the following four methods:

a. Spectrophotometry
Owing to the toxicity of the reagent (potassium ferricyanide and potassium cyanide), the cyanmethemoglobin (HiCN) method is obsolete. However, the method is used as a reference method in standardizing all new methods. It is a simple, convenient, and reproducible method. It is based on the following principle:

$$1.\ \text{Hemoglobin} \xrightarrow[\text{alk. pH}]{\text{pot. ferricyanide}} \text{Methemoglobin}$$

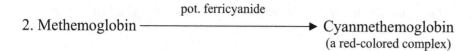

2. Methemoglobin $\xrightarrow{\text{pot. ferricyanide}}$ Cyanmethemoglobin
(a red-colored complex)

Nowadays, automated hematology analyzers use sodium lauryl sulfate (SLS), replacing the toxic reagent used in the cyanmethemoglobin (HiCN) method. Sodium lauryl sulfate (pH of 7.2), a surfactant, plays a dual role:

(i) Causes lysis of erythrocytes to liberate hemoglobin
(ii) Leads to the formation of a colored complex, SLS–MetHb (stable for a few hours)

The absorbance of the complex, SLS–MetHb, is read at a wavelength of 539 nm. The complex obeys Beer-Lambert's law, showing precise linearity between the hemoglobin concentration and the absorbance of SLS-MetHb. Thus, this is an accurate method in the determination of hemoglobin.

b. Electrophoresis
The technique uses cellulose acetate gel, a buffer at pH 8.6, and an electric supply instrument as basic components. Since Hb S and Hb D migrate to the same destination in alkaline cellulose acetate paper electrophoresis, citrate agar-gel electrophoresis at pH 6.2 can successfully separate these two hemoglobins. Hemoglobin D migrates farther from the point of origin than Hb S.

The blood specimen is applied close to a cathode (a negative electrode). Various hemoglobin forms migrate towards the anode (a positive electrode). The nature of an electrical charge and its magnitude carried by an individual form of hemoglobin determines its direction and the speed of migration, respectively during the electrophoretic run. For more information about the technique, the reader is advised to refer to chapter 3 (Fig. 3.6).

Hemoglobin electrophoresis is very valuable in the identification of any abnormal types of hemoglobin in some blood disorders e.g., sickle cell anemia, thalassemia, and polycythemia vera. Also, it is used to screen genetically abnormal variants of hemoglobin in newborns, if any.

c. Chromatography
Recently, high-performance liquid chromatography (HPLC), a form of column chromatography, has been adopted widely in the determination of hemoglobin. The basic components of HPLC include a column, stationary phase, mobile phase, autosampler, detector(s), and a data system. HPLC separates various variants of hemoglobin efficiently. Thus, the measurement of Hb A2 and Hb F by the HPLC is rapid, reproducible, precise, and technically easy.

Glycosylated hemoglobin (A1c) is successfully separated from other hemoglobins (e.g., Hb F) by the HPLC method. The percentage of A1c (Normal= 4-5.6%) reflects the average blood glucose level over the past three months. A1c is formed by the irreversible attachment of glucose to the hemoglobin.

CO-oximeter uses multi-wavelength spectrophotometry and complex computations. In other words, the device measures the absorption of light from a few (2 or 3) to several dozens of wavelengths, thus differentiating between oxyhemoglobin (O_2 Hb) and deoxyhemoglobin (HHb).

Additionally, it enables the device to distinguish between these and carboxyhemoglobin (COHb), methemoglobin (metHb), other hemoglobins, and 'background' light-absorbing species.

A well-mixed arterial blood specimen is injected into the blood gas analyzer (BGA)/CO-oximeter. A portion of the blood specimen is automatically pumped to a measuring cuvette of the CO-oximeter followed by the lysis of erythrocytes, releasing the hemoglobin. Then, hemoglobin species are scanned spectroscopically at multiple wavelengths between 520-620 nm. Finally, the software calculates the concentration of each of the hemoglobin derivatives, namely HHb, O2Hb, MetHb, and COHb. Thus, hemoglobin ctHb[3] is measured within a minute or two, justifying its applications for point-of-care testing (POCT), e.g., emergency rooms.

---

[3] The sum of oxygenated Hb, deoxygenated Hb, carboxyhemoglobin, and methemoglobin.

Chapter 8

Anemias and Hematological Indices

Introduction

Anemia is a blood condition in which the Hb has fallen below the normal for a person. It may be due to fewer normal red cells, or due to less Hb in the normal number of red cells. There may be a fewer red cells, as well as, less Hb in them. Anemias can be classified based on etiology. They are classified as under:

A. Anemia caused by blood loss

Bleeding may be chronic or acute.

1. Chronic bleeding: There is a slow loss of erythrocytes. Newly formed erythrocytes have less hemoglobin because of a gradual loss of iron from the body. Chronic bleeding occurs in the following conditions:

- Hook-worm infection
- Gastrointestinal bleeding (e.g., peptic ulcers, malignant growths)
- Abnormal menstrual bleeding

Chronic bleeding may result in iron-deficiency anemia with hypochromic and microcytic erythrocytes.

2. Acute bleeding: There is a rapid loss of erythrocytes. Acute bleeding may develop shock and heart failure. It occurs in the following conditions:

- Antepartum hemorrhage (APH)
- Postpartum hemorrhage (PPH)
- Accidental injury

Laboratory findings in anemias caused by acute bleeding and chronic bleeding are shown in Table 8.1.

Table 8.1: Laboratory findings in anemias caused by acute bleeding and chronic bleeding

Laboratory finding	Acute bleeding	Chronic bleeding
RBCs	-Normocytic, normochromic	-Microcytic, hypochromic (iron deficiency) -Increased RDW
Reticulocytes	-Increased within 3-5 days	-Normal
Hematocrit and hemoglobin	- Steady during the first few hours. - Hemorrhage is evident within 48-72 hours.	-Decreased
Other	-Nucleated RBCs may be released	-Decreased serum iron and ferritin -Increased TIBC

B. Anemia caused by the destruction of erythrocytes

There are many conditions in which the lifespan of erythrocytes is shortened, leading to hemolytic anemia.

1. Abnormal hemoglobins: Clinically significant abnormal hemoglobins include Hb S, Hb C, Hb D, and Hb E. Hb S causes sickle cell anemia. Hb S, in a reduced state, undergoes crystallization with the formation of sickle cells. Sickle cells so formed have a very short life span and undergo rapid hemolysis. Thus, hemoglobin level decreases. Sickle cell anemia occurs mainly in India, tropical Africa, and amongst African Americans.

2. Glucose-6-phosphate dehydrogenase (G6PD) deficiency: Normally G6PD is present in the erythrocytes. But, inherited abnormality of G6PD deficiency is noticed in certain people, including those of New Guinea, Africa, Greece, and Sardinia. G6PD deficient erythrocytes undergo abnormal hemolysis if they are exposed to certain oxidizing drugs (e.g., primaquine, aspirin, and dapsone). Therefore, a physician advises patients for the G6PD test if they are to be treated with such drugs. Following treatment with the above-mentioned drugs in patients with G6PD deficiency, Heinz bodies can be seen in the erythrocytes.

3. Immune antibodies: In the following three conditions, immune antibodies cause hemolysis with the development of hemolytic anemia.

- a. Incompatible blood transfusions (see chapter 51)
- b. Hemolytic disease of the fetus and newborn (see chapter 51)
- c. Autoimmune hemolytic diseases (Autoimmune antibodies are found in some diseases, e.g., viral pneumonia, congenital syphilis, leukemia, malignant diseases, and lupus erythematosus)

4. Toxic substances: Toxic substances (e.g., snake venom, the toxin of *Clostridium welchii*, and certain drugs, including herbs) bring about lysis of erythrocytes, leading to the development of hemolytic anemia.

5. Malaria: In the course of the development of malarial parasites, trophozoites attack erythrocytes and pass through the stage of schizont. Mature schizonts rupture erythrocytes, liberating merozoites.

The liberated merozoites invade fresh erythrocytes and thus the cycle of erythrocytic schizogony is repeated. In addition to this, erythrocytes without malarial parasites have a narrow lifespan, contributing to the development of anemia. Further details are given in chapter 44.

C. Anemia caused by abnormalities of red cell formation

1. Thalassemia: It is an inherited quantitative abnormality. Hb A is not formed in the normal way. There is a resemblance between Thalassemia (Cooley's anemia) and severe iron deficiency anemia.

2. Iron-deficiency: This causes the commonest type of anemia called iron-deficiency anemia found all over the world. The frequency and severity of this type of anemia is more amongst the poor. Iron deficiency is noticed in 20-40% of the Indians. Causes of iron deficiency anemia can be summarized as follows:

a. Increased demand for iron: e.g., breastfeeding of over 6 months, loss of blood at the time of delivery, and iron transferred to fetus and placenta.

b. Dietary deficiency: The total iron content of the diet for males and females should be 10 mg and 20 mg respectively per day. Iron is present in cereals, wheat, and leafy vegetables. Thus, the average Indian diet contains sufficient iron to meet the needs of non-pregnant women (about 20-22 mg). The author, during his research work, found that excessive phytate in the diet decreases the absorption of iron.

c. Chronic blood loss: There are many conditions in which a gradual loss of blood occurs, e.g., peptic ulcer, colorectal cancer, and hookworm infestation.

d. Failure to absorb iron: Iron and other nutrients are absorbed into the bloodstream through the small intestine. Therefore, intestinal disorders (e.g., celiac disease) influence the intestine's ability to absorb nutrients, including iron.

Laboratory findings are listed below:

    (1) The level of MCHC is less than 30%.
    (2) The peripheral smear reveals hypochromia and microcytosis.
    (3) There is an absence of stainable iron in the marrow.
    (4) There is marked erythroid hyperplasia in the marrow film.
    (5) The serum iron is low (< 60 µg/dL) and the total iron-binding capacity (TIBC) is high (> 300µg/dL).
    (6) There is a low percentage of transferrin saturation (< 15%).

3. Folic acid and vitamin B12 deficiencies: Folic acid and vitamin B12 are important compounds for the formation of nuclear DNA. The most prominent effect of deficiency of these compounds is seen in the bone marrow in which cell turnover is fast. Thus, erythrocytes are unable to develop normally. As a result of this, cells enlarge with poorly developed nuclei and they are called macrocytes. These cells enter the bloodstream where they disappear shortly. Anemia developed in this way is called megaloblastic anemia.

Folic acid deficiency can occur due to dietary insufficiency, malabsorption (e.g., tropical sprue), or increased demands by the body (e.g., pregnancy and sickle cell anemia). Folic acid is present in meat, yeast, spinach, and green vegetables. It is destroyed by prolonged cooking.

Animals cannot form vitamin B12. Moreover, this vitamin is absent in vegetables. The deficiency of vitamin B12 usually occurs due to malabsorption. There should be the presence of intrinsic factor (IF) in the stomach for the absorption of vitamin B12. In other words, vitamin B12 can only be absorbed if combined with IF. Thus, anemia develops in the absence of IF and is called pernicious or Addisonian anemia. This anemia is rarely seen in India. The deficiency of vitamin B12 occasionally occurs by infection with the fish tapeworm *(Diphyllobothrium latum)* which sucks the vitamin from its host. Vitamin B12 is present in animal products, including meat and eggs. There is pancytopenia, hypersegmentation of polymorphs, presence of Howell-Jolly bodies with normal MCHC. Megaloblastic and pernicious anemia show normochromic and macrocytosis. Biochemically, serum vitamin B12 is less than 120 ng/L (normal: >160 ng/L) and mild jaundice (serum bilirubin rarely exceeds 3 mg%). Serum vitamin B12 can be assayed, using *Lactobacillus leichmannii.*

It is advisable to confirm the megaloblastic anemia by examining bone marrow. One can notice the increase of marrow activity (hyperplasia), showing the presence of megaloblasts and large metamyelocytes.

D. Anemia caused by bone marrow inactivity

Normally, the bone marrow produces blood cells, including erythrocytes. Erythropoietin from the kidney is an important factor for the hypercellularity of marrow. But damaged marrow may produce a diminished number of erythrocytes with the development of hypoplastic anemia. When marrow fails to form erythrocytes, the anemia is called aplastic anemia. Conditions, where marrow is damaged, include leukemia, other malignant diseases, the reaction of certain drugs (e.g., chloramphenicol), and exposure to large doses of X-rays.

Paroxysmal nocturnal hemoglobinuria (a type of hemolytic anemia) may be followed by aplastic anemia.

Laboratory findings in aplastic anemia include pancytopenia, increased leukocyte alkaline phosphatase, and absence of nucleated red cells. Furthermore, the size and shape of the erythrocytes are usually normal. In other words, aplastic anemia is normocytic, normochromic anemia.

Packed cell volume (PCV)

The packed cell volume, also called hematocrit, is the volume occupied by the packed erythrocytes in a given volume of anticoagulated blood after optimum centrifugation in a microhematocrit tube. It is expressed as a percentage of the total volume of the blood specimen. It is a simple and very accurate method of ruling out whether a patient is normal, anemic, or polycythemic.

The "rule of 3" states that the hemoglobin (Hb) times 3 should approximate the hematocrit (Hct), e.g., Hb of 10 g/dL x 3 = Hct of 30%.

Microhematocrit method

It can be performed, using capillary blood or anticoagulated venous blood. It is a quick method because of much less centrifugation time.

Procedure

Fill about two-thirds of the tube with blood and seal the other end with plasticine[4] (Capillary blood can be collected directly into a heparinized capillary tube).

1. Centrifuge the capillary or microhematocrit for 5 minutes at 12,000 rpm
2. Read the percentage of packed erythrocytes in the spun capillary tube, placing in the specially provided scale.
3. In the case of a microhematocrit, the percentage can be read directly from the graduations marked on the microhematocrit itself.

The hematocrit value is calculated (i.e., indirect measurement) in modern auto analyzers. It is obtained by multiplying the red cell count by the mean cell volume.

Lowered levels of hematocrit are witnessed in:
- Bone marrow disorders
- Chronic inflammatory disease
- Nutritional deficiencies, e.g., iron, folate, and vitamin B12
- Hemolytic anemia
- Sickle cell anemia
- Internal bleeding
- Kidney failure
- Leukemia
- Lymphoma

Elevated levels of hematocrit are witnessed in:
- Dehydration
- Dengue fever
- Congenital heart disease (CHD)
- Lung diseases
- Kidney tumor
- Polycythemia vera

Hematological indices: {see Appendix IX (a)}

Hematological indices are very useful values in the study of anemias. They are calculated as under:

$$1.\,\text{Color index} = \frac{\text{Hb\%}}{\text{RBC\%}}$$

Normal: 0.9-1.1; **High**: pernicious anemia; **Low**: iron deficiency anemia.

---

[4] It is not necessary to seal the microhematocrit tube because the end is closed when it is screwed into position in the centrifuge machine.

$$2.\,Mean\ corpuscular\ volume\ (MCV) = \frac{PCV \times 10}{RBC\ in\ million/cu\ mm}$$

Normal: 76-96 femtoliters (fL); **High:** macrocytic anemia; **Low:** microcytic hypochromic anemia

$$3.\,Mean\ corpuscular\ hemoglobin\ (MCH) = \frac{Hb/liter\ blood}{RBC/liter\ blood}$$

$$= \frac{Hb \times 10}{RBC\ in\ millions}\ expressed\ in\ micrograms$$

Normal: 29.5 g; **High:** macrocytic anemia; **Low:** hypochromic anemia.

$$4.\,Mean\ cell\ hemoglobin\ concentration\ (MCHC) = \frac{Hb\ in\ g\ \%\ \times 100}{PCV}$$

Normal: 32-36%; **High:** not possible; **Low:** iron deficiency anemia.

Chapter 9

Manual Count of Blood Cells

1. Total leukocyte count

The total number of leukocytes in one cubic millimeter of blood is called the total leukocyte count. It is clinically significant when accompanied by a differential leukocyte count. An improved Neubauer chamber (see Fig. 9.1) is used to perform the manual total count of leukocytes.

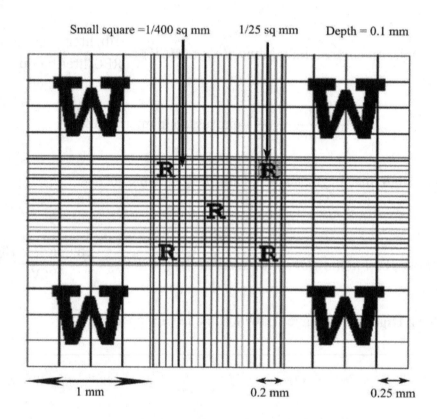

Fig.9.1: Improved Neubauer Chamber.

Reagent

WBC diluting fluid (Turk solution)

	mL
1% aqueous gentian violet solution	1.0
Acetic acid, glacial	2.0
Distilled water	to 98.00

Procedure

1. Pipette 0.38 mL of WBC diluting fluid in a clean and dry test tube.
2. Add 0.02 mL of blood into the diluting fluid and mix well.
3. Attach securely the special coverslip to the counting chamber.
4. Charge the chamber with the diluted blood.
5. Let the cells settle for two minutes.
6. Count the cells in an area of 4 sq mm, using the 10x objective lens with reduced condenser aperture (see Fig. 9.2).

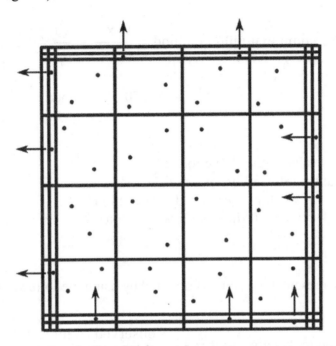

Fig. 9.2: Cells on the lines of any two adjacent sides of the square are included in the count.

Calculation

Area of one large corner square = length x breadth
$$= 1 \text{ mm X } 1 \text{ mm}$$
$$= 1\text{sq mm}$$

Now, the volume of one large corner square = area x depth
$$= 1\text{sq mm x } 0.1 \text{ mm}$$
$$= 0.1 \text{ cu mm}$$

Therefore, the volume of four large corner squares = 0.4 cu mm

Suppose, the total number of cells counted in 4 large corner squares,

$$\mathbf{W} = (W_1 + W_2 + W_3 + W_4)$$

If 0.4 cu mm contains **W** cells. Therefore, 1 cu mm (1 µL) contains (?)

$$= \frac{W \times 1}{0.4}$$

$$= \frac{W \times 10}{4}$$

Since the dilution is 1 in 20,

Therefore, the total WBC count in undiluted blood $= \dfrac{W \times 10 \times 20}{4}$ /µL of blood

$$= W \times 50 /\mu L \text{ of blood}$$

Example

    If **W** = 180
    By plugging this value in the above formula,
    Total WBC count = 180 x 50/µL of blood
                 = 9,000/µL *or* 9.0×10^3/µL of blood
                 = 9.0×10^9/liter of blood (SI Unit)

Note:

1. If nucleated RBCs are present, the count is corrected by using the following formula:

$$\text{Corrected leukocyte count} = \frac{\text{observed count} \times 100}{100 + \text{percent nucleated RBCs}}$$

2. The percent nucleated erythrocyte is obtained from the differential count.
3. The count is reported to the nearest hundred.

Factors affecting total leukocyte count

    1. Age
    2. Exercise
    3. Emotional stress
    4. Epileptic seizure
    5. Gender

Sources of error

    1. Faulty equipment such as poorly calibrated or dirty hemocytometers, and scratched or warped cover-slips may cause erroneous results.
    2. Inadequate mixing of the patient sample causes inaccurate cell distribution.
    3. Excess blood left on the outside of the capillary pipette contaminates the diluting fluid, and falsely increases later determinations using the same fluid.

4. Air bubbles introduced into the pipette during dilution cause over dilution, resulting in decreased counts.
5. Inadequate mixing of the diluted blood causes poor cell distribution.
6. Improper filling of the chamber causes erroneous results.
7. Failure to expel the first few drops of cell-free diluting fluid results in decreased counts.
8. Overfilling the chamber results in increased counts. Filling the chamber using more than one drop may cause poor cell distribution. Also, too hard squeezing of the reservoir may expel the specimen, making an inadequately mixed sample.
9. Evaporation of the diluting fluid from the charged hemocytometer results in the concentration of the specimen, giving high counts.
10. Only mature erythrocytes are hemolyzed by the diluent, but reticulocytes are not lysed.

Both the multiple sources of error and lack of feasibility of a manual leukocyte method, the technique is obsolete. The purpose of the inclusion of a manual method is to simply familiarize the reader with the old method. Fully automated instruments use state-of-the-art technology to achieve quick, accurate, and precise blood counts. The author recognizes this as a "period of transition" in all areas of a clinical laboratory. The reader is advised to refer to chapter 15 for the details.

Clinical significance

Leukocytosis (an increase of leukocytes)
- Pyogenic bacterial infections
- Leukemia

Leukopenia (decrease of leukocytes)
- Typhoid
- Malaria
- Influenza
- Infective hepatitis

2. Absolute eosinophil count

There is considerable variation in the eosinophil count. The lowest counts are found in the morning (10 a.m. to 12 noon) and the highest at night (12 midnight to 4 a.m.).

Principle
The diluent stains the eosinophil granules brightly and distinctly and at the same time lyse the erythrocytes and all other types of leukocytes.

Reagent
Dunger's solution (Diluting fluid)

	mL
Yellow eosin aqueous (200 g/L)	10.00
Acetone	10.00
Water	80.00

The diluting fluid can be stored for 2 to 3 weeks at 4°C. It must be filtered before use. Merthiolate (an antifungal agent) may be added to increase its shelf-life. The manual absolute eosinophil counting is not only erroneous but also tedious and time-consuming.

Automated hematology analyzers (i.e., CBC with five-part WBC differentials) have rendered manual methods obsolete. Thus, the fluorescent flow cytometry is undoubtedly a promising technology that discerns the cell morphology, e.g., nucleus-plasma ratio.

Clinical significance

- Skin diseases, e.g., scabies, eczema, and dermatitis
- Helminth infections, e.g., *Loa loa* and *Wuchereria bancrofti*
- Allergic disorders, e.g., bronchial asthma, hay fever, and urticaria
- Following irradiation
- Following treatment with certain drugs, e.g., penicillin
- Hodgkin's disease
- Brucellosis

3. Total erythrocyte count

Hematocytometer results may not be accurate. Therefore, this method is obsolete. Cell counters can be used for the accuracy of the count. However, it may be requested when investigating an anemic patient.

Reagent
Formol citrate solution

Sodium citrate	3 g
Formalin	1 mL
Distilled water	99 mL

Alternatively, Hayem's diluting fluid can be used.

Procedure

1. Draw well-mixed venous blood to the mark using a 0.02 mL pipette, avoiding air bubbles.
2. Wipe the tip of the pipette, ensuring the blood is still on the mark.
3. Wash the pipetted blood in 4 mL of diluting fluid and mix well.
4. Securely attach the coverslip to the chamber and press it into place.
5. Charge the chamber with the well-mixed diluted blood by using a fine bore Pasteur pipette.

6. Allow the cells to settle for 5 minutes while the chamber sits in a Petri dish that contains a piece of wet filter paper.
7. Count the number of red cells under a 40x objective lens in 1/5 sq mm, including 5 small squares of the large central square as shown in Fig. 9.2.

Calculation

$$\text{Total RBC count} = \frac{\text{red cells counted x dilution factor}}{\text{volume counted}} /\mu L \text{ of blood}$$

$$= \text{red cells counted x } 200 \text{ x } 5 \text{ x } 10/\mu L \text{ of blood}$$
$$= \text{red cells counted x } 10{,}000/\mu L \text{ of blood}$$

Example

$$\text{Red cells counted in 1/5 sq mm} = 400$$
$$\text{Red cells counted in 1 } \mu L = 400 \text{ x } 10{,}000$$
$$= 4{,}000{,}000$$
$$= 4.0 \text{ million } \textbf{\textit{or}} \; 4.0 \text{ x } 10^6$$
$$\text{Total RBC count} = 4.0 \text{ x } 10^6/\mu L \text{ of blood}$$
$$= 4.0 \text{ x } 10^{12}/\text{liter of blood (SI Unit)}$$

Clinical significance

Polycythemia (an increase of red cell count)

- Cyanotic congenital heart disease
- Polycythemia vera
- Renal adenocarcinoma
- Chronic obstructive pulmonary disease
- Carbon monoxide exposure

4. Platelet count

Platelets (thrombocytes) are simply fragments of megakaryocytes. Megakaryocytes, in turn, are produced in the bone marrow. A single megakaryocyte can generate approximately 2000 - 4000 fragments, i.e., platelets. Unlike living cells, platelets lack a nucleus and are unable to divide. The life span of platelets is about 8-10 days. The destruction of platelets occurs in the spleen. These small biconvex disc-like structures play a key role to stop the bleeding of injured blood vessels through the formation of a 'plug'.

Platelets contain two types of important granules: (1) Alpha granules that contain molecules, e.g., glycoprotein IIb/IIIa (GP IIb/IIIa), glycoprotein Ib (GP Ib), and Platelet factor 4 (PF4) (2) Dense body granules contain substances, namely calcium, ADP, thromboxane, and serotonin. The components of these granules directly or indirectly play a major role in stimulating the platelets to mediate adhesion and aggregation. The activated GP Ib serves as an important receptor that helps platelets cross-link von Willebrand's factor located on exposed collagen during subendothelial injury. This process is called adhesion. On the other hand, the activated platelet receptor named GPIIb/IIIa binds the soluble plasma fibrinogen to form a web-like aggregation of the stimulated platelets (i.e., hemostatic plug formation). Interestingly, the damaged endothelial cells also release the most potent inhibitory substance, prostacyclin, capable of acting against the platelet aggregation.

It is required to take precautions while doing platelet counts because they are very small in size, agglutinate, break up easily, and adhere to glassware and particles in the diluent. Three methods namely, immunological, optical, and impedance were compared using phase-contrast microscopy. Phase-contrast microscopy allows biologists to characterize the living cells without staining. Immunological platelet counting (e.g., CELL - DYN 4000 from Abbott) was justified as a method of choice because impedance- and optical-based methods yield inaccurate results in some conditions, e.g., red cell fragments and of giant platelets.

Manual platelet count requires a hemocytometer for some conditions, e.g., the presence of giant platelets and schistocytes.

Procedure
1. Collect blood by making a clean venipuncture and mix gently with EDTA in a small glass tube.
2. Make the standard dilution 1:100, using 1% ammonium oxalate diluent (or Rees Ecker diluting fluid). Therefore, the dilution factor is 100.
3. Charge the chamber with the help of a narrow-bore Pasteur pipette and keep the chamber in a moist petri-dish for 20 minutes to allow the platelets to settle.
4. Using a high power lens and keeping the condenser racked down, platelets appear as highly refractive particles. It is required to count in one or more areas of 1 mm^2. One must count at least 100 platelets.

Calculation

$$\text{Platelet count} = \frac{\text{Number of cells counted x dilution}}{\text{Volume included*}}/\mu L \text{ of blood}$$

$$= \frac{N \times 100}{1 \times 0.1} /\mu L \text{ of blood}$$

*volume = area counted x depth of the chamber

Where,

N = platelets counted
100 = dilution factor
1 = area counted (mm^2)
0.1= depth of chamber (mm)

Example

   Number of platelets counted = 240
   By plugging the value in the above formula,

$$\text{Number of platelets} = \frac{240 \times 100}{1 \times 0.1} \ /\mu L \ (mm^3)$$

$$= 240 \times 1000/\mu L \ \textbf{\textit{or}} \ 240 \times 10^3/\mu L$$
$$= 240 \times 10^9/\text{liter of blood (SI Unit)}$$

Clinical significance

Thrombocytopenia (decrease in platelet count)
- Aplastic anemia
- Leukemias
- Splenic sequestration
- Idiopathic thrombocytopenic purpura

Thrombocytosis (increase in platelet count)
- During infections
- Immediately after the surgery and following severe bleeding.
- Post splenectomy
- Polycythemia Vera

5. Reticulocyte count

Reticulocytes are immature erythrocytes. They contain the remains of ribonuclear-protein. They are found in great numbers in the conditions in which a reduction of erythrocytes take place e.g., hemorrhage. Thus, reticulocyte count is valuable in pernicious anemia. Indirectly, the erythroid activity of bone marrow can be measured.

Principle

Ribonuclear-protein (basophilic substance) is stained by the supravital staining technique and appears as a dark blue-staining network or reticulum.

Reagent
1% brilliant cresyl blue[5]

Brilliant cresyl blue	1 g
Sodium chloride	0.7 g
Sodium citrate	0.6 g
Distilled water	to 100 mL

It is stored in a dark bottle. It is filtered before use.

Procedure

1. Take 1 volume of stain in a clean, dry, and small test tube.
2. Add 1 volume of capillary or venous blood (EDTA anticoagulated) and mix well.
3. Incubate at 37°C for 10 minutes[6].
4. Mix the contents of the tube and prepare a thin smear by putting one drop of stained blood on a clean and dry glass slide.
5. After the smear dries, examine under an oil immersion lens.
6. Count systematically 500 cells, noting the number of reticulocytes.

Calculation

The number of reticulocytes seen while counting 500 red cells is to be multiplied by 2. Then, the value obtained is divided by 10, giving the percentage of reticulocytes.

$$\text{Absolute reticulocyte count} = \text{reticulocyte \% x total erythrocyte count} (\text{ x } 10^{12}/L)$$

Example
If the relative reticulocyte count is 1% and the erythrocyte count is $6 \times 10^{12}/L$,

$$= 1\% \times (6 \times 10^{12}/L)$$
$$= 0.06 \times 10^{12}/L$$
$$= 60 \times 10^{9}/L \text{ (SI Unit)}$$

Conclusion

The manual cell count using a hemocytometer is performed for

1. Specimens with abnormal leukocyte and erythrocyte counts on an automated cell counter
2. Cell count of body fluids, e.g., CSF, peritoneal fluid, and synovial fluid
3. Enumeration of yeast cells and fungal spores

---

[5] Alternatively, new methylene blue can be used. But, it is not easily available.
[6] Allowing the incubation time to exceed 15 minutes increases the possibility of an error due to the stain adhering to mature erythrocytes.

Chapter 10

Staining of Blood Cells

Introduction

It is necessary to stain the blood cells to study them, e.g., morphology, presence of red cell inclusions. Uniform and thin blood smear prepared on the glass surface is stained by a suitable technique and is examined under the oil-immersion lens. The author advises preparing blood smears directly from the patient's blood. In other words, the smear should be prepared from the blood before it is mixed with any anticoagulants. If collected in an EDTA bulb, a satisfactory smear can be prepared within 2 hrs.

The differential leukocyte count calculates the relative proportion of five types of leukocytes. It is expressed as a percentage of each type of 100 leukocytes counted in a suitable area of the smear. This particular investigation provides gross information for many diseases.

Preparation of the smear: (see Fig. 10.1)

1. Place a small drop of blood in the central line of the glass slide about 1 or 2 cm from one end.
2. Put the spreading edge of the spreader at an angle of 45° to the slide just in front of the blood drop. The spreader is smooth-edged and narrower than the slide used for the preparation of smear.
3. Move the spreader back a little until it touches the drop and let the blood run along the edge of the spreader.
4. Prepare the smear by a rapid, smooth, and forward movement of the spreader. (Blood from anemic patients should be spread more rapidly).
5. Allow the smear to air-dry.
6. Label the smear with the patient's name and date or a reference number, using an ordinary lead pencil on the head part.

Well-made blood smear preparations are necessary to report accurate differential counts of WBCs. Therefore, too thick or too thin blood films are unacceptable. The following errors cause too thin blood smears:

1. A small drop of blood
2. Too slow-spreading
3. A low spreader angle

Too thin blood films have increased neutrophils and monocytes in the tail area, thus making incorrect differential count reports. Too thick blood smears have a very small counting area.

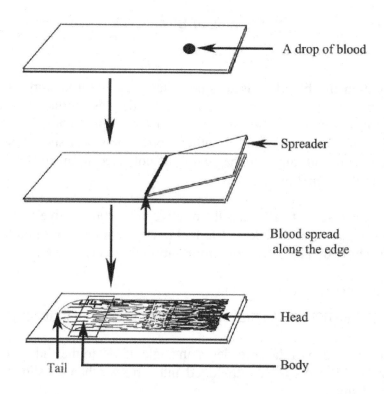

A drop of blood

Spreader

Blood spread along the edge

Head

Tail

Body

Fig. 10.1: Preparation of a blood smear.

Chemical fixation of blood smear

After drying of the blood smear, it is to be fixed chemically to kill the blood cells and to prevent the blood from being washed off the glass slide during staining. Chemical fixatives used here are alcohol and formalin vapor.

1. Alcohol

The most commonly used fixative is methyl alcohol (methanol). 'Methanol Technical' with traces of acetone is as satisfactory as 'Pure Methanol'. Thus, it is advisable to use a less expensive 'Methanol Technical' in routine procedures. If the climate is dry, the blood smear on a rack can be fixed by covering it with alcohol for 2-3 minutes. On the other hand, smear fixation is done by placing the glass slide in a closed jar of methyl alcohol for 2-3 minutes in case of a humid climate. Ethyl alcohol (ethanol) can also be used as a fixative. Methylated spirit is not used as a fixative because it fixes the smear badly due to the presence of water in it.

2. Formalin vapor

A blood smear can be fixed by placing it in a petri dish loaded with a filter paper moistened with a few drops of formalin. It requires 5 minutes for fixation. Thereafter, the smear is well washed with water before being stained.

Staining of blood smear

Blood cells contain basic, acidic, or neutral structures in them. Basic structures (e.g., eosinophil granules and hemoglobin) can be stained by acidic stains (e.g., eosin or azure I and II). These structures appear red after staining. Oppositely, some structures are acidic (e.g., basophilic granules and nucleic acids) by nature. These are stained by basic stains (e.g., methylene blue or toluidine blue) and appear blue. Some structures are neutral in reaction (e.g., neutrophil granules) and can be stained by both acidic as well as basic stains.

Romanowsky (1890) developed stains to stain the blood cells. These Romanowsky stains are mixtures of acidic and basic stains that give beautiful staining results. Furthermore, old stains are far better than fresh stains because ageing brings about the oxidation of old stains.

Based on the method of preparation of Romanowsky stains by various workers, staining powders are named accordingly (e.g., Leishman, Wright, May-Grunwald, Jenner, and Giemsa). The staining powders are dissolved in alcohol[7]. The stability of such staining solutions can be increased by adding glycerin.

The staining solutions must be used at the right pH or reaction to obtain satisfactory results. Highly acidic or alkaline staining solutions make the blood cells too blue or too pink-red, respectively. This is why the stain is diluted by the buffered water with a suitable pH.

For example, pH 6.8 buffered water is added to Leishman's stain while staining the blood smear. But pH 7.2 buffered water is used while staining the smear for malaria parasites and trypanosomes. Buffered water should carefully be added to prevent overflowing from the slide. It is to be mixed with the stain by sucking the mixture into and out of the Pasteur pipette.

---

[7] Field's stain is prepared by dissolving the powder in water.

Causes and corrections of highly acidic or alkaline stains are listed in Table 10.1.

Table 10.1: Causes and corrections of highly acidic or alkaline stains

Concentration of stain	Causes	Corrective steps
A. *Highly acidic* (red) - RBCs: bright red-orange - Nuclei of leukocytes: pale blue - Granules of eosinophils: brilliant orange-red	- Stain/buffer highly acidic - Excess buffer for stain - Insufficient staining time - Very thin films - Old stain(oxidized alcohol)	- Correct pH, remake buffer - Decrease buffer time/amount - Increase staining time/amount - Correct film thickness - Check expiration date/stain
B. *Highly alkaline* (blue) - RBCs: blue-green - Granules of eosinophils: gray/blue - Nuclei of leukocytes: blue/purple - Granules of neutrophils: too dark - The cytoplasm of lymphocytes: gray	- Stain/buffer highly alkaline - Insufficient buffer for stain - Excessive staining time - Very thick films	- Correct pH, remake buffer - Increase buffer time/amount - Decrease staining time/amount - Correct film thickness

A very important factor affecting the staining results is time. It is necessary to optimize the time for each fresh bottle of stain because the properties of a stain vary from batch to batch of the same supplier. Furthermore, staining time decreases as the stain ages. The time can be optimized by preparing 6 smears of normal blood and labeling them from 1 to 6. Each smear is stained for different times and results are recorded. The periods giving satisfactory staining results are used in routine staining.

Properly prepared and well-stained blood smears with Romanowsky stain exhibit the staining characteristics as shown in Table 10.2.

Table 10.2: Staining characteristics of properly prepared and well-stained blood smears with Romanowsky's stain

Structure/Cell	Color
Erythrocytes	Salmon pink
Nuclei of neutrophils	Deep blue-purple
Specific granules of neutrophils	Light purple or violet
Granules of both lymphocytes and platelets	Light purple or violet
Specific granules of basophils	Deep purple
Specific granules of eosinophils	Orange
Chromatin (e.g., Howell-Jolly bodies)	Purple
Dohle bodies	Blue-gray
Granules of promyelocytes and Auer rods	Purple-red
Cytoplasm of lymphocytes	Blue
Cytoplasm of monocytes	Blue-gray
Cytoplasm of neutrophils	Light pink
Cytoplasm of platelets	Purple-blue to lilac

(A) Leishman's staining
Reagents

(i) Leishman's stain

Leishman powder	1.5 g
Methyl alcohol	1 liter

    a. Rinse out a 1-liter bottle with methyl alcohol and keep a few glass beads in it.
    b. Add Leishman's powder and methyl alcohol.
    c. Mix the staining solution intermittently over for one day until the stain is completely dissolved.

(ii) pH 6.8 buffered water: {see Appendix I (a)}

Procedure
1. Cover the blood smear with Leishman's stain for 2 minutes, avoiding drying of the stain.
2. Add pH 6.8 buffered water to the stain. Mix thoroughly and carefully by sucking the diluted stain into and out of the Pasteur pipette and allow it to react for 10 minutes.
3. Wash with tap water and remove any stain on the other side of the slide, using a gauze moistened with alcohol.

(B) Wright's staining
Reagents

(i) Wright's stain

Wright's staining powder	1.6 g
Methyl alcohol (methanol)	1 liter

The method for preparation of Wright's stain is the same as that described for Leishman's stain.
(ii) pH 6.4 buffered water: {see Appendix I(a)}

Procedure
Adopt Leishman's staining procedure.

(C) Giemsa's staining
Reagents

Giemsa's stain

Giemsa's staining powder	3.8 g
Glycerin (glycerol)	250 mL
Methyl alcohol (methanol)	250 mL

The method for preparation of Giemsa's stain is the same as that described for Leishman's stain except for the addition of glycerin to the methanol before Giemsa's staining powder is added.

Procedure
1. Fix the blood smear with acetone-free methyl alcohol for 3-5 minutes.
2. Cover the smear with the diluted (1:10) stain for 20 minutes or more.
3. Wash off the stain with distilled or tap water.
4. Allow the slide to air-dry.

Giemsa's staining method for thick and thin blood smears used to stain malaria parasites and trypanosomes is discussed in chapter 44.

(D) Field's staining
Reagents

(i) Field's stain A (methylene blue)
Dissolve 5 g of Field's stain A powder in 600 mL of boiling water. Mix it until it is completely dissolved and filter it after it is cooled.

(ii) Field's stain B (eosin)
Dissolve 4.8 g of Field's stain B powder in 600 mL of boiling water. Mix it until it is completely dissolved and filter it after it is cooled.

Both stains are available in the market.

Procedure
1. Fix the smear for 2-3 minutes in methanol.
2. Immerse the slide 3 times in a glass jar of Field's stain B.
3. Wash the slide in a beaker filled with tap water.
4. Immerse the slide 3 times in a glass jar of Field's stain A.
5. Wash the slide well with tap water and allow it to air-dry.

Field's staining method for fresh thick blood smears is used to stain malaria parasites and trypanosomes.

Differential leukocyte count

All the leukocytes in the blood are not identical. They are differentiated into five types. The main identifying features are:

1. Size of the cell
2. Size and shape of the nucleus
3. Nature of the granules

The differential count must be carried out on well spread and well stained thin blood smear. One hundred leukocytes are counted in a zigzag fashion as shown in Fig. 10.1 and the proportion of each type is recorded as a percentage. Thus, the proportion of each type is of diagnostic value.

1. Neutrophilia
Neutrophilia is a blood condition in which the absolute number of circulating neutrophils increases to over 7,500/mm^3 of blood:

- Acute hemorrhage
- Malignant[8] diseases (e.g., sarcoma, carcinoma)
- Tissue damage due to surgery or burns
- Severe pyogenic bacterial infection of wounds and abscesses.

2. Lymphocytosis
Lymphocytosis is a blood condition in which the absolute number of circulating lymphocytes exceeds 3,500/mm^3 of blood:

- Infectious mononucleosis (glandular fever) with the formation of atypical lymphocytes
- Pertussis (Whooping cough)
- Bacterial infections, including enteric fever, tuberculosis, and brucellosis
- Viral infections, including measles, mumps, and chickenpox
- Lymphocytic leukemia

---

[8] A malignant growth or tumor is one which, if not removed, will spread and cause similar growths in other parts of the body until the patient dies.

3. Monocytosis

Monocytosis is a condition where the absolute number of circulating monocytes increase to over $800/mm^3$ of blood. A monocytosis occurs in:

- Protozoal diseases, e.g., malaria and trypanosomiasis
- Bacterial diseases, e.g., typhoid fever, tuberculosis, and brucellosis
- Hodgkin's disease
- Tetrachloroethane poisoning
- Monocytic leukemia

4. Basophilia

Basophilia is a blood condition in which the absolute number of circulating basophils increase to over $100/mm^3$ of blood. It is rarely seen. It occurs in:

- Chronic myeloid leukemia
- Polycythemia (an increased number of erythrocytes)
- Ulcerative colitis
- Basophilic leukemia

5. Leukemia

Leukemia is a malignant disease of the tissues which produces the white blood cells. Leukemia shows many immature white blood cells and nucleated red cells in the peripheral smear. According to the type of white blood cell series affected, leukemia is classified as under:

- Myeloid (Granulocytic) leukemia
- Monocytic leukemia
- Lymphatic leukemia
- Myelomonocytic leukemia

Any of the above types of leukemias can be acute or chronic as shown in Table 10.3.

Table 10.3: Differences between acute and chronic leukemias

Acute	Chronic
Sudden onset with rapid progress.	Gradual onset and the patient survives much longer.
The white cell count is variable (maybe near normal or low).	The white cell count is greatly increased.
Peripheral blood shows a high percentage of blast cells.	Peripheral blood shows a low percentage of blast cells.
The platelets are reduced in number.	The platelets are increased in number.

Leukemoid reaction is a blood condition in which the peripheral blood picture resembles that of leukemia, e.g., The blood pictures in miliary tuberculosis, pyogenic infections, diphtheria, gas gangrene, and Hodgkin's disease resembles monocytic leukemia.

Chapter 11

Leukocytes and their Abnormalities

Introduction

It is desirable to have the following three qualities with the laboratory professional while studying leukocytes in the stained smear:

1. Thorough knowledge about the features of normal and abnormal leukocytes
2. Knowledge about the factors affecting the morphology of leukocytes
3. Should have practical experience

There are many diseases where clues are provided from the elementary information about the leukocytes, e.g., lymphocytosis in viral infections. In other words, it is the most common blood test and provides valuable information about general health. This chapter is restricted to the morphological features of normal and abnormal leukocytes as it may help avoiding misreporting.

Key characteristics and functions of normal leukocytes are listed in Table 11.1.

Table 11.1: Several characteristics and functions of the six varieties of normal leukocytes

Leukocyte variety	Characteristics	Function(s)
1. Neutrophils (polymorphonuclear leukocytes)	- Are formed in the bone marrow - Pale pink stained cytoplasm, including fine neutrophil granules - Deeply blue-stained nucleus, consisting of 2-5 lobes connected by thin chromatin strands - The average diameter is 10-12 μm - The relative number is 55-65% - The average life span is less than a day - Able to migrate from the bloodstream - Secrete powerful proteolytic enzymes - Are destroyed by the reticuloendothelial system	- Defense mechanism through phagocytic activity

Table 11.1 (cont.): Several characteristics and functions of the six varieties of normal leukocytes

Leukocyte variety	Characteristics	Function(s)
2. Eosinophils	- Are formed in the bone marrow - Sky blue tinge cytoplasm, including many large bright red granules - Deeply blue-stained bilobed nucleus, resembling the 'spectacle' arrangement - A little larger than a neutrophil (i.e., 13 μm) - The relative number is 1-3% - A circulating half-life of approximately 18 hours and a tissue lifespan of at least 6 days - Able to migrate outside of blood vessels, especially in fluids under the linings of the respiratory and digestive tracts - Granules are lysosomes, containing acid hydrolases, peroxidase, and histamine - Are very fragile and are often ruptured during the preparation of blood films	- Less actively participate in the defense mechanism through phagocytic activity
3. Basophils	- Are formed in the bone marrow - Mauve colored cytoplasm with many large deep purple granules which tend to overlie the nucleus and obscure detail - Kidney shaped or slightly lobulated nucleus or bilobed which stains light purple and hidden by granules - The average diameter is 14-16 μm - Relative number 0-1% - Lifespan is about 60-70 hours (Siracusa et al., 2011) - Least capable of movement - Granules contain heparin, histamine, and 5-hydroxytryptamine	- Appear to react in allergic states, especially atopy
4. Small lymphocytes	- Are formed in the bone marrow, spleen reticular tissues of lymph glands, and nodes - Pale blue-stained cytoplasm with occasional scattered reddish violet granules - Deeply blue-stained and the sharply defined nucleus is generally round, maybe indented at one site - A little larger than a red blood cell (i.e., 9-12 μm) - Relative number 20-25% - Life span is believed to be of several months - Able to migrate in large numbers in connective tissue	- Involved in the formation of immunoglobulin molecule at sites of inflammation

Table 11.1 (cont.): Several characteristics and functions of the six varieties of normal leukocytes

Leukocyte variety	Characteristics	Function(s)
5. Large lymphocytes	- Abundant cytoplasm which is stained pale blue with few round, red-purple granules - Usually, the round nucleus which is stained pale mauve - The average diameter is 12-15 μm - The relative number is 5-10%	- Similar to that of small lymphocytes
6. Monocytes	- Are formed in the bone marrow, lymph glands, and spleen - Abundant cytoplasm staining a gray-blue with occasional small red granular and often seen small vacuoles of varying sizes - The nucleus may be single, lobulated or deeply indented or horseshoe-shaped, and stains even mauve color with a smooth foamy appearance - Average diameter 12-18 μm - Relative number 2-10% - Lifespan is 1-3 days - Able to migrate readily through capillary walls into the connective tissues - Granules are lysosomes containing acid hydrolases and peroxidase	- Act against *Mycobacterium tuberculosis* - Possess a powerful phagocytic action; removing cell debris (e.g., malaria pigment and foreign material)

There are medical conditions that influence the morphological features of leukocytes, e.g., hyper-segmentation of nucleus in neutrophils. Abnormalities of leukocytes and their causes are summarized in Table 11.2.

Table 11.2: Abnormalities of leukocytes and their causes

Abnormality	Characteristics	Cause(s)
1. Toxic granulation	Azurophilic granules	- Bacterial infection - Sepsis
2. Hyper-segmentation	> 5 nuclear lobes	- Pernicious anemia - Folate deficiency
3. Döhle's bodies	Dilated endoplasmic reticulum	- Bacterial infection - May-Hegglin anomaly (also thrombocytopenia)
4. Pelger-Huët anomaly	Hyperchromatic chromatin	- Autosomal dominant disease - Pseudo-Pelger-Huët (leukemia, myeloproliferative disease)

Table 11.2 (cont.): Abnormalities of leukocytes and their causes

Abnormality	Characteristics	Cause(s)
5. Giant lysosomes	Giant lysosomes	- Chédiak-Higashi syndrome
6. Auer rods	Auer rods in the cytoplasm	- Acute myelogenous leukemia
7. Barr body	Barr body	- Inactivated X chromosome (normal women)
8. J. Sézary cell	Nuclear cleft	- Séjary syndrome (malignant T cell disorder)
9. Atypical lymphocyte	Ballerina skirt	- Infectious mononucleosis - Mononucleosis syndromes (CMV, toxoplasmosis) - Viral hepatitis - Phenytoin
10. Alder-Reilly anomaly	Large, intensely azurophilic granules	- A rare autosomal recessive disorder
11. Left shift	Increased number of immature cells	- Active infection - Hypoxia and shock
12. Leukocyte adhesion deficiency	Recurrent bacterial infections, mucositis, and neutropenia	- CD18 deficient
13. Secondary granule deficiency	Recurrent skin and lung infections	- Maturation arrest in neutrophils
14. Bilobed nucleus *-Congenital*	Asymptomatic Variable	- Unknown
-Acquired	Variable	- Myelodysplastic syndromes and leukemia
15. Chronic granulomatous disease (CGD)	Recurrent infections of skin, lung, and bone and granuloma	- NADH oxidase dysfunction

Chapter 12

Erythrocytes and their Abnormalities

Introduction

A normal erythrocyte shows the following features:

1. It has a diameter of about 7.2 μm and a thickness of about 2 μm.
2. It is thinner in the central area.
3. It is biconcave in shape but appears circular in the blood film.
4. It stains pink-red by Romanowsky stains. It appears paler at the center than at the edges.
5. It lacks a nucleus.
6. The average lifespan is about 120 days.
7. All erythrocytes are negatively charged, causing them to repel each other.

A normal erythrocyte is called a discocyte or normocyte. Many types of abnormal erythrocytes are found in various physiological or pathological conditions. They are summarized in Table 12.1.

Table 12.1: Abnormalities of erythrocytes

Features	Designation	Occurrence
A. Variation in cell size (anisocytosis):		
1. Smaller than normal (4-6 μm)	Microcytes (< 80 fL)	- Iron deficiency anemia (most common) - Anemia of chronic disease - Thalassemia trait - Sideroblastic anemia (least common) - Lead poisoning
2. Larger than normal (>10 μm)	Macrocytes or megalocytes (> 100 fL)	- Megaloblastic anemia (e.g., folate or B_{12} deficiency) - Leukemia - Cirrhosis of the liver
3. Heterogenous red cell population (microcytes + macrocytes)	Dimorphic RBCs	- Microcytic/macrocytic anemia - Myelodysplastic syndrome - Post red cells transfusion - Post-iron therapy in iron deficiency anemia (IDA)

Table 12.1 (cont.)**:** Abnormalities of erythrocytes

Features	Designation	Occurrence
B. Variation in cell shape (poikilocytosis)**:**		
1. Spherical like small balls without a pale central area and too little membrane	Spherocytes	- Hereditary spherocytosis - Hemolytic anemias (e.g., ABO incompatibility) - *Clostridium perfringens* septicemia - Burns - Wilson disease
2. Oval* (normal central pallor)	Ovalocytes or elliptocytes	- Hereditary ovalocytosis (membrane structural defect)
3. Rod-shaped or pear-shaped	Exaggerated ovalocytes	- Iron deficiency anemia
4. Central and peripheral areas stain pink with a colorless zone in between (appearance of a shooting target with a bullseye) and too much membrane	Target cells or leptocytes or codocytes	- Thalassemia - Cirrhosis of the liver (alcoholism) - Sickle cell anemia - Following dehydration and splenectomy - Hemoglobin C disease
5. Elongated curved cells with pointed ends	Sickle cells or drepanocytes	- Sickle cell disease** - HbS/β-thalassemia
6. Small cells with sharp-pointed projections	Crenated cells or acanthocytes or spur cells	- *Plasmodium falciparum* infection - Following placement in hypertonic medium - Abetalipoproteinemia - Fulminant liver failure - Spur cell anemia
7. Shrunken cells with rounded and pointed uneven projections	Burr cells or echinocytes	- Chronic kidney disease - Uremia - Liver disease - Malnutrition - An artifact after storage (*in vitro*)
8. Red cell fragments	Schistocytes or Schizocytes	- Disseminated intravascular coagulation (DIC) - Thrombotic thrombocytopenic purpura/hemolytic uremic syndrome - Burns - Hypertension - Prosthetic heart valve

*Very rare elliptocytes (<1%) may be seen in a normal blood smear.
**With sickle cell trait, a mixture of normal and faulty hemoglobin is present in red blood cells.

Table 12.1 (cont.): Abnormalities of erythrocytes

Features	Designation	Occurrence
9. Removal of one or more semicircular portions from the cellular margin (i.e., removal of denatured Hb by macrophages in the spleen)	Bite cell or degmacyte	- Glucose-6-phosphate dehydrogenase deficiency
10. Bone marrow not producing healthy RBCs due to toxins or tumor cells (teardrop cells)	Dacrocytes or dacryocytes	- Primary myelofibrosis - Severe iron deficiency - Myelodysplastic syndromes (MDS) - Megaloblastic anemia - β-thalassemia
11. BiconcaveRBCs with a strip of Hb crossing the clear central area	Knizocytes	- Chronic liver diseases (alcoholic or post-viral causes) - Familial lecithin/cholesterol acyltransferase deficiency
12. A central slit-like pallor (appearance of coffee beans) and cells are biconcave rather than biconcave	Stomatocytes	- Hereditary stomatocytosis - Alcoholism
C. Variation in cell staining:		
1. Blue-mauve (immature cells with residual RNA)	Polychromatic cells or reticulocytes	- Hemolytic anemias - Post-treatment for iron deficiency/ B_{12} deficiency/ folate deficiency - Myelophthisic anemia
2. Large pale staining central area	Hypochromic cells	- Iron deficiency anemia - Thalassemia
3. Blue-black stippling (aggregates of ribosomes)	Basophilic stippled cells	- Lead poisoning (coarse granules) - Thalassemia (fine granules) - Iron deficiency (fine granules) - Anemia of chronic inflammation (fine granules)
4. Basophilia	Shift cell	- Severe hemolytic anemias

Table 12.1 (cont.): Abnormalities of erythrocytes

Features	Designation	Occurrence
D. Presence of inclusions in erythrocytes:		
1. Small, round, and dark blue particles (1-2 μm), maybe one or more in the peripheral area, composed of DNA	Howell-Jolly bodies	- Post-splenectomy (asplenia) - Autosplenectomy caused by HbSS disease - Anemias, especially macrocytic
2. Thin red to violet staining rings or "figure-8 shaped" inclusions (remnants of the mitotic spindle)	Cabot rings	- Hemolytic anemia - Megaloblastic anemia - Leukemia - Effect of medication
3. Small fragments containing Iron (aggregates of ferritin)	Pappenheimer bodies* or siderocytes**	- Lead poisoning - Myelodysplasia - Sideroblastic anemias - Iron overload conditions
4. Refractile crystalline deep purple bodies composed of denatured Hb (up to 1 μm in diameter)	Heinz bodies***	- Chemical poisoning - Glucose-6-phosphate dehydrogenase deficiency
5. An immature red cell with a nucleus	Nucleated red cells (erythroblasts)	- Many blood and marrow disorders
6. Presence of malaria parasites	Invaded erythrocytes	- Malaria
E. Miscellaneous		
1. Aggregations of red blood cells	Rouleaux	- Increased γ-globulins or fibrinogen - Multiple myeloma - Waldenstrom's macroglobulinemia (↑levels of IgM)
2. Clumping of red blood cells	Agglutination	- Presence of isoagglutinin (e.g., blood group antibody)

*Using Prussian blue iron stain, the Howell-Jolly bodies (unstained) can be differentiated from the iron-containing Pappenheimer bodies (blue).
**Neither siderocytes nor sideroblasts are present in normal peripheral blood.
***Visible with supravital staining.

Sickle cell test

Since a solubility-based sickle cell test (2% sodium metabisulphite reagent) fails to distinguish between sickle cell disease and sickle cell trait, the following accurate methods have rendered it obsolete:

 a. Hemoglobin electrophoresis
 b. High-performance liquid chromatography (HPLC)
 c. Deoxyribonucleic acid (DNA) testing

Osmotic fragility of erythrocytes

Erythrocytes have a semi-permeable membrane. Therefore, water can pass freely in and out of these cells. Swelling and subsequent hemolysis occur due to the intake of too much water from the surrounding hypotonic medium. Conversely, shrinkage of cells takes place if they are suspended in the hypertonic solution. But, water content remains almost unaffected if cells are placed in 0.85% NaCl solution (isotonic solution). This explains why 0.85% NaCl solution in water (normal or physiological saline) is used as a diluting fluid in many procedures, e.g., serological tests. The osmotic facility test is obsolete.

Principle
Heparinized or defibrinated blood, in the proportion of 1 to 100, is added to the tubes containing hypotonic solutions of varying concentrations of NaCl buffered to pH 7.4. Hemolysis so produced is measured in a photoelectric colorimeter.

Clinical significance
This test is useful in the investigation of hereditary hemolytic anemias. Increased osmotic fragility is seen in congenital spherocytosis, idiopathic acquired hemolytic anemia, isoimmune hemolytic disease of the newborn, or other hemolytic anemias.

Normal osmotic fragility is seen in symptomatic hemolytic anemia and paroxysmal nocturnal hemoglobinuria.

Decreased osmotic fragility is found in sickle cell anemia and some hemoglobinopathies, showing large flat target cells.

Factors affecting osmotic fragility of erythrocytes
 1. The relative volumes of NaCl solution and blood.
 2. Any considerable degree of jaundice.
 3. The final pH of the saline-blood suspension.
 4. Presence of hemolytic organisms in blood samples.
 5. Age of the blood specimen.

Erythrocyte sedimentation rate (ESR)

The ESR may be defined as the rate at which erythrocytes of anticoagulated blood, filled in a narrow graduated tube, settle in a given time. The height of the column of the clear plasma in mm per hour indicates the ESR. The ESR is a non-specific test.

Estimation
Westergren method (Internationally accepted)

Procedure
1. Dilute the venous blood accurately with trisodium citrate (3.2%) in the proportion of 4 volumes of blood to 1 volume of citrate.
2. Draw the diluted blood in the Westergren pipette (graduated in millimeters from 0-200mm) up to the mark 0.
3. Fix the pipette upright in the ESR stand, lying on the leveled surface.

Results
Record the results at the end of 1 hour or 2 hours.
Nowadays, the modified Westergren method is in use.

Factors affecting ESR
1. Size, shape, and concentration of erythrocytes.
2. Nature and concentration of an anticoagulant used.
3. Length and diameter of Westergren pipette (Optimum length and diameter are 30 cm and 2.5 mm respectively).
4. Age and sex of the patient.
5. Time and temperature of the test.
6. The inclination of the pipette (e.g., Deviation by 3° from vertical accelerates the ESR by as much as 30%).
7. Composition of plasma (e.g., Elevation of globulin and fibrinogen accelerate the ESR. But, the elevation of albumin decreases ESR).
8. Rouleaux formation.

Automated ESR systems use an infrared laser in an optoelectronic sensor that allows the change in the opacity of a column of blood while erythrocytes settle. The results can be available only in 20 minutes because of the positioning of tubes at an angle to accelerate the sedimentation. Additionally, each analysis is temperature corrected to 18.3°C. However, automated ESR analyzers provide biosafety (minimizing contact with blood samples) as well as quicker results, it is recommended that a correction factor be applied for the range of ESR values.

Clinical significance
Conditions in which the ESR is high:
- Anemias
- Tuberculosis
- Malignant diseases
- Acute infectious hepatitis
- Rheumatic fever
- Normal pregnancy after the first three months

Conditions in which the ESR is low
   1. Polycythemia
   2. Congestive cardiac failure (CCF)

Note:
   1. Heparin cannot be used as an anticoagulant.
   2. Clots in the tube invalidate the result.
   3. The tube must be clean and free of scratches.
   4. Do not wash Westergren pipette with detergent but rinse well with tap water.

Chapter 13

Hemostasis

Introduction

The prevention of the flow of blood is termed hemostasis. When a blood vessel is damaged, bleeding takes place. Normally, bleeding is arrested within a few minutes. This is accomplished by the hemostatic mechanism. This involves the following three reactions:

a. Contraction of the damaged blood vessel, thus reducing blood flow.
b. Formation of a platelet plug by aggregation, blocking the damaged blood vessel.
c. Activation of the blood clotting mechanism, forming the fibrin clot. All of these reactions are interdependent and occur in the order shown above.

Blood coagulation

The role of blood coagulation in hemostasis is not fully understood because it is a complicated process.

The essential reaction in the clotting of blood is the conversion of 'fibrinogen' (soluble protein) into 'fibrin' (insoluble protein). Furthermore, an active form of an enzyme 'thrombin' is required for this conversion. It is initially present in an inactive form, called 'prothrombin', and is converted into thrombin in the presence of 'thromboplastin' and Ca^{++} ions. The source of thromboplastin may be either damaged tissues or blood platelets. The schematic presentation of blood coagulation may briefly be given as shown in Fig. 13.1.

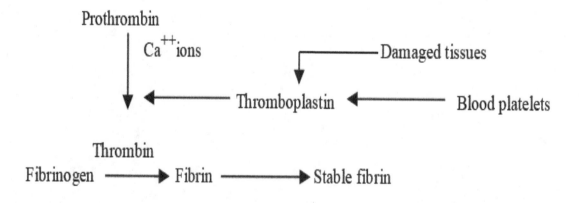

Fig. 13.1: Brief schematic presentation of blood coagulation.

Plasma contains clotting factors that participate in blood coagulation. Most coagulation factors are referred to by the Roman numerals assigned to them by the International Committee for Nomenclature of Blood Clotting Factors. But, fibrinogen and prothrombin are usually referred to by their proper names and not as factors I and II, respectively. The nomenclature of blood clotting factors is given in Table 13.1.

Table 13.1: Nomenclature of blood clotting factors

Factor	Synonym or description
I	Fibrinogen (FI seldom used)
II	Prothrombin (FII seldom used)
V	Proaccelerin, labile factor
VII	Proconvertin, stable factor
VIII: C	FVIII coagulant activity, antihemophilic factor (AHF)
VIII: WF	FVIII activity which corrects prolonged bleeding time in von Willebrand's disease
VIIIR:Ag	Protein precipitated by specific rabbit antiserum
IX	Christmas factor, plasma thromboplastin component (PTC)
X	Stuart - Prower factor
XI	Plasma thromboplastin antecedent
XII	Hageman factor, contact factor
XIII	Fibrin - stabilizing factor (FSF), transamidase
Prekallikrein	Fletcher factor
HMW (high mol. wt.) kininogen (HMWK)	Fitzgerald factor

Coagulation factors act either as substrates or cofactors. Substrates get converted into active enzymes under the influence of enzymes. These enzymatic forms of clotting factors are denoted by the suffix 'a' after the Roman numerals. Cofactors act on enzyme-substrate complexes. There are two systems involved in the coagulation of blood (see Fig. 13.2).

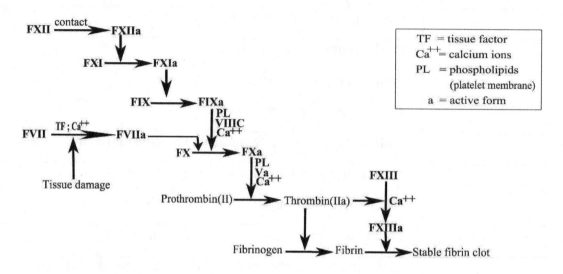

Fig. 13.2: The postulated scheme of the involvement of various clotting factors.

Intrinsic system
This system involves only the blood components necessary for clotting. It occurs when shed blood comes in contact with a foreign surface.

Extrinsic system
This system is dependent on extracts of various tissues (thromboplastins). It accelerates blood clotting. Furthermore, it bypasses the initial time-consuming reactions of the intrinsic system. The distinction between the intrinsic and extrinsic systems is not as crystal clear as previously thought. But, both systems have a final common pathway. Activation of the intrinsic system activates the extrinsic system by the action of factor XIIa on factor VII.

Some properties of clotting factors are listed in Table 13.2.

Table 13.2: Some properties of clotting factors

Factor	Molecular weight	Electrophoretic mobility	Plasma concentration	Adsorbed by	Presence in serum	Vitamin K-dependent	Temp. and time for precipitation	Stability at 37°C
I (Fibrinogen)	340,000	β-globulin	1.5-4.0 g/L	-	absent	No	56°C/10 min	Yes
II (Prothrombin)	72,000	α-globulin	100-150 mg/L	Al(OH)$_3$	trace to <10%	Yes	56°C/10 min	Yes
V	250,000	β-globulin	c 10 mg/L	-	absent	No	56°C/3 min	No
VII	45,000	α-globulin	c 0.5 mg/L	Al(OH)$_3$	present	Yes	56°C/5 min	Yes
VIII: C	c 300,000	?	?	-	absent	No	56°C/5 min	No
VIII: WF	polymers up to 20 x 10^6	β-globulin	c 10-15 mg/L	-	present	No	65°C/10 min	Yes
IX	55,000	α1-globulin	4-7 mg/L	Al(OH)$_3$	present	Yes	56°C/10 min	Yes
X	55,000	α1-globulin	c 5 mg/L	Al(OH)$_3$	present	Yes	56°C/20 min	Yes
XI	200,000	γ-globulin	c 5 mg/L	Celite	present	No	60°C/10 min	No
XII	80,000	β-globulin	c 20 mg/L	glass	present	No	65°C/10 min	Yes
XIII	320,000	β-globulin	10 mg/L	-	trace to < 10%	No	56°C/20 min	Yes

Normal fibrinolytic system
That mechanism which brings about digestion and solubilization of fibrin clot is termed as fibrinolysis. This leads to the formation of soluble amino acids and peptides. Fibrinolysis occurs through the action of the proteolytic enzyme, plasmin (fibrinolysin). Plasmin is formed from an inactive β-globulin precursor, plasminogen (profibrinolysin) present in both plasma and serum. This conversion is caused by the action of a plasminogen activator. This activator is present in many tissues and is secreted into the blood by vascular endothelial cells.

Plasmin degrades fibrin to produce a soluble intermediary product, fragment X. Fragment X, in turn, is degraded with the formation of low molecular weight fragments Y and D. Finally, fragment Y is degraded, thus forming fragments D and E. In this way, one mole of fibrin is converted into two moles of fragment D and one mole of fragment E. These degradation end-fragments are termed fibrin degradation products (FDPs).

The plasminogen activators may be inhibited by anti-activators present in the plasma. There are naturally occurring plasmin inhibitors, α2-antiplasmin, antithrombin III, and inter-α-inhibitor. Furthermore, fibrinolysis is also influenced by the pituitary hormones. Thyroid-stimulating hormone (TSH) and pituitary growth hormone (PGH) promote the fibrinolytic system. On the other hand, adrenocorticotropic hormone (ACTH) inhibits the fibrinolytic system. The different steps in the fibrinolytic system are shown in Fig. 13.3.

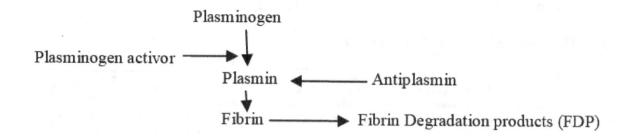

Fig.13.3: The different steps in the fibrinolytic system.

Screening tests of hemostasis

Tests used to screen patients for bleeding disorders are non-specific tests. These simple tests are used to assess the overall hemostatic function. Unfortunately, they lack sensitivity. Therefore, one should not conclude that a patient has a normal hemostatic mechanism if all the following listed test results turn out normal. Under such circumstances, it is advisable to carry out more specific tests after considering the history and the clinical findings of a patient.

To achieve accurate coagulation laboratory findings, an acceptable blood specimen is needed. Therefore, specimens are rejected for the following reasons:

1. The incorrect ratio of blood to anticoagulant (tube less than 90% full)
2. More than 2 hours if stored at room temperature/more than 4 hours if stored at 4°C
3. Exposure to extremely low or high temperature
4. Clotted or hemolyzed specimen
5. Lipemic or pigmented specimen
6. Improper centrifugation

It is advisable to carry out the following screening tests:

1. Bleeding time (BT)
2. Clotting time (CT)
3. Prothrombin time (PT)
4. Activated partial thromboplastin time (APTT)
5. Thrombin time (TT)
6. Platelets
7. Miscellaneous tests

Bleeding time (BT)

Procedure
1. Clean the ear-lobe or the fingertip with 70% alcohol and allow it to dry before pricking.
2. Prick deeply enough with a lancet, and start the stop-watch at the same time.
3. Blot away the drops with the filter paper every half-minute without touching the skin.
4. Stop the stop-watch when the blood ceases to flow.
5. Record the BT to the nearest half minute.

Normal value: 1-3 minutes

Conditions where BT is prolonged:

- Pernicious anemia
- Aplastic anemia
- Acute leukemia
- Chronic lymphocytic leukemia (CLL)
- Multiple myeloma
- Infectious mononucleosis
- Abnormal platelet function

Prothrombin time (PT)

'Quick' one-stage method
"The time taken for the citrated plasma to clot in a glass test tube after adding calcium and tissue thromboplastin is called prothrombin time." PT is prolonged in deficiencies of factors, namely I, II, V, VII, and X.

Procedure:
1. Add 4.5 mL of blood (obtained by a clean venipuncture) into a tube containing 0.5 mL of 3.8% sodium citrate, mix the contents well and centrifuge at 2,000-3,000 rpm for 10 minutes. Transfer the supernatant plasma into a clean and dry test tube. In the same way, obtain a control plasma.
2. Take 0.1 mL of saline thromboplastin suspension and 0.1 mL of 0.15M calcium chloride (CaCl2) into a 10 x 75 mm test tube. Agitate the tube gently and put it in a 37°C water bath.
3. After 1 minute, transfer 0.1 mL of the plasma rapidly into the tube containing calcium chloride (CaCl2) - thromboplastin mixture and start the stop-watch.
4. Stop the stop-watch the moment the clot appears and record the time.
1. Repeat the test twice and report the average value of the two results. Similarly, carry out the PT test with the control plasma. The normal value is 11-13.5 seconds.

Clinical significance
Prothrombin time is used:
1. To assess the bleeding tendency in preoperative patients
2. To diagnose the severity of chronic liver disease
3. To monitor the effectiveness of the blood-thinning medication, e.g., warfarin (Coumadin)

International normalized ratio (INR): INR of 1.1 or below is considered to be normal. For patients taking warfarin, the therapeutic range of 2-3 indicates the effectiveness of the drug. INR is calculated using the following formula:

$$INR=\left(\frac{\text{Patient's PT}}{\text{Mean Normal PT **}}\right)^{\text{ISI *}}$$

*ISI=International Sensitivity Index
(specific for each lot of reagent)
** Mean Normal PT=Mean PT of at least 20 known normal specimens

If INR exceeds the normal range, it signals a slower blood clot formation. Oppositely, a faster blood clot formation is expected when INR falls below the reference value.

Activated partial thromboplastin time (APTT)

It is also called partial thromboplastin time with kaolin (PTTK) or kaolin-cephalin clotting time (KCCT). It is one of those routinely requested screening tests to measure the activity of the intrinsic and common pathways of coagulation. The APTT is prolonged in deficiencies of factors, namely I, II, V, VIII, IX, X, XI, and XII.

Principle: The first part of the test involves incubation of platelet-poor plasma (PPP) at 37°C followed by the addition of a phospholipid substitute and a contact activator. This causes the conversion of factor XI to XIa (activated form). The addition of the pre-warmed (37°C) calcium initiates the clotting reaction in the second part of the test. The length of time (in seconds) taken to form a fibrin clot after recalcification is called APTT.

Reagents: 1. Contact activator: e.g., micronized silica, celite, ellagic acid, or kaolin
2. Platelet phospholipid substitute: e.g., cephalin
3. Calcium: the initiator of coagulation

Mixing studies: In 4:1 mixing studies, APTT is interpreted as shown in Table 13.3.

Table 13.3: Interpretation of APTT in 4:1 mixing studies

Immediate correction, %	Correction post-incubation, %	Indication
≥50	>10	factor deficiency
<50	>10	mild factor deficiency
≥50	≤10	factor inhibitor
<50	≤10	lupus anticoagulant

According to Garcia Moreira V et al. (2018), serum acute-phase proteins contribute to overestimating the concentration of albumin, especially at lower concentrations in the BCG-based method.

D-dimer test

It is a blood test employed to rule out the presence of a serious blood clot. Normally, several reactions take place post clotting to break the clot down. After all that, there are some leftover fibrin split fragments in the blood. The D-dimer is one of those leftover fragments. The D-dimer test serves the following purposes:

a. to rule out deep vein thrombosis, pulmonary embolism, and stroke
b. to diagnose and monitor the efficacy of treatment in disseminated intravascular coagulation (DIC) disorder
c. to determine if a follow-up testing is required to help in the diagnosis of diseases associated with hypercoagulability or a tendency to clot abnormally, e.g., systemic lupus erythematosus (SLE) flare and systemic infection

The D-dimer assay can be performed by a latex agglutination test (poor sensitivity), ELISA, or western blot method.

Thrombin time (TT)

The thrombin time test is useful to measure the availability of functional fibrinogen. Thus, it helps identify the cause of a prolonged APTT.

Platelet function tests

There are several platelet function tests to date. This fast-growing list of tests has become possible because of new facts accumulated through research studies, flow cytometry, and software technology. It is noteworthy that a single platelet function test cannot furnish information over multiple platelet dysfunction causes. However, platelet adhesion and platelet aggregation tests are routinely performed.

a. *Adhesion test*: To evaluate the property of adhesiveness in platelets, a specimen is passed through a glass bead filter. Here, some platelets adhere to glass beads. Then, the platelet count is performed on a filtered specimen and compared with the venous platelet count (control). The resulting decrease in platelet count depends upon the proportion of platelets trapped in the filter. The percentage of platelets retained by a glass bead filter indirectly reflects the degree of adhesiveness of platelets. In other words, the assay helps identify von Willebrand's factor (vWF) disorder, if present.

b. *Aggregation test*: Aggregometer works on the principle of "change in optical density". Since platelets undergo aggregation in the presence of a specific stimulating agent (e.g., collagen). This results in the formation of large clumps, decreasing the optical density of the platelet-rich plasma (PRP). The platelet aggregation pattern can be either monophasic (e.g., collagen, arachidonic acid, and ristocetin) or biphasic (e.g., ADP, thrombin, and epinephrine), depending upon the characteristics of a wave response. The test is used to diagnose platelet disorders and monitor antiplatelet therapy.

Abnormal results with stimulants, namely collagen, arachidonic acid, ADP, thrombin, and epinephrine are found in Glanzmann's thrombasthenia and hypofibrinogenemia (low fibrinogen).

However, results remain normal with all the above said stimulating agents except ristocetin in cases of Bernard-Soulier syndrome and von Willebrand's disease.

Stypven time

The Stypven time test is used to detect deficiencies of factors, namely I, II, V, and X. Unlike the prothrombin time test, it fails to detect the deficiency of factor VII.

Reptilase time

The test name is coined from the snake venom, Reptilase (thrombin–like an enzyme). The Reptilase time test is prolonged in fibrinogen abnormalities, increased levels of fibrinogen/fibrin split products (FSPs), and exogenous fibrinolytic agents. In other words, it measures the rate of conversion of fibrinogen to fibrin. It is used to evaluate a prolonged TT. The normal range is from 16-22 seconds.

Fibrinogen assay

Fibrinogen (factor I), a glycoprotein, is synthesized in the liver. Its role in the formation of a blood clot is critical. Normally, soluble plasma fibrinogen is converted into insoluble fibrin strands. This conversion is catalyzed by thrombin. Then, fibrin strands undergo cross-linking in the presence of a factor XIII, resulting in the stabilization of a fibrin clot. The fibrinogen assay is useful in the diagnosis of fibrinogen-related disorders e.g., afibrinogenemia (total absence of fibrinogen), hypofibrinogenemia (low level of fibrinogen), and dysfibrinogenemia (normal level with its malfunction). Also, the test is requested to evaluate the prolonged PT and aPTT test results. The enzyme-linked immunosorbent assay (ELISA) technique is very convenient and sensitive in assaying the plasma fibrinogen.

Antithrombin III (AT-III) assay

Antithrombin III is a protease that can neutralize thrombin (factors IIa, IXa, and Xa). Thus, thrombin is rendered inactive to block the process of the blood clotting mechanism. This is how antithrombin III helps maintain the equilibrium between bleeding and clotting. The test is used to detect the deficiency of antithrombin III.

Protein C and protein S assay

Protein C is a vitamin-K dependent glycoprotein. Normally, Protein C and/or Protein S cleave factors Va and VIIIa, making them inactive. So, deficiency of Protein C or Protein S leads to a decreased ability to inactivate factors Va and VIIIa, leading to a hypercoagulable state.

Lupus anticoagulant test

It is also called a lupus inhibitor test. Lupus anticoagulant test is a coagulation-based qualitative test that helps detect the functional status of the phospholipids (aPL) present in the outer layer of the cell membrane. Phospholipids (aPL) are substances that play a crucial role to prevent the process of blood clotting. Lupus anticoagulant (autoantibodies) can inactivate phospholipids, thus leading to the formation of clots. The test is used in case of a prolonged APTT, thrombotic episodes, and frequent miscarriages. It needs to be remembered here that this test is not useful in the laboratory diagnosis of systemic lupus erythematosus (SLE).

Some coagulation tests and their clinical significance are listed in Table 13.4.

Table 13.4: List of common coagulation-related laboratory tests and their clinical significance

Coagulation test	Clinical significance
Bleeding time (BT)	– Prolonged with platelet abnormalities – Prolonged by aspirin
Clot retraction	– Decreased with thrombocytopenia and platelet defects
Platelet aggregation	– To detect qualitative defects in platelets e.g., von Willebrand's disease
Prothrombin time (PT)	– To detect deficiencies in extrinsic and common pathways – To monitor Coumadin therapy
Activated partial thromboplastin time (APTT)	– To detect deficiencies in intrinsic and common pathways – To monitor heparin therapy
Fibrinogen (quantitative)	– Diminished in DIC
D-Dimer*	– Positive in DIC, pulmonary embolism, deep vein thrombosis, and following lytic therapy
Plasminogen	– Decreased following DIC, lytic therapy, and primary fibrinolysis
Antithrombin III (AT- III)	– To detect thrombosis-related deficiencies
Protein C and Protein S	– To detect thrombosis-related deficiencies

* Are degradation products of cross-linked fibrin following the plasmin action.

Laboratory findings of coagulation tests in primary fibrinolysis *versus* disseminated intravascular coagulation (DIC) are listed in Table 13.5.

Table 13.5: Understanding the laboratory findings of coagulation test in Primary fibrinolysis *versus* disseminated Intravascular Coagulation (DIC)

Test	Primary Fibrinolysis	Disseminated Intravascular Coagulation (DIC)
Platelet count	Normal	Decreased
Red cell morphology	Normal	Schistocytes
PT	Extended	Extended
APTT	Extended	Extended
Fibrinogen (quantitative)	Diminished	Diminished
FDPs	Present	Present
D-dimer	Negative	Positive
AT-III	Normal	Diminished

Furthermore, some coagulation tests shown in Table 13.6 have proven to be gold standards in the laboratory diagnosis of some selected diseases.

Table 13.6: Summary of selected diseases and coagulation laboratory results

Disease	Coagulation laboratory results
Hemophilia A	Factor VIII = ↓ APTT = ↑ PT = N Bleeding time = N Platelet count = N
Hemophilia B	APTT = ↑ PT = N Bleeding time = N Platelet count = N
von Willebrand's disease	Bleeding time = ↑ Platelet aggregation with ristocetin = Abnormal Factor VIII = Maybe ↓ APTT = Maybe ↑ PT = N Platelet count = N

Table 13.6 (cont): Summary of selected diseases and coagulation laboratory results

Disease	Coagulation laboratory results
Bernard-Soulier syndrome	Bleeding time = ↑ Platelet count = ↓ Giant platelets = Present Clot retraction = N
Glanzmann's thrombasthenia	Bleeding time = ↑ Platelet count = N Clot retraction = Abnormal Platelet aggregation with* = Abnormal

Key: N = Normal, ↑ = Elevated, ↓ = Decreased
* ADP, collagen, thrombin, epinephrine.

Anticoagulants namely, heparin and Coumadin (warfarin) are in widespread use as blood thinners. Some salient features of these two medicines are summarized in Table 13.7.

Table 13.7: Some salient features of anticoagulant therapy

	Heparin	Coumadin (warfarin)
Route of administration	Subcutaneous or IV	Oral
Mode of action	Antithrombin effect	Vitamin K antagonist
Effect	Immediate	Delayed
Duration	Short	Long
Test to monitor	APTT	PT/INR
Reversal agent	Protamine sulfate	Vitamin K
Other	Requires AT-III to be effective	Decreases production of II, VII, IX, X

Conclusion

The author believes that introduction of new tests in the future will not be surprising. This positive tendency is due to the accumulation of new research findings, highly sophisticated instrumentation technology, and the latest software update. Therefore, some old tests could disappear with the advent of new tests that offer more accuracy and feasibility. For example, the fibrinogen/ fibrin degradation products (FDPs) test is less commonly used than a newly developed D-Dimer test. Apart from the screening tests, the need for follow-up studies (e.g., correction studies) will remain unavoidable.

Chapter 14

Examination of Bone Marrow

Introduction

Bone marrow is a primary site for the production of new blood cells (hematopoiesis). It produces about 500 billion blood cells of both myeloid and lymphoid lineages. It is a semi-solid tissue present inside the spongy areas of the bones. It consists of the hematopoietic cells, marrow adipose tissue, and supportive stromal cells. Bones of a newly born baby are rich in active "red" marrow. The "red" marrow progressively turns "yellow" with age. The characterization of marrow as "red" or "yellow" depends upon the prevalence of hematopoietic cells versus fat cells. In adults, bone marrow is located in the ribs, vertebrae, sternum, and bones of the pelvis. It accounts for 4% of the total body mass. For example, approximately 5.7 lbs of bone marrow can be found in an adult weighing 143 lbs. With many blood disorders, important changes in the bone marrow could be noticed. Therefore, careful microscopic examination and intelligent evaluation of the blood cells produced by the bone marrow as to the number, appearance, development, and presence of infection are of great importance.

Aspiration

1. Select a suitable site to aspirate active bone marrow (The upper part of the body of the sternum is usually preferred).
2. Sterilize the skin with spirit, iodine, and spirit again.
3. Anesthetize the skin, subcutaneous tissue, and periosteum with a 1% solution of procaine.
4. Insert the needle[9] into the center of the bone with a boring motion after the effect of anesthesia.
5. Remove the stylet and attach a 2 or 5 mL syringe after the cortex is pierced.
6. Apply the suction withdrawing not more than 0.3 mL of the marrow pulp into the syringe.
7. Place a sterile bandage over the sternal puncture wound.

Note: It is of utmost importance to use aseptic technique.

Preparation of the smear

1. Transfer the contents of the needle onto a clean and dry slide immediately after aspiration.
2. Suck off as much blood as possible with the help of a needle, leaving yellowish irregularly shaped fragments on the slide.
3. Pick up several of these fragments accompanying a small amount of blood in the pipette.
4. Put small drops near the end of several clean and dry slides from the charged pipette.
5. Put the remaining material in 10% neutral formol-saline for histological sections.
6. Prepare the films the same way as the blood films with the help of a spreader.
7. Allow the films to air dry.
8. Fix some of the films in absolute methanol for 20 minutes immediately after drying and stain them with Romanowsky stains, e.g., Giemsa's method, Leishman's method, May-Grunwald's method, and so on.
9. Fix the rest of the films in formal-ethanol and perform cytochemical staining.

---

[9] Short, stout, and beveled 18-gauge needles equipped with an adjustable guard are used.

Examination

1. Select the slides with well-spread films containing easily visible marrow particles.
2. Examine the marrow particles with a low-power objective and study their cellularity, i.e., normoblastic, hypoblastic, or hyperblastic.
3. Study a highly cellular area of the film with well spread and stained nucleated cells under a low-power objective. Also, look for megakaryocytes.
4. Study the type of erythropoiesis (e.g., normoblastic, megaloblastic, or dyserythropoietic) and the general maturity of the erythropoietic and leukopoietic cells.
5. Find out the myeloid: erythroid ratio.

Precursor cells (blast cells and their progeny) are predominantly found in normal bone marrow as shown in Table 14.1.

Table 14.1: Cells found in normal bone marrow (myelogram)
(Courtesy of Fence Creek Publishing, LLC, Madison, Connecticut)

Cells	Percent
Proerythroblasts	0.5-5.0
Erythroblasts	
basophilic	1.0-3.0
polychromatic	2.0-20.0
reticulocyte	2.0-10.0
Megakaryocytes	0.1-0.5
Lymphocytes	5.0-20.0
Plasma cells	0.0-3.5
Monocytes	0.0-0.2
Macrophages	0.0-2.0
Myeloblasts	0.1-3.5
Promyelocytes	0.5-5.0
Myelocytes	
neutrophilic	5.0-20.0
eosinophilic	0.1-3.0
basophilic	0.0-0.5
Metamyelocytes and bands	10.0-30.0
Segmented cells	
neutrophils	7.0-25.0
eosinophils	0.2-3.0
basophils	0.0-0.5

Clinical significance

- Demonstration of megaloblasts in pernicious and iron deficiency anemias
- Diagnosis of aleukemic leukemia and multiple myeloma
- Detection of certain parasites, e.g., Leishman-Donovan bodies in Kala-azar
- Diagnosis of carcinomatosis, myelomatosis, and disorders of lipoid-storage such as Gaucher's disease
- Demonstration of iron by Perls's staining method

Chapter 15

Hematology and Automation

Introduction

The most outstanding and overwhelming contribution of Wallace H. Coulter (1913-1998) in the automated hematology laboratory is unforgettable. Applying the principle of electrical impedance (resistance), he successfully designed and manufactured the first automated cell counter and named it the Coulter cell counter (sold out to Beckman Company). Later, other cell counters came into existence using a different principle called the light scatter. Though automated cell counters are efficient and cost-effective, a tedious manual method remains as an inevitable technique in case of aberrant results. A brief account of the principles and measurement of different parameters of blood cells is included in this chapter.

Principle

1. Electrical impedance (see Fig. 15.1)

The suspended cells pass from an outer chamber into an inner chamber through an aperture called the "sensing zone". Both chambers are equipped with submerged electrodes to sense the electric current (direct current) flowing through the aperture. When a stream of cells is pulled through the aperture by creating a vacuum, an electric impedance is created. In other words, there is a change in electrical conductivity because cells are nonconductors (act as an insulator). The electric impedance produced is recorded as a voltage pulse (cell counting). Additionally, the degree of resistance developed helps in the measurement of the size of the cells (cell sizing). The impedance-based instruments sometimes use radio frequency (RF) to produce a high-voltage electromagnetic current (alternating current) resistance and provide information about internal structure.

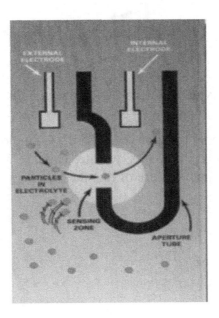

Fig. 15.1: Electrical impedance principle.
(Courtesy of Coulter International Corporation, 1996)

The pitfalls of electrical impedance methodology include coincidence counting, non-axial passage, and deformability of cells (different cell shapes) affecting the size of the cell.

2. Light scatter (see Fig. 15.2)

Light scatter-based automated hematology counters use a laser or tungsten halogen lamp facing at the sensing zone. The channel used in these machines is very narrow to let the cells pass one by one. This is accomplished with the help of hydrodynamic focusing, called *sheath flow*. When a cell passes through a beam of light, the light gets scattered into a specific direction according to the size of the cell. Then, a photodetector converts the scattered light to an electrical impulse. The number of these electrical impulses is directly proportional to the number of cells passing through the sensing zone in a specific period. These machines need to be calibrated using human blood specimens.

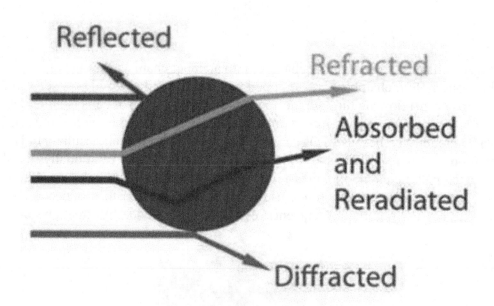

Fig. 15.2: Four types of interaction between light and a surface.
(Courtesy of HORIBA Scientific)

The Multi-Angle Polarized Scatter Separation (MAPSS™) technology (see Fig. 15.3) from Abbott uses four optical scatter detectors to assess various cellular features. The application of a depolarized light detector is a unique feature of this methodology, enabling the identification of eosinophilic granules.

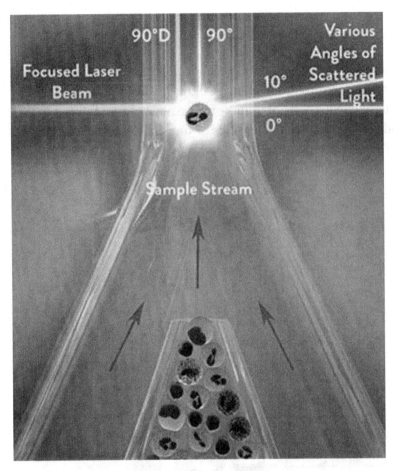

0° or axial light loss: related to size
0° to 10° intermediate angle scatter: related to cellular complexity
90° polarized side scatter: related to nuclear lobularity/segmentation
90° depolarized side scatter: related to eosinophilic granules

Fig. 15.3: Multi-Angle Polarized Scatter Separation (MAPSS™) technology.
(Courtesy of Abbott Diagnostics)

The sum of diffraction (bending around corners), refraction (bending due to a change in speed), and reflection (turning back of light rays by obstruction) enables in the characterization of the cells.

These four signals discern cell morphology that is closely similar to the microscopic evaluation of a stained smear. The WBC subpopulations are classified based on various combinations of these four measurements. MAPSS™ technology provides:

1. Identification and counting of WBCs and subpopulations
2. Identification of abnormal cell types
3. Identification of interferents, thereby giving:
   - first pass identification of nRBCs
   - accurate identification of platelet clumps

101

3. Flow cytometry (see Fig. 15.4)

Flow cytometry is a technique in which individual cells or other biological particles in a single file (fluidics system) are passed through a beam of light. It allows the rapid sorting of large numbers of cells within a heterogeneous cell population and provides simultaneous multiparametric analysis of the physical and/or chemical characteristics at the single-cell level. The key components of a flow cytometer are briefly discussed below:

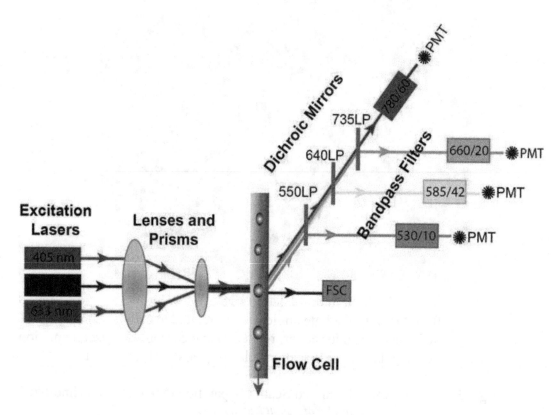

Fig. 15.4: Flow cytometry principle.
(Courtesy of Bitesize Bio)

(i) *Fluidics system:* focuses the flow of a sample to deliver the suspended cells or particles at the interrogation point as a single file and keep them on the same axis. This can be achieved using a fast-moving cell-free sheath stream (normal saline) to induce a laminar flow. Because both streams (sample and sheath) travel at different rates, they do not intermingle.

(ii) *The light source and focusing optics:* LASER stands for "light amplification by stimulated emission of radiation". The laser light beam is used to generate light at one specific wavelength, e.g., 633 nm (red laser). Besides, it provides the energy to excite fluorophore (fluorochrome) of interest. This explains why it is necessary to make sure the fluorophore of interest is excited by the wavelength intended to use. The lenses are used to shape and focus the laser beam. The wavelength of the excitation spectrum (high energy) is shorter than the emission spectrum (low energy).

(iii) *Dichroic mirrors:* direct certain wavelengths of light one way and deflect other wavelengths. There are two main types, namely the long pass, and the short pass. A long pass filter allows light equal to or longer than their marked wavelength to pass through. Conversely, short pass filters allow light that is equal to or shorter than their marked wavelength to pass through. For example, a fluorophore on a 600 LP dichroic mirror allows only wavelengths longer than 600 nm to reach the next filter and detector while shorter wavelengths are deflected.

(iv) *Bandpass filters:* Following the deflection caused by the dichroic mirror, the light path passes through bandpass filters. Such filters only allow a narrow range of wavelengths to be sent to the final detector. Usually, they are marked with two numbers. For example, a filter labeled as 450/50 can allow the wavelengths of the first number within 50 nm, i.e., 425 to 475 nm. Therefore, it is important to make sure that emission wavelength lies within these bandpass filter limits for successful detection.

(v) *Photomultiplier tubes* (PMT)*:* Once the optical signal passes through the bandpass filter, the emitted weak fluorescent light is amplified through a photomultiplier tube before measurement. This is accomplished through the conversion of photons of light to electrons. So formed electrons produce a voltage pulse that is converted to a digital readout (the computer screen display).

To learn more, the reader is advised to watch the crystal clear presentation video (WEBINAR, May 24, 2018) about "Multicolor flow cytometry-Understanding the basics" by Dr. Guerric Epron (Miltenyi Biotec).

Sample

Ideally, EDTA-anticoagulated and clot-free whole blood samples are accepted and processed within 4 hours of collection at room temperature. The open sample module requires the minimum sample volume of 0.5 mL. However, the machine aspirates 30 µL of the blood sample. The hematology analyzer can be operated in one of the following two analysis modes:

a. Whole blood mode: After proper mixing of the whole blood sample, the tube cap is removed followed by the aspiration of the sample through the sample probe one after another. The auto rinsing in between the samples keeps the sample probe ready for the next sample in the row.

b. Pre-diluted mode: So-called pre-diluted mode because the whole blood sample is diluted into 1:26 before analysis (i.e., 500 µL of diluent + 20 µL of a well-mixed whole blood sample). Once the whole blood sample is diluted, it is recommended to analyze the diluted samples within 30 minutes of dilution to avoid platelet clumping. There is no need to apply the calculation factor since the dilution is predetermined. This mode is used in cases of low sample volumes, e.g., pediatric sample or capillary blood sample. There is no output of absolute and differential WBC counts.

Apparatus (see Fig. 15.5)

A variety of hematology analyzers are available from different manufacturers, e.g., Sysmex Corporation (Kobe, Japan), Beckman Coulter, Inc. (California, USA), Siemens Medical Solutions USA, Inc. (PA, USA), and Abbott Diagnostics (Illinois, USA). These automated hematology analyzers are mainly based on Coulter impedance, light scatter, or both.

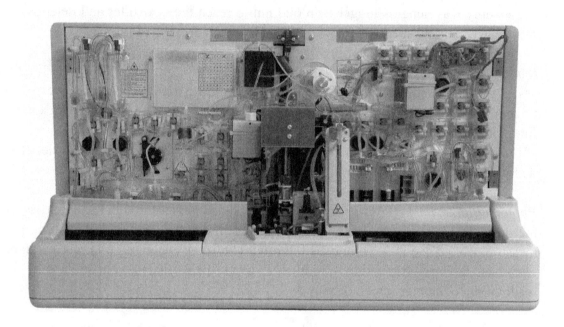

Fig. 15.5: Detailed inner view of an automated hematology analyzer.
(Reproduced with permission from Abbott Diagnostics)

In one study by Baccini, Veronique, and her associates (France, 2020), the optical-based analyzers were found to be more reliable and of higher clinical relevance than the impedance-based counters.

Small-scale hospitals need a truly compact table/benchtop instruments that can process low- to mid-volume. For example, CELL-DYN Emerald 22 (Abbott Diagnostics) is a compact hematology analyzer that delivers a 5-part differential for low-volume laboratories. It is the ideal solution for any small healthcare site, namely emergency rooms, surgical suites, and physician office laboratories.

Analyzers with two analytical modules capable of processing 200 samples per hour are available for high-volume laboratories. For example, Sysmex XN 2000 provides advanced clinical parameters, namely nucleated RBCs with every complete blood count (CBC), immature granulocytes with every differential, and immature platelet fraction.

Some automated systems combine light scatter with fluorescence, enabling analysis of RNA/DNA content of the reticulocytes, reticulated platelets, and nucleated RBCs. Alinity hq, a state-of-the-art hematology analyzer, utilizes MAPSS™ technology and includes 7 light detectors positioned at different angles, a fluorescence detector, and advanced software algorithms to count cells and report 29 different measurands.

Many automated systems include an additional feature of automated smear preparation and subsequent staining, and several machines can review the smears (Sysmex SP-1000i).

Working

The hematology analyzers consist of the following three basic chambers:

1. Platelet (PLT) and red blood cell (RBC) chamber (see Fig. 15.6)

a. PLT count

Both the PLT and RBC populations are measured in a single chamber. Like RBC and WBC counts, platelet count also utilizes the same principles. Therefore, the platelet count is equivalent to the sum of platelet impulses and are individually detected by Coulter's principle. The amplitude of the pulse corresponds to the size of the individual cell. The analyzers generate a platelet volume histogram on which log normal curves are fitted and final data are calculated. Thus, the machine extrapolates the platelet count in the area between 2-30 fL, circumventing interference with small erythrocytes. However, inaccuracies of platelet count obtained from methods relying on cell size can result in overestimation or underestimation of the platelet count.

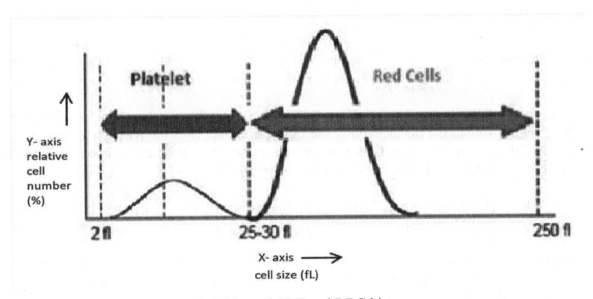

Fig. 15.6: Normal PLT and RBC histograms.
(Courtesy of the U.S. National Library of Medicine)

Light scatter-based analyzers (e.g., ELT®800) to count platelets were patented in the eighties. In ELT®800, the laser light scattering and hydrodynamic focusing improve platelet counting. The scattered light is directly related to the size, surface irregularities, and refractive index of the illuminated cell or particle. At a low angle of scattered light detection, the area of the cell represents the highest input source to extrapolate cell volume. At a high angle of scattered light detection, the refractive index is the major determinant. Based on this principle, the low angle scattered-light measurements provide better discrimination of particles with the same volume but different contents. If low and high angle scattered-light measurements are used, the platelet size is represented by the low angle scattered-light measurement whereas the platelet density is represented by the high angle scattered light measurement.

Other platelet-related parameters include:

    a. MPV = Pct (%) /PLT $(x10^3/\mu L)$ count.
    b. Platelet crit = MPV x platelet count.
    c. Platelet distribution width (PDW): PDW is measured at a 20% relative height of the total height of the curve (9-4 fL).
    d. Platelet large cell ratio (P-LCR): P-LCR is the percentage of giant platelets with a volume of greater than 12 fL (normal: 15-35%).
    e. Immature platelet fraction (IPF): The immature platelet fraction (%IPF) is a calculated parameter by automated hematology analyzers. It measures the relative count of immature (reticulated) platelets in the blood smear. The normal range is approximately 1-5% of the total platelet count. The platelet size influences this parameter. It is a valuable parameter in the differential diagnosis of thrombocytopenia. For example, a high% of IPF value with thrombocytopenia is indicative of increased destruction of platelets. e.g., Idiopathic thrombocytopenic purpura (ITP) and disseminated intravascular coagulation (DIC). Conversely, a low/ normal IPF value with a low platelet count signals bone marrow disorders, e.g., aplastic anemia.

b. RBC count

Different diluents are used for both RBC and WBC counts. Electrolyte solution (isotone) can be replaced by phosphate-buffered physiological saline (pH 7.4) as a diluting fluid for RBC count.

The total count of RBCs uses the principle that is similar to the platelet count except for the threshold values. Unlike the platelet count, the machine extrapolates the RBC count in the area between 30-250 fL as shown in Fig. 15.6. Some analyzers have two flexible discriminators, namely lower discriminator (25-75 fL) and upper discriminator (200-250 fL).

The normal RBC distribution curve is the Gaussian (bell-shaped) curve. The peak of a curve should fall within the normal MCV range of 80-100 fL.

Apart from the total RBC count, RBC indices are directly measured by using a mathematical principle called Lorenz-Mie theory. It provides an equation to analyze the light scattering from a homogeneous spherical particle.

RBC-related parameters include:

    a. PCV/MCV: determined based on the amplitude of the pulse height.
    b. MCV (fL) = Hct (%) /RBC $(x10^6$ cells /$\mu L)$ count.
    c. MCH (pg) = Hb (g/dL) /RBC $(x10^6$ cells/$\mu L)$ count.
    d. MCHC (g/dL) = Hb (g/dL) /Hct (%).

e. Red cell distribution width (RDW): is equivalent to the microscopic assessment of anisocytosis. It is calculated as a coefficient of variation of the distribution of RBC volumes (histograms) divided by the MCV.

c. Reticulocyte count

Fluorochromes (auramine O, ethidium bromide) used for staining of reticulocytes combine with RNA, enabling them to fluoresce. Immature reticulocytes fluoresce more strongly than mature reticulocytes, allowing them to assess the maturity of reticulocytes. Fluorescent cells are counted using a nucleated red cell count flow cytometry.

The Bayer/Miles technology uses a polymethine dye, oxazine 750, and cells are analyzed for cell size and hemoglobin concentration. The helium-laser light absorption and light scatter at a low angle (2° to 3°) and high angle (5° to 15°) are measured. An absorption threshold aids in the separation of stained reticulocytes from unstained mature red blood cells.

2. WBC chamber (see Fig. 15.7)

a. Total count

Fully automated hematology systems work on the same principles as that of the RBC count. But, WBC total count method makes use of a different diluent to lyse RBCs (selective lysis). It requires setting up a threshold for WBC to exclude platelets because giant platelets, nucleated RBCs, and agglutinated WBCs lead to erroneous results. Some instruments have floating (flexible) discriminators. For WBC total count, a floating lower discriminator (LD) fluctuates between 30-60 fL whereas the upper discriminator (UD) remains fixed at 300 fL. Also, there are two troughs, namely T1 (between 78-114 fL) and T2 (< 150 fL). The number of cells between the UD and the LD is the total count of WBCs.

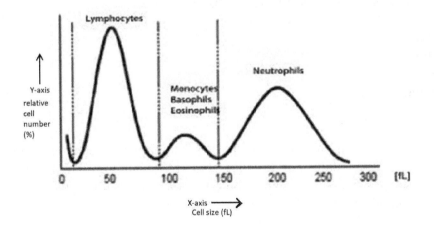

Fig. 15.7: Normal WBC histogram.
(Courtesy of the U.S. National Library of Medicine)

b. Differential count

In the WBC channel, the aspirated blood is mixed with stromatolyser (a lytic reagent) for selective lysis of RBCs before a blood specimen is directed towards the WBC chamber for counting. Following the lysis of all RBCs, the leftover WBCs have only a thin rim of cytoplasm remains. As a result of this, the size of WBCs corresponds to the size of their nuclei. This explains why neutrophils are the biggest after treatment with a lytic reagent even though originally monocytes are the largest among leukocytes as shown in Table 15.1.

Table 15.1: Sizes of different leukocytes before and after treatment with a lytic reagent
(Courtesy of "Labs for life, a partnership project of MoHFW and CDC)

Leukocyte (before treatment)	Size, μ	Leukocyte (after treatment)	Size, fL
Monocytes	12-20	Neutrophils	120-250
Neutrophils	10-15	Eosinophils	80-140
Eosinophils	11-16	Basophils	70-130
Basophils	9-14	Monocytes	60-120
Lymphocytes	7-12	Lymphocytes	30-80

There are two types of differential counts available, namely 3-part and 5- to 7-part.

A 3-part differential count classifies WBCs in the following three categories:

1. Neutrophils
2. Lymphocytes
3. Mixed cells

A 5-part differential count classifies WBCs into five categories:

1. Neutrophils
2. Eosinophils
3. Basophils
4. Lymphocytes
5. Monocytes

A 5-part differential count employs two principles, namely flow cytometry (volume, conductivity, and scatter) and peroxidase stain. For instance, ADVIA technology has a peroxidase channel (cytochemistry) that uses peroxidase stain. The peroxidase stain is the gold standard that helps differentiate white blood cells as under:

1. Eosinophils: strongly stained
2. Neutrophils: medium stained
3. Monocytes: weakly stained
4. Lymphocytes and basophils: unstained
5. Large unstained cells (LUCs)

Then, a tungsten-based optical system measures the absorbance (i.e., stain intensity) and cell size (forward light scatter) for each cell. Finally, the peroxidase activity and cell size parameters are represented on the X- and Y-axes of the cytogram, respectively. This brings about the formation of different populations or clusters. By applying the cluster analysis, different cell populations can be identified. Furthermore, some automated analyzers can recognize large unstained cells without peroxidase activity as atypical lymphocytes and other abnormal cells.

The basophil channel (also called lobularity/nuclear density channel) uses surfactant and phthalic acid (lysis reagents) to separate basophils from all other leukocytes. These cell-specific lysis reagents not only lyse red blood cells and platelets but also strip away the cytoplasmic membrane from all leukocytes except basophils. Then, cells are counted and classified according to size, providing a secondary total white cell count as an integral QC check to monitor the sample integrity.

A 7-part differential count (e.g., Sysmex XE Technology) adds immature granulocytes (IGs) and nucleated red blood cells (nRBCs) to a 5-part differential count list.

3. Hemoglobin chamber

At the beginning of automation, automated cell counters made use of a modified spectrophotometric manual cyanmethemoglobin (HiCN) method in the direct measurement of Hb. Nowadays, cyanide is replaced by a non-toxic reagent, sodium lauryl sulfate (SLS) in automated cell counters.

A photodetector measures (540 nm) the amount of transmitted light through the lysed sample against the blank hemoglobin reagent. The transmitted light signal of a lysed sample is lower than a blank reagent because the imidazole-hemoglobin complex (colored) absorbs light. The concentration of hemoglobin is derived based on the absorbance difference using the following formula:

$$Absorbance = log10 \left(\frac{V_R}{V_S}\right)$$

Where,
V_R = Reference voltage
V_S = Sample voltage

Newly designed instruments can perform the testing of HbA1c using HPLC, increasing the hematology laboratory efficiency.

Understanding histograms

The histograms are graphical representations of the blood cell populations. A histogram is generated by plotting the size of a specific blood cell on X-axis (femtoliters) and its relative number (percent) on Y-axis. They can be used to determine

1. The average size of the blood cells

2. Distribution of size
3. Detection of the subpopulation

The histograms together with other CBC parameters may be abnormal in various hematological disorders and provide clues in the diagnosis and treatment of blood cell disorders. The histograms should be used as the screening tools and should not be considered diagnostic for any particular condition. The following typical examples will help us understand the value of histograms:

a. Abnormal PLT histograms: Spurious PLT count may occur in the presence of platelet clumps and cell fragments as depicted in Fig. 15.8 (a), (b).

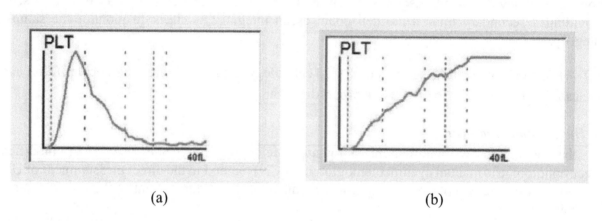

(a)   (b)

Fig. 15.8: (a) Interferences caused by PLT clumps. (b) Interferences caused by cell fragments.
(Courtesy of Sysmex Europe GmbH:Seed Haematology, Aug. 2016)

b. Abnormal RBC histograms: (see Fig. 15.9)

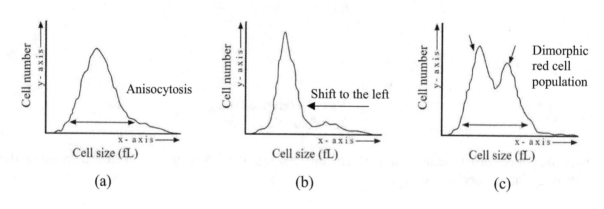

(a)   (b)   (c)

(a) Normal MCV and high RDW
(b) Low MCV and RDW
(c) High RDW
Fig. 15.9: Abnormal RBC histograms.

c. Abnormal WBC histograms: (see Fig. 15.10):

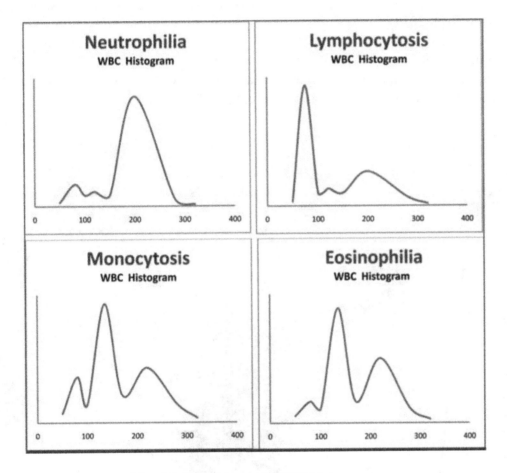

Fig. 15.10: Abnormal WBC histograms.
(Courtesy of the U.S. National Library of Medicine)

Interpretation of scattergrams (scatter plots, dot plots, or cytograms)

The scattergram is a two-dimensional (2 D) pictorial display of blood cell distribution based on their size and inner complexity (i.e., lobularity/granularity) characteristics represented by the X- and Y-axes, respectively. The magnitude of the forward scatter is roughly proportional to the size of the cell whereas the side scatter corresponds to the overall intracellular complexity of the cell. The points fall along the curve when both variables are correlated. The better the correlation, the tighter the points, enabling them to touch the curve.

The scattergrams furnish valuable information based on the findings of blood cell distribution. Some important clinical implications are:

(i) Immature granulocytes (IGs) are not seen in the scattergram of a healthy individual. In contrast, 2.5% of IGs are found in the scattergram of the patient with sepsis (Shanaz Khodaiji, 2019).

(ii) The cell population data (CPD) along with scatter plots and flags may be used in the screening of acute myeloid leukemia (AML) as a rapid and cost-effective method (Varma N. and her associates, Sept. 2018).

(iii) Leukemias can be classified as acute or chronic based on the relative positioning of the cells with respect to the mature lymphocyte population on the CD45 side scatter (SS) scattergram (Handoo, A. and Dadu, T., 2018) as shown in Fig. 15.11.

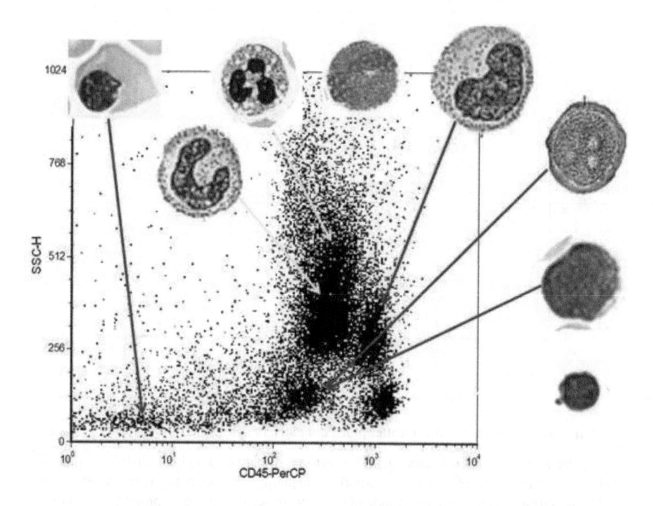

Fig. 15.11: The CD45-SS scattergram showing the presence of blast cells.
(Courtesy of Indian pediatrics)

(iv) Provide a clue for malaria infestation through hemozoin detection (see Fig. 15.12). Most studies (Sehgal, S. 2013, and German Campuzano-Zuluaga et al., 2010) indicate sensitivities that comply with WHO malaria-diagnostic guidelines (i.e., $\geq$ 95% in samples with >100 parasites/μL). Currently, only a handful of manufacturers (e.g., Coulter® GEN•S, LH 750, Sysmex® XE-2100, and Abbott® Cell-Dyn) have incorporated a "malaria alert" as an adjuvant diagnostic tool.

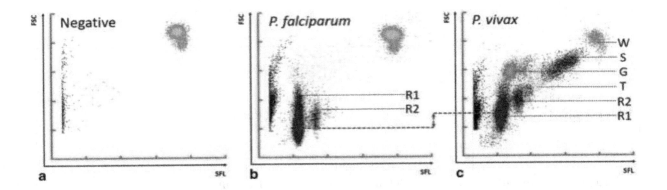

Fig. 15.12: The scattergrams of malaria-negative and -positive cases.
(Courtesy of Springer Nature)

Sources of error

There are times where automated systems in hematology show flags in the case of abnormal blood specimens. These conditions and their possible resolutions are summarized in Table 15.2.

Table 15.2: Sources of error and their resolutions

Source of error	Results affected	Resolution
Cold agglutinins	– Decreases RBC count – Increases MCV, MCH, and MCHC – Inaccurate Hct	– Prewarm blood to 37°C and rerun
Lipemia	– May increase Hb, MCH, and MCHC	– Follow the manufacturer's manual directions to obtain accurate Hb – Recalculate indices
Nucleated RBCs	– Increases WBC count	$Corrected\ WBC = \dfrac{Uncorrected\ WBC \times 100}{100 + nRBCs\ per\ 100\ WBCs}$
WBCs over 50,000	– Increases RBC count – May increase Hb – Inaccurate Hct and indices	– Dilute blood and rerun – Subtract RBC from WBC count – Follow the manufacturer's manual directions to obtain accurate Hb – Do spun Hct – Recalculate indices
Giant platelets, platelet clumps, or satellitism	– Decreases platelet count – Increases WBC count	– Perform microscopic examination of blood film for platelet clumps or satellitism – Recollect in sodium citrate – May need manual counts or smear estimates
Hemolysis	– Decreases RBC count and Hct – Increases MCH and MCHC	– Recollect if hemolysis is *in vitro*

Table 15.2 (cont.): Sources of error and their resolutions

Source of error	Results affected	Resolution
Old specimens	– Increases MCV – Decreases platelet count – Automated differential count maybe inaccurate	– Recollect
Schistocytes, microcytes	– Decreases RBC count – May be Hct and indices inaccurate	– Manual counts – Do spin Hct – Recalculate indices
Resistant RBCs	– Increases WBC count – Inaccurate Hb	– Manual Hb, adding water to lyse RBCs – Manual WBC count – Recalculate indices
Fragile WBCs	– Decreases WBC count – May increase platelet count	– Manual counts

Advantages and disadvantages

Advantages

1. No manual intervention required but simple presentation of an appropriate blood sample.
2. Ensure a high level of precision for cell counting as well as cell sizing.
3. Generally, results are accurate, provided instruments are calibrated and regular maintenance protocols are followed.
4. More efficient (120-150 specimens in one hour) and cost-effective in the long run.
5. No slide cell distribution error.
6. Many parameters are available (8-20 parameters).
7. No statistical sampling error.
8. Modern computers and networking help store patients' data.
9. "Flagging" of abnormal results for subsequent review.

Disadvantages

1. High capital investment.
2. Cell counting errors (e.g., cell clumps, bubbles, and particles).
3. Need daily maintenance and calibration.

Available automated hematology analyzers

1. Abbott Cell-Dyn 300 CS
2. Beckman Coulter LH 500
3. Siemens Advia 2120i
4. Sysmex XN 350
5. ABX Horiba Pentra 60 C+

Conclusion

Undoubtedly, automation in hematology has been making innovative technological advances since the invention of the original Coulter counter in 1954. The roles played by the fluorescence flow cytometry (a device developed by Wolfgang Gohde in 1968), monoclonal antibodies, and flow cytometry software programs are unique.

Several parameters are determined (measured and calculated) on every CBC analysis (e.g., indices, histograms, scatterplots, and interpretive comments). The results must be explicitly reported. Unfortunately, about 70% of technologists have no clues as to the cause of some abnormal CBC results, e.g., interpretation of graphic displays.

The University of York (United Kingdom) has recently developed cytoflex platform flow cytometers for research applications. These flow cytometers demonstrate remarkable sensitivity and reproducibility with six excitation wavelengths, namely 355 nm, 375 nm, 405 nm, 488 nm, 638 nm, and 808 nm. According to Dr. Karen Hogg, these analyzers are powerful for the isolation and analysis of blood, bacteria, algae, yeasts, microparticles, and even nanoparticles.

Section II: Clinical Chemistry

Chapter 16

Introduction to Clinical Chemistry

Introduction

This chapter deals with the determination of the content of various components in blood. These chemical estimations are valuable in the diagnosis and treatment of diseases (e.g., elevated levels of blood glucose are suggestive of Diabetes mellitus). They have a prognostic value too.

Specimens

The type of blood to be used depends upon the blood compound to be estimated. The specimens required for chemical determinations include whole blood and plasma or serum (plasma and serum are almost interchangeable). The following two factors are relevant to the choice of serum or plasma:

1. If immediate separation of the cells is required, plasma is preferred for the test.
2. Avoidance of hemolysis.

To avoid hemolysis, the following precautions are taken:

a. Avoid mechanical breakdown of erythrocytes and movement of water out of the cells.
b. Draw blood specimens slowly and steadily into the syringe.
c. Detach the needle from the syringe.
d. Expel blood from the syringe slowly and gently into the container.
e. Avoid the use of an excessive amount of anticoagulants.
f. Mix blood with anticoagulant by gentle rotation of the container.
g. Centrifuge decanted serum at low to moderate speeds.

Claims have been made that it is somewhat easier to obtain hemolysis-free serum than plasma. But, it appears much less important with heparin. Therefore, serum or heparinized plasma would be the sample of choice for most compounds.

No anticoagulant is added to the container to obtain serum from blood. Usually, clotting occurs in 15-30 minutes at room temperature. The yield of serum is directly proportional to the time given to clot for retraction. Normally, 5 mL of blood yields 2.0-2.5 mL of serum. The clot is loosened as gently as possible with the help of a clean, dry, thin glass rod. Specimens required for various routine biochemical tests are listed in Table 16.1:

Table 16.1: Specimen requirement for routine biochemical tests

Specimen	Biochemical tests
Oxalated whole blood	– Hemoglobin, glucose, urea, NH_3, lactate, pyruvate, pH, lead.
Serum	– Bilirubin, cholesterol, creatinine, total protein, urate, urea, most enzymes, sodium, calcium, and hormones.
Plasma	– NH_3, ascorbic acid, bicarbonate, chloride, and fibrinogen.
Red cells	– G6PD, abnormal hemoglobins, pyruvate kinase, and acetylcholine esterase.

Precautions to be taken while performing biochemical estimations

It is of utmost importance to take the following precautionary measures during biochemical determinations to obtain accurate and precise results and sometimes to avoid accidents. They are summarized below:

1. The glass-wares to be used in the estimations should be checked for calibration markings and capacity.
2. The glass-wares should be clean and dry. In the case of determinations involving enzymes, enzyme inhibitors should be absent.
3. The test tubes should be labeled properly before the test is begun.
4. All the test reagents should be brought to assay temperature before their use.
5. Serum/plasma should be free from hemolysis, non-lipemic, and clear.
6. The test reagents showing bacterial/fungal growth should be discarded.
7. Mouth pipetting should be avoided in the case of corrosive chemical reagents (e.g., sulfuric acid and sodium hydroxide).
8. The contents of test tubes should be incubated at the correct assay temperature and time. Furthermore, the level of water inside the water-bath should be at least up to the level of the reaction mixture in the test tube.
9. In some determinations (e.g., triglycerides by acetylacetone method), test tubes should be covered with aluminum foil to prevent evaporation.
10. A sufficient quantity of colored solution should be taken in the cuvette for measuring its optical density (OD), e.g., 3 mL in a colorimetric measurement.
11. Instruments used for photometric measurement should be calibrated before use.
12. Readings of colored solutions should be taken within the specified time limit because some colored complexes are unstable.

In addition to these precautions, a medical technologist should have enough experience in carrying out biochemical tests.

Normal biochemical values

One can report the clinical laboratory results using either SI units or traditional units. SI units are predominantly used in the United States. Unlike the United States, other countries adapt traditional units for reporting the test results. Test values depend on:

1. test methodology
2. age and sex
3. diet
4. time of collection (e.g., cortisol)

The normal values of some common biochemical components are given in Table 16.2.

Table 16.2: Normal values of common biochemical tests

Test	Specimen	SI unit	Traditional unit
Albumin	serum	35 – 50 g/L	3.5 – 5.0 g/dL
Ammonia (NH₃)	blood	11 – 35 µmol/L	15 – 50 µg/dL
Anion Gap $[Na-(Cl^- + HCO_3^-)]$	plasma (heparin)	7–16 mmol/L	7–16 mEq/L
$[(Na + K) – (Cl + HCO_3)]$		10 – 20 mmol/L	10 – 20 mEq/L
Amylase	serum	0.41 – 2.13 µkat/L**	24 –125 U/L
Bicarbonate (HCO₃)	serum	23 – 29 mmol/L	23 – 29 mEq/L
Bilirubin: Neonates: - Conjugated	serum	0 – 10 µmol/L	0 – 0.6 mg/dL
- Total		1.7 – 180 µmol/L	1.0 – 10.5 mg/dL
Adults: - Conjugated		0 – 5 µmol/L	0 – 0.3 mg/dL
		3 – 22 µmol/L	0.2 – 1.3 mg/dL
Calcium: Total	serum	2.10 – 2.50 mmol/L	8.4 – 10.6 mg/dL
Ionized		1.15 – 1.35 mmol/L	4.6 – 5.1 mg/dL
	urine	<6.2 mmol/d	<250 mg/d
Carcinoembryonic Antigen (CEA)	serum	<3.0 µg/L	<3.0 ng/mL
Carbon Dioxide, Total (t CO2)²	serum or plasma (heparin)	22 – 29 mmol/L	22 – 29 mEq/L
Chloride	serum or plasma (heparin)	96 – 106 mmol/L	96 – 106 mEq/L
Infant	urine	2 – 10 mmol/d	2 – 10 mEq/d
Child		14 – 50 mmol/d	14 -50 mEq/d
Adult		110 – 250 mmol/d	110 - 250 mEq/d
	cerebrospinal fluid	118 – 132 mmol/L	118 – 132 mEq/L
Cholesterol, Total: Adult	serum or plasma (heparin or EDTA)	<5.2 mmol/L	<200 mg/dL
Cortisol: 8AM	serum or plasma (heparin)	170 – 635 nmol/L	6 – 23 µg/dL
4AM		82 – 413 nmol/L	3 – 15 µg/dL

Abbreviation:
**µkat = microkatal

Table 16.2 (cont.): Normal values of common biochemical tests

Test	Specimen	SI unit	Traditional unit
Creatinine	serum or plasma	50 – 110 µmol/L	0.6 – 1.2 mg/dL
Male	urine	8.8 – 17.6 mmol/d	1.0 – 2.0 g/d
Female		7.0 – 15.8 mmol/d	0.8 – 1.8 g/d
Creatinine Clearance (endogenous)	serum or plasma and urine	0.72 – 1.2 mL/s/m²	75 – 125 mL/min/1.73m²
Creatine Kinase (CK, CPK): Male (race dependent)	serum	0.34 – 3.65 µkat/L**	20 – 215 U/L
Female (race dependent)		0.34 – 2.72 µkat/L**	20 – 160 U/L
Ferritin	serum or plasma	20 – 200 µg/L	20 – 200 ng/mL
Follicle-Stimulating Hormone (hFSH, follitropin): Male	serum or plasma (heparin)	1 – 10 IU/L	1 – 10 mIU/mL
Female (premenopausal)		20 – 50 IU/L	20 – 50 mIU/mL
Female (postmenopausal)		40 – 250 IU/L	40 – 250 mIU/mL
Glucose: Fasting	serum	3.9 - 6.1 mmol/L	70 – 110 mg/dL
2 hrs. Postprandial		< 6.7 mmol/L	<120 mg/dL
	cerebrospinal fluid	2.2 – 4.4 mmol/L	40 – 80 mg/dL
Glucose - 6 - phosphate dehydrogenase (G-6-PD)	red blood cell	0.65 - 0.90 U/mol of Hb	10 – 14 U/g of Hb
γ- Glutamyltransferase (GGT)	serum	≤ 0.85 µkat/L**	≤ 50 U/L
Glycated hemoglobin (HbA1c)	whole blood (EDTA, heparin, or oxalate)	4.5 – 5.7 % of total Hb	0.045 – 0.057 Hb fraction
Growth hormone (hGH): Adult (fasting)	serum	0.0 – 10 µg/L	0 – 10 ng/mL
High - Density Lipoprotein-Cholesterol (HDL-C) (recommended range)	serum or plasma (EDTA)	>0.91 mmol/L	>35mg/dL
Human chorionic gonadotropin (hCG) Adult: Female (nonpregnant)	serum	<3 IU/L	<3 mIU/mL
International normalized ratio (INR)		0.9 – 1.1	0.9 – 1.1
Lactate Dehydrogenase (LDH): Adult	serum	1.7 – 3.2 µkat/L**	100 – 190 U/L
Child	1.9 – 5.0 µkat/L**	110 – 295 U/L	1.9 – 5.0 µkat/L**
>60 years old	1.9 – 3.6 IU/L	110 – 210 U/L	1.9 – 3.6 IU/L
Lactose	serum	<14.6 µmol/L	<0.5 mg/dL
	urine	350 – 1168 µmol/L	12 – 40 mg/dL
Low - Density Lipoprotein-Cholesterol (LDL-C) (recommended range)	serum or plasma (EDTA)	<3.4 mmol/L	<130 mg/dL

Abbreviation:

**µkat = microkatal

Table 16.2 (cont.): Normal values of common biochemical tests

Test	Specimen	SI unit	Traditional unit
Luteinizing Hormone (LH): Male	serum	1 – 9 mIU/L	1 – 9 IU/L
Female (follicular)		2 – 10 mIU/L	2 – 10 IU/L
(Mid-cycle)		15 – 65 mIU/L	15 – 65 IU/L
(luteal)		1 – 12 mIU/L	1 – 12 IU/L
(postmenopausal)		12 – 65 mIU/L	12 – 65 IU/L
Magnesium	serum	0.65 – 1.05 mmol/L	1.3 – 2.1 mg/dL
	urine	3.0 – 4.3 mmol/d	6.0 – 8.5 mEq/d
Oxygen Saturation	whole blood arterial (heparin)	94 – 99%	94 – 99%
Parathyroid Hormone (hPTH)	serum	10 – 65ng/L	10 – 65 pg/mL
Carbon Dioxide, Partial Pressure (*p*CO2)	whole blood arterial (heparin)	35 – 45 mm Hg	35 – 45 mm Hg
pH	arterial blood	7.35 – 7.45	7.35 – 7.45
Phosphatase, alkaline	serum	0.5 – 1.5 µkat/L**	36 – 92 U/L
Phosphatase, acid: Total	serum	5 – 199 µkat/L**	0.3 – 11.7 U/L
Tartrate – inhibited fraction		0 – 60 µkat/L**	0 – 3.5 U/L
Phosphate: Adult	serum	1.0 – 1.5 mmol/L	3.0 –4.5 mg/dL
Child		1.3 – 2.3 mmol/L	4.0 – 7.0 mg/dL
Oxygen, Partial Pressure (*p*O2)	whole blood, arterial (heparin)	80 – 100 mm Hg	80 – 100 mm Hg
Potassium: Newborn	serum	3.7 – 5.9 mmol/L	3.7 – 5.9 mmol/L
Infant		4.1 – 5.3 mmol/L	4.1 – 5.3 mmol/L
Child		3.4 – 4.7 mmol/L	3.4 – 4.7 mmol/L
Adult		3.5 – 5.1 mmol/L	3.5 – 5.1 mmol/L
Potassium	urine	25 – 125 mmol/d	25 – 125 mEq/d

Abbreviation:

**µkat = microkatal

Table 16.2 (cont.): Normal values of common biochemical tests

Test	Specimen	SI unit	Traditional unit
Progesterone: Adult-Male	serum	0.0 –1.3 nmol/L	0.0 – 0.4 ng/mL
Female (follicular)		0.3 – 4.8 nmol/L	0.1 – 1.5 ng/mL
(luteal)		8.0 – 89.0 nmol/L	2.5 – 28.0 ng/mL
Prolactin: Male	serum	1 – 20 µg/L	1 – 20 ng/mL
Female		1 - 25 µg/L	1 – 25 ng/mL
Prostate - Specific Antigen (PSA)	serum (freeze)	0.0 – 4.0 µg/L	0.0 – 4.0 ng/mL
Protein: Total	serum	60 – 80 g/L	6.0 – 8.0 g/dL
	cerebrospinal fluid (lumbar)	150 - 400 mg/L	15 – 40 mg/dL
Sodium	serum or plasma (heparin)	135 – 145 mmol/L	135 – 145 mEq/L
Testosterone: Male	serum or plasma	9.5 – 30 nmol/L	275 – 875 ng/dL
Female		0.8 - 2.6 nmol/L	23 – 75 ng/dL
Female (Pregnant)		1.3 – 6.6 nmol/L	38 – 190 ng/dL
Thyroid-Stimulating Hormone (hTSH): Adult	serum or plasma	0.4 – 4.8 mU/L	0.4 – 4.8 µIU/L
Term infant: (0-1 day)		1 – 39 mU/L	1 – 39 µIU/L
(1-4 days)		1 – 17 mU/L	1 – 17 µIU/L
(2-20 weeks)		1.7 – 9.1mU/L	1.7 – 9.1µIU/L
(21 weeks to 20 years)		0.7 – 6.4 mU/L	0.7 – 6.4 µIU/L
Thyroxine, Total (T4)	serum	66 – 155 nmol/L	5 – 12 µg/dL
Thyroxine, Free (FT4)	serum	13 – 27 pmol/L	1.0 – 2.1 ng/dL
Transaminase: AST (SGOT)	serum	0 – 0.58 pkat/L*	0 – 35 U/L
ALT (SGPT)		0 – 0.58 pkat/L*	0 – 35 U/L
Transferrin	serum	2.0 – 4.0 g/L	200 – 400 mg/dL
Triiodothyronine (T), Total	serum	1.1 - 2.9 nmol/L	70 – 190 ng/dL
Triiodothyronine, Free (FT)	serum	4.0 – 7.4 pmol/L	260 - 480 pg/dL

Abbreviation:
*pkat = picokatal

Table 16.2 (cont.)**:** Normal values of common biochemical tests

Test	Specimen	SI unit	Traditional unit
Triglycerides (TG): ≥12hrs. fast	serum	0.45 – 1.71 mmol/L	40 – 150 mg/dL
Urea	serum or plasma	4.0 – 8.2 mmol/L	24 – 49 ng/dL
Urea nitrogen (BUN)	serum or plasma	2.9 – 8.2 mmol/L	8 – 23 mg/dL
Uric acid (uricase)	serum	0.15 – 0.42 mmol/L	2.6 – 7.2 mg/dL
Vitamin B (Cyanocobalamin)	serum	118 – 701 pmol/L	160 – 950 pg/mL
D-Xylose Absorption Test Adult: 2hrs.(25g dose)	whole blood (NaF)	>1.67 mmol/L	>25 mg/dL
	urine, 5hrs.	>26.64 mmol/5 hrs.	>4.0 g/5 hrs.

Chapter 17

Blood Glucose and Diabetes Mellitus

Introduction

Diabetes mellitus may be defined as a metabolic disorder that is secondary to an absolute or relative deficiency of insulin secretion by the beta cells of the islets of Langerhans in the pancreas.

The global incidence of diabetes mellitus is 1.5 to 2.0% of the population. There are about 150 million known diabetic patients in the world. It has been reported that there is one unknown case of diabetes for every known diabetic. Diabetes mellitus is manifested by elevated blood glucose levels and renal glycosuria. The diabetic patient may belong to one of the following four classes:

A. Insulin-dependent diabetes mellitus (IDDM)
B. Non-insulin-dependent diabetes mellitus (NIDDM)
C. Impaired glucose tolerance (IGT), or prediabetes
D. Gestational diabetes mellitus (GDM)

Etiology

Causes of Diabetes mellitus are summarized as shown in Fig. 17.1:

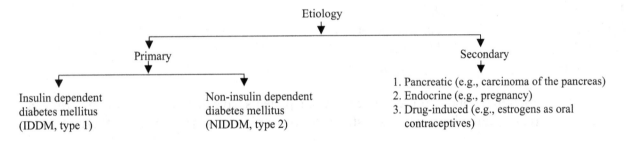

Fig. 17.1: Causes of Diabetes mellitus.

The distinctive features of insulin-dependent diabetes mellitus (IDDM, type 1) and non-insulin-dependent diabetes mellitus (NIDDM, type 2) are listed in Table 17.1.

Table 17.1: Distinctive features of insulin-dependent diabetes mellitus (IDDM, type 1) and non-insulin-dependent diabetes mellitus (NIDDM, type 2)

Distinctive feature	IDDM, type 1*	NIDDM, type 2**
prevalence, %	5-10	90-95
the usual age of onset	below 15 years	over 40 years
state of nutrition	underweight	usually obese
tendency to ketosis	ketosis-prone	ketosis resistant
onset of symptoms	usually rapid	usually insidious
insulin secretion	low	low/normal/high
response to oral hypoglycemic agents	poor	satisfactory

*formerly classified as juvenile diabetes
**formerly classified as maturity-onset diabetes

Hyperglycemic cases present with polyuria, polydipsia, polyphagia, loss of weight, excessive fatigue, and pruritus (itchy skin). Complications associated with various body tissues and certain conditions are listed as under:

1. Eyes
2. Ears
3. Mouth
4. Heart
5. Lungs
6. Nervous system
7. Vascular system
8. Skin
9. Kidneys
10. Genital organs
11. Infections
12. Pregnancy

Since diabetes mellitus cannot be cured but controlled, patients have to be very careful to normalize blood glucose (e.g., regular blood glucose estimation as per physician's advice, diet, exercise, etc.).

Insulin

Insulin is a protein hormone. Human insulin has a molecular weight of 5808 g/mol. Insulin enhances the entry of glucose into muscles and adipose tissue. In addition to this action, it plays a key role in the regulation of the blood glucose level by:

1. Increased utilization of carbohydrates in tissues.
2. Deposition of glycogen in the liver and muscles.
3. Deposition of fat in adipose tissue by inhibiting the breakdown of triglycerides and by favoring glucose entry.

Hormones, namely glucagon, cortisol, epinephrine, growth hormone, and thyroxine contribute to the increase in blood glucose levels. Both cortisol and growth hormone work as insulin antagonists. Glucagon and epinephrine promote glycogenolysis and gluconeogenesis, thus adding more glucose to the blood.

Classification of carbohydrates

Carbohydrates are compounds containing carbon, hydrogen, and oxygen in the proportion of $1:2:1(CH_2O)$. For example, glucose has 6 carbon elements, 12 hydrogen elements, and 6 oxygen elements. Thus, the proportion of 1:2:1 for carbon, hydrogen, and oxygen is fulfilled. They are classified as under:

1. *Monosaccharides* (simple sugars): Sugars that cannot be further hydrolyzed, e.g., glucose, fructose, galactose (six-carbon sugars or hexoses), and xylose (five-carbon sugar or pentose). D-xylose is used as a diagnostic agent to evaluate malabsorption disorders.
2. *Disaccharides:* Sugars that can be hydrolyzed into two monosaccharide units, e.g., sucrose (glucose + fructose), lactose (glucose + galactose), and maltose (glucose + glucose). Lactose is present in milk. Lactose is used for a lactose tolerance test to evaluate lactase activity.
3. *Trisaccharides:* Sugars that can be hydrolyzed into three monosaccharide units, e.g., raffinose (glucose + fructose + galactose). Raffinose is present in sprouts, broccoli, beans, other vegetables, and whole grains.
4. *Polysaccharides:* Sugars that yield many monosaccharide units upon hydrolysis, e.g., glycogen (many glucose units) and starch (many glucose units). Glycogen is present as the storage form of glucose in animal tissues. Starch is present in most green plants as energy storage.

Blood glucose

Sources of blood glucose are:

a. *Dietary carbohydrate:* Digestive enzymes (e.g., amylase from the pancreas, maltase, invertase, and lactase from the intestine) bring about hydrolysis of dietary carbohydrates with the formation of glucose, fructose, and galactose. Glucose forms the bulk of these monosaccharides. These sugars are transported from the intestine to the liver by portal circulation. Fructose and galactose are converted into glucose in the liver.
b. *Hepatic glycogenolysis:* Normally, an excessive amount of glucose is converted into glycogen (glycogenesis) in the liver. Glycogen is stored in the liver and converted back into glucose, when needed, by a glycogenolytic mechanism.
c. *Gluconeogenesis:* Glucose is derived by gluconeogenic mechanism when dietary carbohydrate is not available in sufficient quantities in the animal body. There are two classes of gluconeogenic compounds:

1. Those which involve a direct net conversion into glucose, e.g., amino acids.

$$\text{Amino acids} \longrightarrow \text{glucose}$$

2. Those are the products of the partial metabolism of glucose in certain tissues, e.g., lactate.

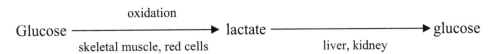

127

Measurement of carbohydrate tolerance ascertains the ability of the body to utilize carbohydrates. It is indicated by the nature of the blood glucose curve following the administration of an appropriate dose of glucose. The test developed for this purpose called the glucose tolerance test (GTT) is a valuable diagnostic laboratory test for diabetes mellitus.

Standard oral glucose tolerance test

This test is performed under standard conditions in the morning. It is performed in cases when the clinical history is atypical or if borderline results are difficult to interpret. It is of greater significance to exclude rather than to confirm diabetes.

Preparation of the patient:
1. The patient must be given a full carbohydrate diet for about a week.
2. Any drugs which might affect the test result are withdrawn for 3 days.
3. Physical activity is unrestricted.
4. The patient is advised to go for testing in the morning after a 10-12-hour fast during the night. A cup of mild tea without sugar may be allowed before the test.
5. The patient is instructed not to smoke, move, and drink any liquids except water during the test.

Procedure:
1. Collect blood and urine specimens from the patient (i.e., FBS and FUS) and record the time.
2. Orally give 75 g[10] of glucose dissolved in about 250-300 mL of drinking water flavored with lemon juice.
3. Collect blood and urine specimens at the end of ½ hr., 1 hr., 1 ½ hrs., 2 hrs. and 2 ½ hrs. after glucose administration.
4. Analyze all the blood and the urine specimens quantitatively for glucose.
5. Plot a graph by taking time (hours) on the X-axis versus concentration of blood glucose (mg/dL) on the Y-axis as shown in Fig. 17.2.

Results:
a. Normal glucose tolerance curve

Time, hour(s)	Fasting	½	1	1 ½	2	2 ½
		After glucose administration				
Blood glucose, mg/dL	75	130	140	100	65	70
Urine glucose	-	-	-	-	-	-

---

[10] For children, the dose of glucose is weight-related: 1.75 g/kg body weight. The maximum load is 75 g.

b. Diminished glucose tolerance curve

Time, hour(s)	Fasting	½	1	1 ½	2	2 ½
		After glucose administration				
Blood glucose, mg/dL	235	300	345	365	355	335
Urine glucose	+ +	N/A	+ + +	N/A	+ + +	N/A

c. Increased glucose tolerance curve

Time, hour(s)	Fasting	½	1	1 ½	2	2 ½
		After glucose administration				
Blood glucose, mg/dL	75	90	105	95	85	80
Urine glucose	-	-	-	-	-	-

Interpretation:
a. Normal tolerance curve (see Fig. 17.2a):
It has been observed that the fasting blood glucose value lies within a normal range (70-110 mg/dL). There is a maximum rise after ½ to 1 hr. of oral glucose administration but, the blood glucose level becomes normal again at the end of 1½ -2hrs. Moreover, all the urine samples are negative when tested for glucose.

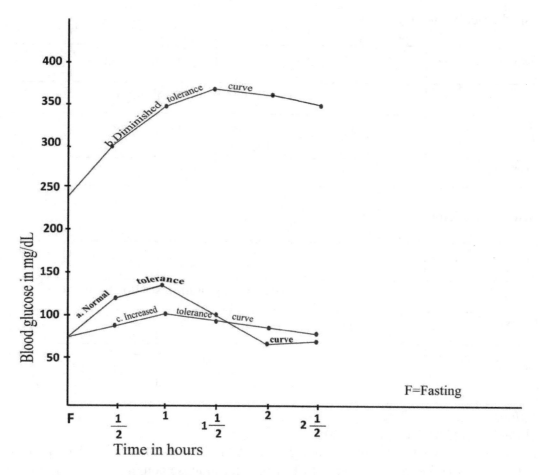

a.Normal glucose tolerance curve.
b.Diminished glucose tolerance curve.
c.Increased glucose tolerance curve.

Fig. 17.2: Glucose tolerance curves.

Abnormal tolerance curves:
b. Hyperglycemia (see Fig. 17.2b):
Hyperglycemia is a blood condition in which the blood glucose level reaches above the higher limit of the normal range. It is usually equated with diabetes mellitus. It may occur as:

1. *Mild hyperglycemia* (120-130 mg/dL): found in Cushing's syndrome, hyperthyroidism, hyperpituitarism, and liver disease.
2. *Moderate hyperglycemia* (300-500 mg/dL): usually encountered in diabetes mellitus.
3. *Marked hyperglycemia* (>500 mg/dL): noticed in uncontrolled diabetes mellitus associated with ketoacidosis, anoxemia, and advanced vascular disease. The last two entities are non-ketotic and non-acidotic.

c. Hypoglycemia (see Fig. 17.2c):
Hypoglycemia is a blood condition in which the blood glucose level falls below the lower limit of the normal range. It is encountered in hyperinsulinism, hypothyroidism (myxedema, cretinism),

hypoadrenocorticism (Addison's disease), hypopituitarism (Simmonds' disease), and acquired extensive liver disease.

Raised renal threshold:
It is a condition in which the blood glucose level exceeds 200 mg/dL without glucose being found in the urine. This confusing situation is encountered with advancing age, in many diabetics (250-300 mg/dL) and arteriosclerosis.

Lowered renal threshold (renal glycosuria):
It is a symptomless and harmless condition in which the tolerance curve is normal but shows the presence of glucose in some or all urine specimens. It is discovered accidentally (e.g., at the medical examination for life insurance) because of some abnormality in the reabsorption of glucose.

Intravenous glucose tolerance test

This test is advised in subjects who might have abnormal digestive absorption of glucose (e.g., hypothyroidism). The quantity of glucose to be injected intravenously ranges from 20-30 g over a few minutes. The blood specimens collected during the procedure include fasting and samples being withdrawn at half-hour intervals for 2 hours after injecting glucose. Soskin (1944) studied intravenous glucose tolerance in several cases and drew the following conclusions:
1. The level of blood glucose returns to normal in less than 1 hour in normal humans.
2. The level of blood glucose returns to the initial value only after 2 hours in diabetics.

Fasting blood sugar and 2-hours postprandial or post glucose test

It is advisable to carry out two determinations of blood glucose (i.e., FBS and PP2BS/PG2BS) in cases of known diabetics. It is also necessary to collect urine specimens (FUS and PP2US/PG2US). Thus, diabetics undergo this investigation regularly and take the doses of hypoglycemic agents, including insulin proportionately to control diabetes mellitus.

Results:
1. If fasting and postprandial/post-glucose values are below 140 mg/dL and 180 mg/dL, respectively, it suggests a non-diabetic case.
2. If fasting and postprandial/post-glucose levels are above 140 mg/dL and 200 mg/dL, respectively, it confirms diabetes mellitus.

Gestational diabetes

The American College of Obstetricians and Gynecologists makes a recommendation to perform a one-hour blood glucose challenge test (after taking 50 g of glucose) to screen for gestational diabetes in pregnant women (between 24-28 weeks of pregnancy) at low-risk. In case of pregnant women at high risk of developing gestational diabetes (e.g., obesity and family history of diabetes), it is recommended to undergo an earlier screening test to prevent complications.

If the plasma glucose level is greater than 140 mg/dL after a one-hour test, the health care provider recommends the three-hour glucose tolerance test. Normal three-hour GTT (after taking 100 g of glucose) results are shown in Table 17.2.

Table 17.2: Normal three-hour glucose tolerance test results

Time, hour(s)	fasting	1	2	3
		After glucose administration (100 g)		
Plasma glucose, mg/dL	<95	<185	<155	<140

If one of these results turns out a higher than normal value, a second blood test needs to be performed in a month. If two or more test results exceed the normal value, it confirms gestational diabetes.

Sample

Plasma or serum (separation from red cells within 30 minutes) is the specimen of choice. There is a decrease in the concentration of glucose by 7% per hour if the separation of red cells is delayed. Whole blood may also be used as a sample. However, the concentration of glucose in whole blood is approximately 15% lower than in plasma/serum. This is due to the higher water content of the cellular portion. Glycolysis is inhibited by collecting a blood specimen in sodium fluoride (NaF) vacutainer. Normally, the ratio of CSF/plasma glucose ranges between 0.3-0.9.

Estimation of glucose

Many methods have been developed to estimate blood glucose. They are classified as under:

    a. Enzymatic methods (e.g., glucose oxidase peroxidase and hexokinase)
    b. Condensation methods (e.g., ortho-toluidine)
    c. Reducing methods (e.g., Folin-Wu)

Compared to condensation- and reduction-based methods, enzymatic methods are highly specific and more accurate. However, all enzymatic methods are pH- and temperature-dependent. Each method has its advantages and disadvantages. The selection of a particular method depends upon the situation posed to the laboratory. Some methods are discussed below:

1. Glucose oxidase peroxidase (GOD-POD) method:
It measures true glucose, β-D-glucose. Nowadays, it is routinely used because it is easy to perform, consuming much less time than the other methods. Also, this method is suitable to measure glucose in CSF.

Principle: The aldehyde group of glucose is oxidized in the presence of glucose oxidase[11] (β-D-glucose: oxygen 1-oxidoreductase; EC 1.1.3.4) to give gluconic acid and hydrogen peroxide:

$$\text{(i)} \quad \text{D-Glucose} + O_2 + 2H_2O \xrightarrow{\text{glucose oxidase}} \text{gluconic acid} + 2H_2O_2$$

---

[11] Some commercial preparations of glucose oxidase contain mutarotase to expedite the reaction.

Glucose oxidase (sometimes called notatin, GOD, or GOx) optimally reacts at a pH of 5.5 and a temperature of 40°C.

$$\text{(ii)} \quad 2H_2O_2 + \text{4-aminophenazone} + \text{phenol} \xrightarrow{\text{peroxidase}} \text{quinone imine} + 4H_2O$$

oxygen acceptor   pink colored dye

The hydrogen peroxide, in turn, is split into water and oxygen in the presence of horseradish peroxidase (phenolic donor: hydrogen-peroxide oxidoreductase; EC 1.11.1.7) with the formation of a pink-colored dye which can be measured at 500 nm. The intensity of the color developed is proportional to the concentration of glucose.

Several substances, namely uric acid, ascorbic acid, bilirubin, hemoglobin, and glutathione can interfere with the assay, producing false low plasma glucose results. Unlike CSF samples, the higher concentrations of these interferents in urine make this method unsuitable for urinary glucose measurement.

Alternatively, the liberated hydrogen peroxide (H_2O_2) may also be quantified by reacting with luminol ($C_8H_7O_3N_3$) in the presence of $K_3[Fe(CN)_6]$ to produce luminescence (visible blue light). The amount of emitted light is measured by a chemiluminometer and is directly proportional to the amount of glucose in the sample.

2. Hexokinase method:

Principle: This is a coupled enzyme-mediated method with increased specificity (Ayyanar K. et al., 2019). Initially, hexokinase (ATP: D-hexokinase 6-phosphotransferase; EC 2.7.1.1) catalyzes the phosphorylation of D-glucose in the presence of an energy-rich molecule, adenosine triphosphate (ATP). In other words, one group of inorganic phosphate (Pi) is transferred from ATP to a carbon numbered 6 of a D-glucose molecule. In the second step, glucose-6-phosphate dehydrogenase (D-glucose-6-phosphate: NAD(P)$^+$ 1-oxidoreductase; EC 1.1.1.29) catalyzes the oxidation of D-glucose-6-phosphate to 6-phospho-D-glucono-1,5-lactone with a simultaneous reduction of a cofactor, nicotinamide adenine dinucleotide phosphate NADP$^+$ (or NAD$^+$) to NADPH (or NADH):

$$\text{(i) D-Glucose} + \text{ATP} \xrightarrow{\text{hexokinase; Mg}^+} \text{D-glucose-6-phosphate} + \text{ADP}$$

$$\text{(ii) D-glucose-6-phosphate} + \text{NADP}^+ \xrightarrow{\text{glucose-6-phosphate dehydrogenase (G6PD)}}$$
(or NAD$^+$)

                         6-phospho-D-glucono-1,5-lactone + NADPH+ H$^+$
                                        (or NADH)

The amount of NADPH (or NADH) formed is directly proportional to the concentration of glucose in the specimen. The absorbance reading of NADPH (or NADH) is measured at 340 nm. The greater the absorbance, the higher the glucose level in the sample. This is an endpoint reaction that is specific for glucose.

3. Glucose dehydrogenase method:

Principle: This is a one-step enzymatic assay. Glucose 1-dehydrogenase (β-D-glucose:NAD (P)$^+$ 1-oxidoreductase; EC 1.1.1.47) catalyzes the oxidation of β-D-glucose to D-glucono-1,5-lactone (also called glucono-delta-lactone) while donating electrons to an electron acceptor, NADP$^+$ (or NAD$^+$):

$$\beta\text{-D-Glucose} + NADP^+ \xrightarrow{\text{glucose 1-dehydrogenase [NAD(P)}^+]} \text{D-glucono-1,5-lactone} + NADPH + H^+$$
$$\text{(or NAD}^+) \qquad\qquad\qquad\qquad\qquad\qquad\qquad\qquad \text{(or NADH)}$$

The amount of formed NADPH (or NADH) is directly proportional to the concentration of glucose in the specimen. This method is less frequently used in the United States.

4. Polarographic oxygen electrode method:

Principle: The method is so-called because it employs a polarographic oxygen electrode to measure the rate of oxygen consumption. Glucose oxidase (β-D-glucose: oxygen 1-oxidoreductase; EC 1.1.3.4) catalyzes the oxidation of D-glucose to D-glucono-1,5-lactone with the formation of hydrogen peroxide:

$$\text{(i)} \quad \text{D-Glucose} + O_2 \xrightarrow{\text{glucose oxidase}} \text{D-glucono-1,5-lactone} + H_2O_2$$

The peroxide undergoes an iodide-mediated reduction. This reaction is enhanced using an ammonium molybdate:

$$\text{(ii)} \quad 2I^- + H_2O_2 + 2H^+ \xrightarrow{\text{ammonium molybdate}} I_2 + 2H_2O$$

The added ethanol to the enzyme reagent causes any remaining hydrogen peroxide to be destroyed by catalase (H_2O_2:H_2O_2 oxidoreductase, EC 1.11.1.6) to form acetaldehyde instead of the release of oxygen:

$$\text{(iii)} \quad H_2O_2 + \text{ethanol} \xrightarrow{\text{catalase}} \text{acetaldehyde} + H_2O$$

This reaction consumes oxygen. So the rate of oxygen consumption is measured with the help of a polarographic oxygen electrode and is in proportion to the concentration of glucose in the sample. It is a rapid, sensitive, and accurate method that can be used at the bedside. A novel approach of glucose oxidase (dimeric enzyme) assay is widely used in electrochemical glucose sensors designed for diabetics.

Note

1. The glucose oxidase-polarographic is not suitable for whole blood because red blood cells consume oxygen.
2. D-Glucose is present in two forms, namely α and β. Therefore, kits contain mutarotase to convert the α form to the β form because glucose oxidase is specific for β-D-glucose.
3. The usual interferences inherent in the colorimetric glucose oxidase procedures are circumvented.

5. Ortho-toluidine method:

It is a simple and very economical method. This is a rarely used chemical method with poor specificity. Also, this method is toxic and highly corrosive.

Principle: Glucose, in the presence of hot acetic acid, reacts with ortho-toluidine, and gives a blue-green colored complex:

Ortho-toluidine   Glycosylamine   Schiff base

Other chemical methods include alkaline ferricyanide, Folin-Wu, and Somogyi-Nelson. Like the *o*-toluidine method, these methods have poor specificity. Therefore, they are considered obsolete.

Conclusion

According to Lynnsay M. Dickson et al. (2018), there is no recognized gold standard reference method for plasma glucose. The enzymatic methods, namely glucose oxidase, and hexokinase are the ones frequently used internationally. However, a few clinical laboratories do use the glucose dehydrogenase method for glucose determination.

Chapter 18

Serum Urea

Introduction

The formation of urea (H_2N —$\overset{\overset{\displaystyle O}{\displaystyle \|}}{C}$— NH_2) primarily takes place in the liver and, to a lesser extent, in the kidneys. Krebs and K. Henseleit studied urea-forming reactions using liver sections. Thus, they formulated a series of chemical reactions to explain the biosynthesis of urea in the liver. Primarily, free amino acids are derived from ingested proteins through enzymatic hydrolysis:

Ingested protein $\longrightarrow$ Proteoses $\longrightarrow$ Peptins $\longrightarrow$ Peptones $\longrightarrow$ amino acids

These amino acids are then transported to the liver. Five amino acids are directly involved in the formation of urea, namely aspartic acid, N-acetylglutamic acid, arginine, ornithine, and citrulline. Arginine has been shown to markedly increase the formation of urea:

$$\text{Arginine} \xrightarrow[\text{(liver)}]{\text{arginase}} \text{ornithine} + \text{urea}$$

This explains why the formation of urea is accelerated by a high protein diet. Urea is also one of the chief products of tissue protein metabolism in humans. Thus, it is the principal end-product of protein metabolism. It forms the bulk of non-protein nitrogenous (NPN[12]) compounds. Urea, a waste-product, travels through the blood and is excreted by the kidneys into the urine. This is how body manages to get rid of highly toxic ammonia. Blood urea nitrogen (BUN) is calculated from urea value:

$$\text{BUN (mg/dL)} = \frac{\text{Urea (mg/dL)}}{2.14}$$

Clinical significance

Conditions causing azotemia (increase in blood urea) may be prerenal, renal, or postrenal.
Prerenal: Congestive cardiac failure (CCF), shock, vomiting, diarrhea, intestinal obstruction, extensive burns, pancreatic necrosis, and hemorrhage.
Renal: Acute, subacute, and chronic renal failure, tuberculosis of kidneys, and pyelonephritis (marked).
Postrenal: Bilateral obstructing kidney stones and tumors.

---

[12] NPN compounds consist of urea, uric acid, creatinine, creatine, free amino acids, ammonia, and a small amount of residual nitrogen.

BUN: Creatinine ratio

The ratio helps determine the cause of an elevated blood urea nitrogen (BUN). The laboratory finding of urea, particularly blood urea nitrogen (BUN), is significant if serum creatinine measurement is taken into consideration (e.g., serum urea nitrogen/serum creatinine ratio). The normal reference range of ratio is between 12 -20 mg/dL in a normal individual on a normal diet. Abnormal ratios are interpreted as under:

(i) Excessively low ratios: starvation, severe liver disorder, or acute tubular necrosis
(ii) High ratios (with normal levels of creatinine): high protein intake, prerenal azotemia (elevated blood urea), or tissue breakdown
(iii) High ratios (with increased levels of creatinine): postrenal obstruction or prerenal azotemia.

Note: The ratio may also be influenced by the degree of accuracy of the involved methodologies for the measurement of urea and creatinine. Therefore, it is only a crude parameter.

Sample

Urea is a freely diffusible compound in all body fluids. However, the use of serum or plasma is preferable to whole blood. The concentration of urea in serum or plasma is slightly higher than in whole blood (Martinek, 1969). For urease-based estimation techniques, anticoagulants containing ammonium salts and/or fluoride cannot be used for sample collection. Also, lipemic and hemolyzed samples spuriously increase the result.

Sometimes it is necessary to measure the urinary urea. Urinary urea measurement is performed by the same methods used for estimating serum urea. However, it may be required to dilute with water or isotonic saline (usually 1:10 or 1:20) to bring the urea concentration within a range for the test technique. Urine specimens need to be protected from bacterial degradation of urea. Failure of appropriate preservation of urine specimens gives falsely low values.

Estimation of urea

The estimation methods that involve urease are indirect because they are based on preliminary hydrolysis of urea by urease, followed by the quantitation of the ammonium ions by a suitable technique. Except for the diacetyl monoxime (DAM) method, all methods discussed here are indirect methods.

1. Urease nesslerization method:
It is a widely used manual method. It is a sensitive, specific, and simple method.

Principle: Urease (urea: amidohydrolase; EC 3.5.1.5) catalyzes the hydrolysis of urea with the formation of carbon dioxide and ammonia. Ammonia so formed reacts with Nessler's reagent[13], developing a yellowish-brown colored complex. Urease (from urease active meal) acts optimally at 55°C and a pH between 7.0-8.0.

---

[13] Alkaline solution of potassium tetraiodomercurate (II) (K_2HgI_4) is called Nessler's reagent.

(i)

$$H_2N - \overset{\overset{\displaystyle O}{\|}}{C} - NH_2 + H_2O \xrightarrow{\text{urease}} NH_3 + H_2N.COOH \longrightarrow 2NH_3 + CO_2$$

Urea — ammonia

(ii) $NH_3 + 2K_2HgI_4 + 3KOH \longrightarrow H_2NHgOHgI \downarrow + 7KI + 2H_2O$

Nessler's reagent — iodide of Millon's base (brown ppt.)

The intensity of the colored complex is proportional to the amount of urea in the specimen. It is measured colorimetrically.

2. Coupled enzymatic method:

Principle: This method employs urease (urea: amidohydrolase; EC 3.5.1.5) and glutamate dehydrogenase (L-glutamate: NAD^+ oxidoreductase; EC 1.4.1.2) in a coupled enzymatic reaction:

(i)

$$H_2N - \overset{\overset{\displaystyle O}{\|}}{C} - NH_2 + H_2O \xrightarrow{\text{urease}} NH_3 + H_2N.COOH \longrightarrow 2NH_3 + CO_2$$

Urea — ammonia

(ii) $NH_3 + \alpha\text{-ketoglutarate} + NADH + H^+ \xrightarrow{\text{glutamate dehydrogenase}} L\text{-glutamate} + NAD^+ + H_2O$

Using a spectrophotometer, a decrease in absorbance occurs because NADH is oxidized to NAD^+. This decrease in absorbance, measured at 340 nm, is directly proportional to the concentration of urea in the sample.

The enzymatic method of glutamate dehydrogenase is a reference method.

3. Conductometric method:

Principle: There is the formation of ammonium ions (NH^{4+}) and carbonate ions (CO_3^{2-}) from ammonium carbonate as shown in a coupled enzymatic method. The ammonium ions cause a change in the conductivity, reflecting the concentration of urea in the specimen.

4. Berthelot (endpoint) method:

Principle: This method depends on the formation of an intense blue-colored compound, indophenol. The formation of a blue-colored indophenol compound takes place when ammonia (NH_3) reacts with phenol and sodium hypochlorite (NaOCl) in alkaline conditions. The proposed steps, leading to the formation of indophenol, are:

(i) Ammonia (NH_3) + hypochlorite $\xrightarrow{\text{alkaline pH}}$ monochloramine

(ii) Monochloramine + phenol $\longrightarrow$ benzoquinone chlorimine

(iii) Benzoquinone chlorimine + phenol $\longrightarrow$ indophenol
(an intense blue-colored compound)

The intensity of the formed indophenol blue color is measured spectrophotometrically at 631-720 nm. This reaction can be used in the determination of both urea and blood ammonia. Any ammonia contamination (distilled water, glassware, or room) must be avoided to prevent a false increase in urea or blood ammonia values. The Bertholet method is a simple, rapid, and accurate colorimetric method.

5. Diacetyl monoxime (DAM) method:
It was developed by Ormsby (J. Biol. Chem., 1942, 146:595). It is a simple, highly sensitive, and one-step method. Chemical methods (e.g., diacetyl monoxime method) are based on the Fearon reaction where diazine is formed.

Principle: Urea condenses directly with hot acidic diacetyl monoxime in the presence of thiosemicarbazide and Fe^{3+} ($FeCl_3$) to form a rose-purple colored complex. It is required to keep the reaction mixture test tubes in a boiling water bath (100°C) for 10 minutes. The intensity of the color produced is proportional to the concentration of the urea in the test specimen and its absorption is measured at 540 nm by a spectrophotometer.

(i)

| Urea | diacetyl monoxime | diazine |

(ii) Diazine + thiosemicarbazide $\longrightarrow$ rose-purple colored complex

This reaction is photosensitive, fails to follow Beer's law, and requires special precautions for reproducing the results. In one study by Momose et al., D-glucuronolactone or D-glucuronic amide was found to minimize the photosensitivity of the reaction. Therefore, thiosemicarbazide is used to produce an intense and photostable color of a reaction mixture.

Chapter 19

Serum Creatinine and Creatinine Clearance

Introduction

Creatinine is the anhydride of creatine. The creatinine-forming reaction is non-enzymatic and irreversible:

Creatine phosphate → Creatinine

Thus, they are closely related nonprotein nitrogenous compounds.

Creatine is formed in the liver. Then, it enters the circulation from where it is almost entirely transported to the muscle. Here, it is present as creatine phosphate and in the free state (i.e., creatine). Thus, the formation of creatinine largely occurs in the muscle. The conversion of creatine phosphate to creatinine occurs spontaneously. But, the total amount formed spontaneously each day is about 2%. This spontaneous formation is dependent upon the total muscle mass. Thus, creatinine is a waste product of creatine. Generally, men have a greater mass of skeletal muscle than women. This explains why higher levels of creatinine are produced in men.

Clinical significance

An increase in serum creatinine above the higher limit of normal range occurs in all renal diseases in which 50% or more of the nephrons are destroyed. In addition to renal diseases, elevated levels of serum creatinine and creatininuria may occur in extensive muscle destruction.

Creatinine clearance

The creatinine clearance test measures the rate at which creatinine is excreted from blood/plasma by the kidneys. It is a valuable renal function test. It is calculated by using the formula:

$$C_{creat.} = \frac{U \times V}{P} \text{ mL/minute}$$

Where,

$C_{creat.}$ = Clearance of creatinine (mL/minute)
U = Urinary creatinine (mg/dL)
V = Volume of urine (mL/minute)
P = Plasma creatinine (mg/dL)

For corrected clearance, the body surface area is taken into account:

Therefore,

$$\text{Corrected } C_{creat.} = \frac{U \times V}{P} \times \frac{1.73\text{m}^2}{A}$$

Where,

      1.73 m² = standard body surface area

      A = patient's body surface area

The glomerular filtration of creatinine occurs without its secretion and reabsorption by the renal tubules in healthy conditions. Thus, creatinine clearance[14] is a useful measure to obtain the glomerular filtration rate (GFR[15]). The GFR is related to body size or more accurately the surface area. Unfortunately, creatinine is often secreted by renal tubules and may be reabsorbed in some pathological conditions (e.g., CCF), giving an inaccurate measure of GFR. This difficulty can be overcome using a non-toxic, metabolically inactive exogenous substance (e.g., inulin, mannitol, or [51](r-EDTA) in place of endogenous creatinine. A test substance is to be injected intravenously.

Sample

Hemolysis-free serum/plasma

Urine (1:25 dilution): timed (24-hour ideal)

Estimation of serum creatinine

Folin-Wu developed a manual method. Brod and Sirota (1948) applied the method of Bonsnes and Taussky (estimation of urine creatinine) to determine serum creatinine. Later on, Owen et al. (1954) and Ralston (1955) developed a technique for determining 'true creatinine'. In all these methods, the principle is the same (i.e., Jaffe reaction).

Organic compounds (e.g., protein, ascorbic acid, acetone, and glucose) and some antibiotics (e.g., cefoxitin) interfere in the determination of creatinine by Jaffe's reaction and thus overestimate plasma true creatinine value.

1. Alkaline picrate method:

Though the alkaline picrate method is simple and economical, it lacks specificity.

Principle: Creatinine in a protein-free solution reacts with alkaline picrate with the development of a red-colored complex. The intensity of the developed color is measured colorimetrically. Kinetic methods involving the Jaffe reaction are adapted to centrifugal analyzers.

Some coupled enzymatic methods with increased specificity are available for the estimation of creatinine.

---

[14] The normal creatinine clearance value ranges from 95-105 mL/minute. It may decrease in old age.

[15] The normal GFR is about 120 mL/min/1.73 m² body surface area.

2. Creatinine deaminase:

Creatinine deaminase (creatinine:iminohydrolase; EC 3.5.4.21) catalyzes the degradation of creatinine to N-methyl-hydantoin and ammonium ion (NH_4^+). So formed NH_4^+ is quantitated spectrophotometrically using the indicator chromogen, bromophenol blue (BPB):

(i) $Creatinine + H_2O \xrightarrow{\text{creatininase}} C_4H_6N_2O_2 + NH_3$
$\quad N$-methyl-hydantoin

(ii) $NH_3 + bromophenol\ blue \longrightarrow blue\ colored\ dye$

NH_4^+ may also be measured with an ammonium ion-selective electrode. A commercial nylon coil with immobilized creatininase in conjunction with a potentiometric ammonia probe is used in a continuous flow apparatus. The estimation of creatinine in plasma is viable, provided that samples are processed quickly and that plasma ammonia is evaluated just before the creatinine estimation. Analyses of urine samples require prior separation of ammonia.

3. Creatininase:

Creatininase (creatinine: amidohydrolase; EC 3.5.2.10) catalyzes the hydrolysis of creatinine to creatine. This enzymatic assay for creatinine involves a series of coupled enzymatic reactions:

(i) $Creatinine + H_2O \underset{\text{creatininase}}{\overset{\longrightarrow}{\longleftarrow}} creatine$

(ii) $Creatine + H_2O \xrightarrow{\text{creatinase}} sarcosine + urea$

(iii) $Sarcosine + H_2O + O_2 \xrightarrow{\text{sarcosine oxidase}} glycine + HCHO + H_2O_2$

(iv) $H_2O_2 + 4$-aminophenazone + 2,4,6-triiodo-3-hydroxybenzoic acid (HTIB) $\xrightarrow{\text{peroxidase}}$
$\quad\quad\quad\quad$ oxygen acceptor

$\quad\quad\quad\quad\quad\quad\quad\quad\quad\quad\quad\quad\quad\quad\quad\quad$ quinone imine $+ H_2O + HI$
$\quad\quad\quad\quad\quad\quad\quad\quad\quad\quad\quad\quad\quad\quad\quad\quad\quad\quad\quad$ dye

The colored reaction product is measured at 540 and 700 nm. The intensity of the color is proportional to the amount of creatinine in the sample. The method is simple, specific, sensitive, and reliable.

Any endogenous creatine present in the sample is eliminated by creatinase and sarcosine oxidase during the pre-incubation phase.

4. Isotope-dilution mass spectrometry (IDMS): This method makes use of isocratic ion-exchange high-performance liquid chromatography. Ultraviolet light at 234 nm is used for the detection. It is used as a reference method.

Collection of urine sample and
Estimation of urinary creatinine

A 24-hour creatinine clearance test is usually performed in the morning. The following precautions are to be taken while collecting urine for 24 hours:

1. Ask the patient to empty his or her bladder at the beginning of the test. In other words, urine stored in the bladder overnight is excluded.
2. Collect all aliquots of urine passed during 24 hours by the patient in a big container carefully.
3. Include the last aliquot of urine (i.e., at the end of 24 hours).
4. Measure the total volume of urine with the help of a measuring cylinder to the nearest mL.
5. Store the urine container at room temperature. Do not refrigerate it.
6. Take a representative specimen of urine after sufficient mixing for urinary creatinine.
7. Dilute the urine sample 1:25 and proceed with the estimation of urinary creatinine as per the method for estimating serum creatinine.

Chapter 20

Serum Uric Acid

Introduction

Uric acid is the end-product of the catabolism of purines (adenine and guanine) in humans. The metabolic pathway of purines is:

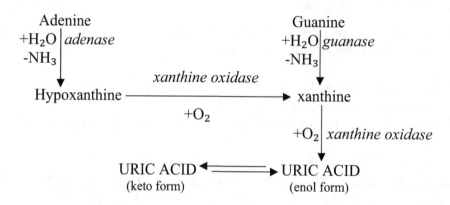

Purines are present in DNA and RNA. There are two sources of purines:

1. *Endogenous:* Cellular nucleoprotein
2. *Exogenous:* Dietary nucleoprotein

Organ meats such as liver, kidneys, and heart are purine-rich foods whereas cereals and vegetables contain poor amounts of nucleoprotein. Uric acid can exist in two forms: ketonic and enolic. It is dibasic and is slightly soluble in water. It forms soluble salts with alkali. Thus, it is present as a monosodium salt in the plasma.

The body contains about 1200 mg of miscible urate. There is a turnover of about 50% of total urate daily. In other words, the daily formation of about 600 mg of uric acid occurs with the loss of about the same amount. About 3/4 parts of the body urate are lost through urinary excretion[16] and colon bacteria destroy 1/4 part.

In sub primate mammals, allantoin is the end-product of the catabolism of purines owing to the presence of an enzyme called uricase:

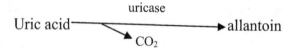

Allantoin is much more soluble than uric acid.

---

[16] Urate is filtered through the glomerulus and is fully reabsorbed by the proximal tubule. So, urate in the urine is excreted in the distal tubule.

Clinical significance

Hyperuricemia (elevated level of urate):
- Heart disease: severe congestive heart failure
- Liver disease: acute hepatitis
- Metabolic diseases: rheumatoid arthritis and gout (Gouty arthritis is the commonest in humans over 50 years of age)
- Renal diseases: acute and chronic nephritis, renal tuberculosis, pyelonephritis, hydronephrosis, pyonephrosis, and reflex anuria
- Other conditions: lympho- and myeloproliferative disorders (e.g., multiple myeloma, acute or chronic leukemia), polycythemia, prostatic obstruction, intestinal obstruction, lead poisoning, hypertension, lobar pneumonia, Lesch-Nyhan syndrome, some cases of chronic dermatitis, and diuretics

Hypouricemia (lowered level of urate):
- Hypouricemia is rarely encountered, e.g., Wilson's disease, malabsorption states

Sample

Serum or plasma (heparin as an anticoagulant) can be used in the determination of uric acid. Anticoagulants containing ammonium salts and/or fluoride cannot be used. Uric acid is stable for several days at 2-8°C.

Urine (1:10) is frequently tested for evaluating kidney function. Like urinary creatinine assay, a 24-hour urine sample is preferred.

Estimation of uric acid

1. Phosphotungstate method:
It was developed by Brown. Thereafter, numerous modifications were made. It is an economical, highly reproducible, and non-specific method. Interferents, namely glucose, and ascorbic acid falsely increase the result.

Principle: Uric acid, in an alkaline medium, reduces phosphotungstic acid to 'tungsten blue'. The intensity of a blue colored complex is proportional to the concentration of uric acid in a test specimen. It is measured colorimetrically.

The phosphotungstate method suffers from its accuracy as compared to the enzymatic method. For example, cystine and thiols in urine samples contribute to the total measured color. Therefore, a correction factor needs to be applied before reporting the uric acid results.

2. Uricase-peroxidase method (indirect uricase method):
It is a highly specific, sensitive, and widely used method. Phosphotungstic acid methods have been replaced with uricase-based methods.

Principle: Uricase[17] (urate: oxygen oxidoreductase; EC 1.7.3.3) catalyzes the oxidation of uric acid with the concurrent production of a by-product, hydrogen peroxide (H_2O_2). The horseradish peroxidase catalyzes the oxidation of 2,4-dichlorophenol sulfonate by accepting oxygen from H_2O_2:

(i) Urate + $2H_2O$ + O_2 $\xrightarrow{\text{uricase}}$ 5-hydroxyisourate + H_2O_2

5-hydroxyisourate + H_2O $\longrightarrow$ allantoin + H_2O_2

(ii) H_2O_2 + 4-aminoantipyrine + 2,4-dichlorophenol sulfonate $\xrightarrow{\text{peroxidase}}$
                  oxygen acceptor

quinine imine + H_2O
(a red colored complex)

The intensity of the color developed is proportional to the concentration of uric acid and is measured photometrically.

Alternatively, catalase (an auxiliary enzyme) can be used to catalyze the oxidation of alcohols (e.g., ethyl alcohol) to produce corresponding aldehydes in the presence of H_2O_2. So formed aldehydes are further oxidized to carboxylic acids in the presence of aldehyde dehydrogenase with the concomitant formation of a reduced nicotinamide adenine dinucleotide (NADH). Finally, the absorbance of NADH is measured at 340 nm.

The first method of quantifying hydrogen peroxide by the use of peroxidase is widely used instead.

The uricase-peroxidase method has a minimum interference because the dialyzing system in the manifold removes the possible interferences of the sera such as lipemic, hemolytic, and icteric. Ascorbic acid (interferent) is removed by using ascorbate oxidase (L-ascorbate: oxygen oxidoreductase; EC 1.10.3.3) in the donor stream of an autoanalyzer. The method is in very good agreement with the manual uricase-catalase and the uricase-ultraviolet method.

This classical method is efficient. However, it is sensitive to common interferences, e.g., endogenous bilirubin, hemoglobin, reduced glutathione, ascorbic acid, and lipids.

---

[17] Uricase (also called factor-independent urate hydroxylase) is absent in humans.

3. Direct uricase method:

Principle: So-called direct (one-step) method is based on the fact that uric acid absorbs light in the ultraviolet region of 290-293 nm. When uricase is mixed with serum, degradation of uric acid to allantoin and CO_2 occurs, thus decreasing the absorbance. This principle of differential spectrophotometry is used on centrifugal fast-analyzer techniques.

This is a highly sensitive and specific method for the analysis of both serum and urine. Sampling errors and spontaneous changes in the turbidity of a sample cause variations in light scattering and apparent changes in UV light absorbance. Thus, the accuracy and precision of the method are influenced.

Chapter 21

Serum Cholesterol

Introduction

Cholesterol is a sterol because it is composed of a steroid and alcohol. It is soluble in fat solvents. Structurally, it has four fused hydrocarbon rings to which a hydrocarbon is attached at one end and a hydroxyl group at the other. It occurs in two forms: free cholesterol and cholesteryl esters (approximately 70% of total cholesterol). In the latter form, cholesterol combines with fatty acids. Key factors that affect cholesterol levels include diet, weight, exercise, gender, and genetics (familial). It serves four functions:(1) structural component of cell membranes (2) precursor for steroid hormones (3) allowing the body to generate vitamin D (4) making the digestive bile acids in the intestine.

Cholesterol is used in the body to form cholic acid in the liver. Cholic acid, in turn, is converted to bile salts which play an important role in the digestion of fats. Cholesterol is transported through the circulation in two forms of cholesterol parcels: low-density lipoprotein (LDL) also called "bad" cholesterol and high-density lipoprotein (HDL) also called "good" cholesterol. Thyroid hormones and estrogens decrease the concentration of cholesterol. On the other hand, androgens increase their concentration.

Biosynthesis of cholesterol

A small quantity of cholesterol (about 0.3g/day) is provided by the diet. But, the greater part of it (about 1g/day) is synthesized from acetyl-CoA. Tissues involved in the biosynthesis of cholesterol are the liver, adrenal cortex, skin, intestines, testes, and aorta. The actual site of synthesis in all these tissues is the microsomal fraction of the cell. There are several stages in the synthesis of this complex molecule. They are diagrammatically represented in Fig. 21.1.

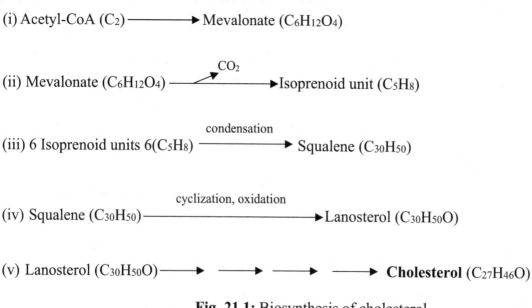

(i) Acetyl-CoA (C_2) ⟶ Mevalonate ($C_6H_{12}O_4$)

(ii) Mevalonate ($C_6H_{12}O_4$) $\xrightarrow{CO_2}$ Isoprenoid unit (C_5H_8)

(iii) 6 Isoprenoid units 6(C_5H_8) $\xrightarrow{condensation}$ Squalene ($C_{30}H_{50}$)

(iv) Squalene ($C_{30}H_{50}$) $\xrightarrow{cyclization,\ oxidation}$ Lanosterol ($C_{30}H_{50}O$)

(v) Lanosterol ($C_{30}H_{50}O$) ⟶ ⟶ ⟶ ⟶ **Cholesterol** ($C_{27}H_{46}O$)

Fig. 21.1: Biosynthesis of cholesterol.

Clinical significance

Hypercholesterolemia:
- Uncontrolled diabetes mellitus
- Obstructive jaundice
- Nephrotic syndrome
- Biliary cirrhosis
- Hypothyroidism
- Pregnancy
- Atherosclerosis

Hypocholesterolemia:
- Malnutrition
- Gaucher's disease
- Acute hepatitis
- Hyperthyroidism

Sample: Unlike samples for estimation of triglycerides, overnight fasting is not a requirement while submitting samples for total cholesterol and HDL-C assays. It is of utmost importance that one considers lipemia-, icterus-, hemolysis-, or turbidity-related interferences while adapting direct methods. Indirect methods (chemical or enzymatic) require initial extraction to remove the interferents.

Before assay, serum or plasma can be stored for four days and one month at 2-8°C and -20°C, respectively.

A. Estimation of total cholesterol

1. Chemical method:
It is a non-specific, relatively simple, and inexpensive method. The modified Abell Kendall method is a standard reference method approved by the National Institute of Standards and Technology (NIST, USA). It is a multi-step classical chemical method.

Principle: Alcoholic potassium hydroxide (KOH) is used during the saponification step to cause hydrolysis of cholesterol esters followed by extraction of hydrolyzed cholesterol with hexane and the subsequent evaporation of the solvent. Finally, the cholesterol is allowed to react with sulfuric acid and acetic anhydride (Liebermann-Burchard reaction) for color development. The development of color is due to the reaction of a hydroxyl group (-OH) present in the cholesterol:

Cholesterol + sulfuric acid + acetic anhydride ———————⟶ bluish green

The intensity of the color developed is commonly measured by ultra-violet (UV) spectrophoto-meter at 410 nm.

Nowadays, this method is *not* acceptable as a routine clinical method in the measurement of total cholesterol because it involves the use of highly corrosive reagents.

2. Enzymatic method:

The enzymatic assay was developed by Richmond (1972), Flegg (1973), and Allain et al. (1974). The enzymatic methods have increased specificity as well as reproducibility. Therefore, chemical methods have been replaced with enzymatic methods.

Principle: Cholesterol esters undergo hydrolysis in the presence of cholesterol esterase (steryl-ester acylhydrolase; EC 3.1.1.13) to release free cholesterol from esterified cholesterol. Then, cholesterol oxidase (cholesterol: oxygen oxidoreductase; EC 1.1.3.6) catalyzes the oxidation of free cholesterol to cholest-4-en-3-one with the concurrent formation of hydrogen peroxide (H_2O_2).

(i) Cholesterol esters + H_2O $\xrightarrow{\text{cholesterol esterase}}$ cholesterol + fatty acids

(ii) Cholesterol + O_2 $\xrightarrow{\text{cholesterol oxidase}}$ cholest-4-en-3-one + H_2O_2

Hydrogen peroxide so formed, in the presence of peroxidase, reacts with 4-aminoantipyrine and phenol (Trinder's reagent) to develop a pink colored complex (quinone imine dye).

(iii) $2H_2O_2$ + 4-aminoantipyrine + phenol $\xrightarrow{\text{peroxidase}}$ quinone imine + H_2O
oxygen acceptor

The intensity of the color is proportional to the concentration of cholesterol and is measured colorimetrically or spectrophotometrically (maximum absorption at 500 nm). The method requires no pretreatment of serum samples. The linearity of the calibration curve is up to 600 mg/dL.

Alternately, consumption of oxygen can be measured amperometrically by an oxygen-sensing electrode.

Compared to classical chemical methods, routine enzymatic assays have the following advantages and disadvantages:

Advantages:

1. Preliminary extraction step not required
2. Lesser interferences due to ascorbic acid, bilirubin, and hemoglobin
3. Non-corrosive reagents
4. An accurate, precise, and expeditious method
5. The linearity of the calibration curve up to 600 mg/dL
6. Can be employed to estimate non-esterified cholesterol

Disadvantages:

1. Not absolutely specific for cholesterol
2. Interferences due to bilirubin and ascorbic acid

3. Gas chromatography-mass spectrometry (GC-MS):
It is used as a reference method because it is a sensitive and accurate method. However, it is an expensive and time-consuming technique. It measures selectively cholesterol, excluding related sterols, and requires low volumes (tens of μL) of samples for analysis.

4. Isotope dilution mass spectrometry (ID-MS):
It is a definitive method.

B. Estimation of high-density lipoprotein-cholesterol (HDL-C)

It is measured directly in a serum sample.

Principle: Estimation of HDL-cholesterol (HDL-C) by an enzymatic method requires pretreatment of a plasma specimen to precipitate cholesterol components of VLDL and LDL out of the plasma. The precipitating mixture includes heparin, manganese chloride, and dextran sulfate. Thus, the resulting HDL-C rich supernatant is a suitable specimen for the test, to begin with.

The blocking reagent (Roche/Boehringer-Mannheim Diagnostics) used during an enzymatic assay of HDL-C successfully omits the detection of apo B containing lipoproteins. In other words, the assay selectively measures HDL-C. Except for the initial pretreatment step, all the remaining steps are exactly similar to that of an enzymatic cholesterol assay:

(i) Apo B containing lipoproteins + α-cyclodextrin + Mg^{+2} + dextran SO_4 $\longrightarrow$

$$\text{a complex with apo B containing lipoproteins}$$
$$\text{(soluble and non-reactive)}$$

(ii) HDL cholesteryl esters $\xrightarrow[\text{cholesteryl esterase}]{\text{polyethylene glycol (PEG) -}}$ HDL-unesterified cholesterol + fatty acid

(iii) Unesterified cholesterol + O_2 $\xrightarrow{\text{PEG-cholesterol oxidase}}$ cholestenone + H_2O_2

(iv) H_2O_2 + 5-aminophenazone + N-ethyl-N-(3-methylphenyl)-N'-succinyl ethylenediamine

$$+ H_2O + H^+ \xrightarrow{\text{peroxidase}} \text{quinone imine dye} + H_2O$$

C. Calculation of low-density lipoprotein-cholesterol (LDL-C)

Most of the cholesterol in the bloodstream is found in three major fractions, namely very low-density lipoproteins (VLDL), HDL, and LDL. It is calculated by using the relationship:

$$LDL\text{-}C = (total\text{-}C) - (HDL\text{-}C) - (TG)/5$$

Where,
> total-C, HDL-C, and triglycerides (TG) are measured values
> (TG)/5 is an estimate of VLDL-C and all values are expressed in mg/dL.

Conclusion

Several golden standard methods are available to date. Nevertheless, new analytical platforms, e.g., ambient ionization mass spectrometry, are being developed and employed. According to Hsieh et al. (2019), direct analysis in real-time mass spectrometry (DART-MS) is a promising tool for rapid and cost-effective preliminary screening of endogenous free cholesterol in serum samples which may be used in POCT.

Chapter 22

Serum Lipids and Lipoproteins

Introduction

Triglycerides belong to plasma lipoproteins. They are esters of glycerol with the group formula given below:

$CH_2.O.CO.R_1$

$CH.O.CO.R_2$

$CH_2.O.CO.R_3$
A triglyceride

Where,
R_1, R_2, and R_3 are fatty acid radicals.

The three fatty acids may be the same or different. Chylomicrons contain 85% of triglycerides. The concentration of triglycerides increases with the increase in age. Fredrickson et. al. proposed a range of 10-190 mg/dL in various age groups.

Formation

Glycerol is phosphorylated at one of the α-positions by glycerol kinase in the presence of ATP. Glycerophosphate can then react with 2 molecules of fatty acyl-CoA with the formation of α, β-3-diacetyl phosphatidic acid. The phosphate molecule is eliminated in the presence of an enzyme. Hydroxyl (-OH) group thus set free is finally esterified with a third molecule of acyl-CoA. The chemical reactions leading to the formation of a triglyceride (also called triacylglycerol) are shown in Fig. 22.1.

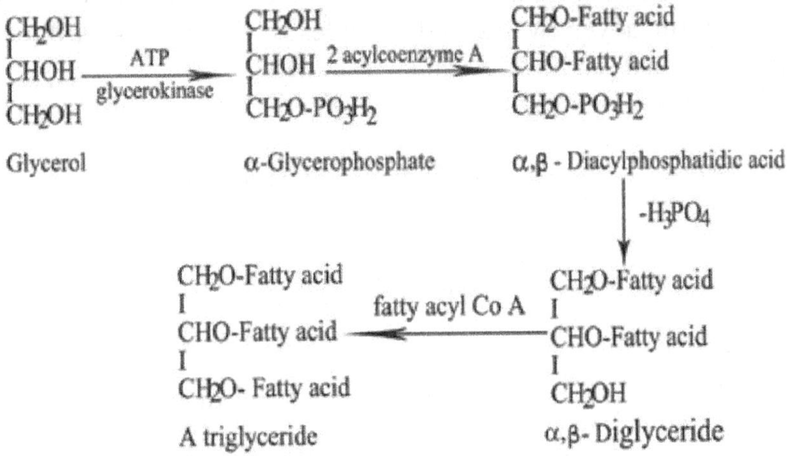

Fig. 22.1: The chemical reactions leading to the formation of a triglyceride.

153

The main three tissues involved in the formation of triglycerides are the small intestine, liver, and all the adipose tissues.

Clinical significance

Estimation of triglycerides in conjunction with other lipid parameters has diagnostic significance in the following conditions:

- Diabetes mellitus
- Biliary obstruction
- Nephrosis
- Atherosclerosis
- Various endocrine-related metabolic disturbances

Sample: It is recommended to do 12-14 hours fasting during night-time before sample collection. The triglyceride levels rise to their peak value between 4 and 6 hours post-meal. Either serum or EDTA-anticoagulated plasma can be used in the estimation of triglycerides. Specimens can be stored at 2°-8°C and -20°C for three days and several weeks, respectively.

Estimation of triglycerides

1. Chemical method:

Van Handel and Zilversmit D B. (1957) developed a nonspecific chemical method for the estimation of serum triglycerides. Although the method is very economical, it involves a time-consuming pretreatment (i.e., extraction) step before analysis. This pre-analytical step helps remove free glycerol, phospholipids, and other interferents. The extraction of serum triglycerides can be accomplished by using isopropanol (solvent) and the subsequent adsorption by zeolite/Llyod's reagent.

Principle: The triglycerides, in the presence of alcoholic potassium hydroxide (KOH), are hydrolyzed to glycerol and fatty acids during the saponification step. So formed glycerol is then oxidized by reacting with periodate to form formaldehyde. Finally, formaldehyde is quantitated through the Hantzsch condensation reaction where formaldehyde reacts with acetylacetone and ammonium acetate to form a yellow colored complex, 3,5-diacetyl-1,4-dihydrolutidine. The sequence of chemical reactions can be represented as under:

(i) Triglycerides + KOH $\longrightarrow$ glycerol + fatty acids

(ii) Glycerol + periodate $\longrightarrow$ formaldehyde

(iii) Formaldehyde + NH_4^+ + acetylacetone $\longrightarrow$ 3,5-diacetyl-1,4-dihydrolutidine
(a yellow colored complex)

The intensity of yellow color of 3,5-diacetyl-1,4-dihydrolutidine is proportional to the concentration of triglycerides and is measured colorimetrically or spectrophotometrically.

2. Enzymatic method:

The glycerol kinase method is a specific, simple, and expeditious method. The initial hydrolysis of triglycerides to form glycerol and fatty acids is a common step in all enzymatic methods.

Principle: Lipase (triacylglycerol: acylhydrolase; EC 3.1.1.3) catalyzes the hydrolysis of triglycerides with the formation of glycerol and three molecules of fatty acids. The glycerol, in turn, undergoes glycerol kinase-(ATP: glycerol 3-phosphotransferase; EC 2.7.1.30) mediated phosphorylation to form glycerol-1-phosphate. Glycerol-1-phosphate is further catalyzed by glycerophosphate dehydrogenase (sn-glycerol-1-phosphate: NAD (P)$^+$ 2-oxidoreductase; EC 1.1.1.261) to produce a by-product, NADH. So formed NADH is measured by using INT[18] (an electron acceptor) in the presence of diaphorase (NADH: (quinone-acceptor) oxidoreductase; EC 1.6.5.11). The sequential enzymatic reactions can be represented as under:

$$\text{(i) Triglycerides} + 3H_2O \xrightarrow{\text{lipase}} \text{glycerol} + 3 \text{ free fatty acids}$$

$$\text{(ii) Glycerol} + \text{ATP} \xrightarrow{\text{glycerol kinase}} \text{glycerol-1-phosphate} + \text{ADP}$$

$$\text{(iii) Glycerol-1-phosphate} + \text{NAD}^+ \xrightarrow{\text{glycerophosphate dehydrogenase}}$$

$$\text{dihydroxyacetone phosphate} + \text{NADH} + \text{H}^+$$

$$\text{(iv) NADH} + \text{INT} \xrightarrow{\text{diaphorase}} \text{formazan} + \text{NAD}^+$$
$$\text{(red)}$$

The intensity of red color of formazan so developed is proportional to the concentration of triglycerides in the specimen and is measured spectrophotometrically at 510 nm.

3. An accurate single-run enzymatic method:

It is called an accurate method because free glycerol is removed by preincubation with glycerol phosphate oxidase and peroxidase. Thereafter, lipase and 4-aminoantipyrine (chromogen) are added.

---

[18] Iodonitrotetrazolium chloride (INT)=2-(4-iodophenyl)-3-(4-nitrophenyl)-5-phenyl -2H-tetrazolium chloride (used for quantitative redox assays)

Principle: Unlike the quantitation of NADH described in the earlier enzymatic method, this enzymatic method differs in the last two steps: (iii) and (iv) while the first two steps: (i) and (ii), remain unchanged. Glycerophosphate oxidase (sn-glycerol-3-phosphate: oxygen 2-oxidoreductase; EC 1.1.3.21) catalyzes the oxidation of glycerol-1-phosphate with the formation of a by-product, hydrogen peroxide (H_2O_2). The horseradish peroxidase (phenolic donor: hydrogen-peroxide oxidoreductase; EC 1.11.1.7) catalyzes a reaction between H_2O_2 and the Trinder's reagent with the formation of quinone imine dye:

(iii) Glycerol-1-phosphate + O_2 $\xrightarrow{\text{glycerophosphate oxidase}}$ dihydroxyacetone phosphate + H_2O_2

(iv) $2H_2O_2$ + 4-aminoantipyrine + phenol $\xrightarrow{\text{peroxidase}}$ quinone imine + H_2O
(a pink complex)

Finally, the intensity of a pink complex is measured which is proportional to the number of triglycerides present in the sample. The absorbance is read at 500 nm. According to Sullivan D.R. et al. (1985), the method is more accurate and precise as compared to that of an NADH-based monitoring method.

Note:
1. The accuracy of the triglyceride assay demands that each enzymatic reaction step be complete and homogenous.
2. Since freshly drawn serum samples contain a small amount of free glycerol, enzymatic methods yield triglyceride values of 10-20 mg/dL higher than colorimetric methods.

4. Gas chromatography-mass spectrometry (GC-MS):
It involves the hydrolysis of fatty acids on triglycerides and the measurement of glycerol. It is used as a reference method.

Cholesterol (see chapter 21):

Lipoproteins

Lipoprotein particles consist of a central hydrophobic core (triglycerides and cholesteryl esters) and a hydrophilic monolayer membrane (free cholesterol, phospholipids, and apolipoproteins). These complex particles vary in their sizes, densities, and chemical properties (see Table 22.1). They play a significant role in transporting lipids from the intestine and liver to the peripheral tissues and vice versa. Considering the physicochemical and immunological properties of lipoproteins, various methods, namely ultracentrifugation, selective precipitation, and electrophoresis are used to fractionate them. Because ultracentrifugation is a reference method, electrophoresis is routinely used in the separation of various lipoprotein fractions. Electrophoretic fractionation of lipoproteins from the same day collected serum/plasma (EDTA) is successfully carried out at a pH value of 8.6 using agarose gel, followed by the staining of electrophoretogram with Fat red 7B or oil red O.

Table 22.1: Some important physicochemical properties of lipoprotein particles

Lipoprotein	Size, nm	Density, g/mL	Electrophoretic Mobility (agarose)	Major lipids, % by weight	Major apolipoproteins
Chylomicron	>75	0.93	origin	triglyceride (exogenous):84	Apo B-48, Apo C, Apo A
VLDL	30-80	0.97	pre-beta	triglyceride (endogenous): 44-60 *(cholesterol): 16-22	Apo B-100, Apo E, Apo C-II
IDL	22-24	1.003	broad beta (between beta and pre-beta)	triglyceride:30 cholesterol:30	Apo B-100, Apo C, Apo E
LDL**	18-25	1.034	beta	*cholesterol:52	Apo B-100
HDL***	4-10	1.121	alpha	*cholesterol:19 phospholipids:28	Apo A, Apo C, Apo E

*cholesterol (unesterified) and cholesterol (esterified) combined
**pro-atherosclerogenic
***anti-atherosclerogenic

Various electrophoretic lipoprotein fractions are briefly discussed below:

Chylomicrons: Among the lipoprotein particles, chylomicrons are the largest ones with the lowest density. These particles form a creamy layer at the top of the specimen, particularly at 4°C. They remain at the point of serum application (i.e., origin) following the electrophoretic run. In other words, they are the closest to the cathode. They are synthesized by the enterocyte (small intestine). Chemically, they consist of exogenous triglycerides (dietary lipids) as a major component with 10% of cholesterol and Apo B-48, Apo C, and Apo A. They transport the endogenous triglycerides in the form of free fatty acids from the intestinal tract to the peripheral tissues. Thus, chylomicrons resemble VLDL in their functionality.

Very low-density lipoproteins (VLDL): VLDL synthesis occurs in hepatocytes (liver), containing triglycerides and Apo B-100. Apo B-100 is synthesized by the rough endoplasmic reticulum. Then, VLDL particles enter into the bloodstream as nascent VLDL and interact with HDL particles. During this interaction, HDL transfers Apo C-II and Apo E to nascent VLDL and transforms to mature VLDL. Finally, mature VLDL delivers triglycerides-split products, free fatty acids, to muscle tissues (energy) and adipose tissues (storage). They measure 30-80 nm in diameter and have migration ability in the pre-beta region.

Intermediate-density lipoproteins (IDL): IDL is formed (intravascular) following the hydrolysis of VLDL catalyzed by lipoprotein lipase (LPL), leading to a substantial loss of triglycerides as under:

$$\text{VLDL} \xrightarrow{\text{lipoprotein lipase}} \text{IDL} + \text{glycerol} + \text{free fatty acids}$$

This catabolic process leaves IDL with approximately similar quantities of cholesterol and triglycerides because triglycerides are partially cleaved to glycerol and free fatty acids. Moreover, IDL is associated with major apolipoproteins, namely Apo B-100 and Apo E. Thus, it is a short-lived precursor of low-density lipoproteins (LDL). IDL particles migrate in a broad beta region (i.e., between beta and pre-beta).

Low-density lipoprotein (LDL): LDL particles transport cholesterol to peripheral tissues because cholesterol serves as not only a precursor for steroid hormones and vitamin D but also a cell membrane component. But, excessive plasma cholesterol undergoes oxidation, leading to the uptake process by macrophages of the arterial wall and subsequent formation of foam cells (a hallmark of plaque). Thus, LDL being the pro-atherosclerotic factor, it is referred to as "bad" cholesterol. They migrate in the beta region. Urine and electrophoretic separation of serum proteins as shown in Fig. 22.2.

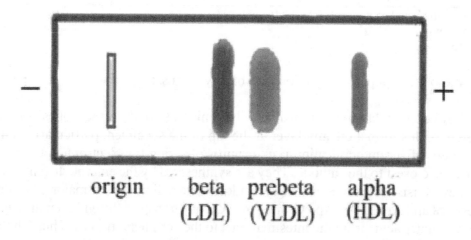

Fig. 22.2: Electrophoretic assay of serum lipoproteins.

High-density lipoprotein (HDL): HDL particles play two important roles: (1) to bring excess cholesterol from peripheral tissues to the liver by a reverse cholesterol transport mechanism and (2) to prevent the oxidation of LDL-cholesterol by under its antioxidant property. Thus, both these functions help lower the cholesterol levels in arterial walls. In other words, HDL being the anti-atherosclerotic factor, it is popularly known as "good" cholesterol. They are the smallest particles with the highest density among the lipoproteins. They migrate to the alpha region near the anode.

Apolipoproteins

It is beyond the scope of this manual to elaborate on apolipoproteins in great detail. Apoproteins are the protein components of the lipoprotein conjugates. Since lipids are insoluble in plasma, apolipoproteins play a crucial role in their transportation and catabolism. They are grouped as A, B, C, and E. Some of them are further sub-grouped, using the Roman numbers, e.g., I, II, and so on. Methods of measurement for apolipoproteins include radioimmunoassay (RIA), enzyme-linked immunosorbent assay (ELISA), radial immunodiffusion (RID), and immunonephelometry (INA).

Apo A: Apo A is sub-divided as Apo A-I, Apo A-II, Apo A-IV, and Apo A-V. Synthesis of Apo A-I, Apo A-II, and Apo A-V takes place in the liver whereas the intestine produces Apo A-IV and some amount of Apo A-I. Both Apo A-I (70%) and Apo A-II (20%) contribute as a structural protein for HDL. In addition to this, Apo A-I is an activator of lecithin cholesterol acyltransferase (LCAT) and Apo A-V facilitates the lipolysis catalyzed by lipoprotein lipase (LPL).

Apo B: There are two species namely, Apo B-48 and Apo B-100. Apo B-48 synthesized in the intestine is a structural backbone of chylomicron particles. On the other hand, liver-made Apo B-100 is an integral part of VLDL, IDL, and LDL. Except for HDL, each lipoprotein particle is equipped with only one Apo B moiety. Therefore, increased levels of Apo B are implicated with increased risk of atherosclerosis.

Apo C: Apo C-II plays a significant role in the catabolism of triglycerides packaged in VLDLs. This is accomplished through the activation of lipoprotein lipase (LPL) by Apo C-II. Thus, triglycerides are cleaved (lipolysis) to liberate free fatty acids needed by peripheral tissues.

Apo E: Apo E is present in more or less quantity in all lipoproteins except LDLs. It is primarily produced in the liver and intestine. It plays a significant role in the recognition and subsequent catabolism of chylomicron remnants and IDLs. Furthermore, Apo E serves as a ligand for LDL hepatic receptors. The deficiency of Apo E is associated with dysbetalipoproteinemia and Alzheimer's disease.

Hyperlipoproteinemias (hyperlipidemias)

Hyperproteinemias are disorders associated with the accumulation of lipids. They are predominantly inherited (primary) ones. These Hyperlipoproteinemias are divided into five types according to Fredrickson classification. Except for Type I, all other types are implicated with an increased risk of coronary artery disease (CAD). These phenotypes are briefly characterized in Table 22.2.

Table 22.2: Characteristics of different types of hyperlipoproteinemias

Type	Triglycerides	Total cholesterol	Chylomicrons	VLDLs	IDLs	LDLs
I	↑		+			
IIA		↑				↑
IIB	↑	↑		↑		↑
III	↑	↑		↑	↑	
IV*	↑			↑		
V	↑	↑	+	↑		

* = frequent occurrence
+ = present
↑ = increased

Some lipid storage diseases are Gaucher's disease, Niemann-Pick disease, and Tay-Sachs disease.

Chapter 23

Plasma Amino Acids and Proteins

Introduction

Amino acids contain both a carboxyl group (-COOH) and an amino group (-NH$_2$). Also, there is a side chain(R) specific to each amino acid:

General formula　　　　Glycine　　　　Alanine

There are 20 alpha-amino acids to build peptides and proteins. Amino acids are linked together principally through their alpha-amino and carboxyl groups, forming a peptide bond:

Glycyl-alanine

Here, the –COOH of one amino acid combines with the –NH$_2$ of the other with the elimination of a water molecule. Oppositely, proteins may be hydrolyzed by strong acids, strong alkalies, or specific enzymes, resulting in the production of a mixture of -amino acids. This is how the hydrolysis of proteins results in a complete loss of colloidal properties.

Aminoacidurias

Primary aminoacidurias (inborn error of metabolism) occur due to inherited defective enzymes. Symptoms vary from benign to lethal e.g., maple syrup urine disease (MSUD). In some cases, clinical symptoms, e.g., persistent vomiting and neurological disorder, are evident. Therefore, routine prenatal screening is required to prevent further damage to an infant. Some selected primary aminoacidurias are listed in Table 23.1.

Table 23.1: Some selected aminoacidurias

Disorder	Cause	Effect(s)	Tests(s)
Alkaptonuria	- Deficiency of homogentisic acid oxidase	- Cartilage pigmentation - Degenerative arthritis	- Urine develops blue color if mixed with $FeCl_3$
Cystinuria	- Increased output of cysteine	- Renal calculi	- Urine develops red-purple color with cyanide nitroprusside
Phenylketonuria	- Deficiency of phenylalanine hydroxylase	- Neurological disorders	- Guthrie bacterial inhibition assay - HPLC to confirm
Tyrosinemia	- Defect in fumarylaceto-acetate hydrolase	- Renal damage - Mental retardation	- Ion-exchange column chromatography
Maple syrup urine disease (MSUD)	- Deficiency of branched-chain keto acid decarboxylase - A buildup of leucine, isoleucine, and valine	- Hypoglycemia - Mental retardation - Convulsions	- Modified Guthrie test

Sample: Plasma is preferred to serum. Heparin is the anticoagulant of choice. The plasma sample is subjected to deproteinization if sulfur-containing amino acids (e.g., cysteine) are to be analyzed. The urine samples are widely used in amino acid-related disorders.

Estimation of amino acids

Amino acids can be identified by thin-layer chromatography (TLC) or paper chromatography. Separated amino acids can be visualized using a staining reagent, e.g., ninhydrin. Rf value is the ratio of the distance traveled by the compound to the distance moved by the solvent. For details, readers should refer to chapter 3.

Other tests include chemical tests of urine, e.g., ferric chloride test to detect phenylpyruvate (dark blue-green) in patients with phenylketonuria and the Guthrie test (uses *Bacillus subtilis*). The $FeCl_3$ test, a non-specific test, can be used to monitor the efficacy of dietary treatment for phenylketonuria (PKU).

An expensive screening by gas chromatography-mass spectrometry (GC-MS) is used by some institutions for accuracy.

The high-performance liquid chromatography (HPLC) is a highly sensitive technique. It is used for the quantitative analysis of amino acids. Other chromatographic techniques, namely ion-exchange column chromatography and gas-liquid chromatography (GLC) are also employed to confirm the screening test results.

Plasma Proteins

Introduction

Plasma contains a very complex mixture of proteins. Plasma proteins include simple proteins as well as mixed or conjugated proteins (e.g., lipoproteins and glycoproteins). These plasma proteins differ from each other in physicochemical properties. The important proteins are listed below:

1. Albumin
2. Globulins
3. Fibrinogen
4. Prothrombin

Formation

The liver is the chief site for the biosynthesis of albumin (9-12 g/day), fibrinogen, and prothrombin. Most of the alpha (α) and beta (β) globulins are also of hepatic origin. Gamma (γ) globulins are formed in plasma cells, lymphoid tissue, and reticuloendothelial cells (phagocytic cells of the bone marrow, spleen, liver, lymph nodes, and subcutaneous tissue). The enzymes are formed in various organs. Dietary proteins serve as the precursors of the plasma proteins.

Functions

1. Nutritive:
The formation of amino acids occurs during the metabolism of proteins. So formed amino acids enter the amino acid pool and some of these are used for the formation of new proteins or other nitrogenous compounds. On the other hand, other amino acids undergo deamination with the formation of compounds that are either completely degraded to carbon dioxide and water or used for the formation of glucose.

2. Maintenance of osmotic pressure:
The plasma proteins, by their colloidal dimensions, cannot diffuse through the membrane of the capillaries. Thus, plasma proteins exert osmotic pressure which acts as a force tending to hold a certain volume of water in the blood. The colloid osmotic pressure (oncotic pressure) is about 25 mm Hg. of the total osmotic pressure of the plasma. It counteracts the hydrostatic pressure of blood, thus maintaining the required circulating blood volume. Albumin is the most important protein in this connection. Each g% exerts an osmotic pressure of 5.54 mm Hg. because of its higher concentration and lower molecular weight than most of the globulins. On the other hand, each g% of serum globulin exerts an osmotic pressure of only 1.43 mm Hg.
The accumulation of excess fluid in the tissue spaces is called edema. This condition is common in nephrosis. It is associated with the loss of plasma proteins, thus changing the balance between colloid osmotic and hydrostatic pressure.

3. Buffering action:

The plasma proteins partly play to maintain the plasma pH. The isoelectric points of albumin and globulin are 4.8 and 5.5, respectively. At the normal pH of the blood (i.e., 7.4), these proteins act as anions and combine with cations (mainly sodium) with the formation of buffer pairs.

4. Transporting agents:

Albumin can transport many compounds. The plasma proteins combine with lipids, fat-soluble vitamins, steroid hormones (e.g., cortisol and thyroxine), antibodies, metals, and possibly carbohydrates with the formation of soluble complexes. These complexes are easily transported.

5. Reserve of body proteins:

The circulating plasma proteins are not static. But, they constantly interchange with the labile tissue proteins of the body and can be used at the time of protein starvation. This interchange is termed as 'dynamic equilibrium'.

6. Blood coagulation:

Many of the factors participating in the coagulation are proteins.

7. As catalysts:

Plasma contains a wide range of enzymes (e.g., blood clotting enzymes, aldolase, lactate dehydrogenase, transaminases, and phosphatases).

8. Protective:

Plasma contains antibodies (immunoglobulins) that protect the body against infections.

Clinical Significance

Hypoproteinemia and hypoalbuminemia:
- Nephrotic syndrome
- Malnutrition (Kwashiorkor)
- Increased catabolism (e.g., Cushing's syndrome)
- Severe liver diseases

Hyperproteinemia:
- Dehydration
- Diarrhea

Hypergammaglobulinemia: There is a normal total protein with low normal albumin and a raised globulin, thus reversing the A/G ratio (normal 1.5 to 2.5:1). It is necessary to quantify zone-electrophoretic patterns.
- Multiple myeloma
- Carcinoma
- Lymphoma
- Chronic granulomatous infectious diseases (e.g., tuberculosis, brucellosis, and collagen disease).

Sample: Hemolysis-free serum or plasma can be used in the estimation of total protein and albumin. The acceptable anticoagulants include heparin and EDTA. Ideally, the serum should be immediately separated from blood cells after centrifugation. Some facilities use plasma to reduce turnaround time (TAT). Since plasma contains fibrinogen, its total protein value is higher (0.2-0.4 g/dL) than serum concentrations. Lipemic (>2+) samples demonstrate a negative interference.

Since the concentration of total protein in blood is nearly 1000 times that of normal CSF, it is strictly recommended that one uses a blood-free CSF sample in the test. Separated serum or plasma can be stored for two days and two months at 2°-8°C and -20°C, respectively.

Estimation of total protein

1. Biuret method (Reinhold, 1953):

Interestingly, biuret [$H_2NC(O)NHC(O)NH_2$] is neither used in the preparation of a biuret reagent nor the test procedure:

$$
\begin{array}{ccc}
NH_2 & NH_2 & \\
| & | & \\
C=O & + & C=O \\
| & | & \\
NH_2 & NH_2 & \\
\text{Urea} & \text{urea} &
\end{array}
\xrightarrow{\ 180°C\ }
\begin{array}{c}
NH_2 \\
| \\
C=O \\
| \\
NH \\
| \\
C=O \\
| \\
NH_2 \\
\text{biuret}
\end{array}
$$

Both reagent and test methods are so named because the response of biuret is similar to proteins if allowed to react with a biuret reagent. The following chemical formulation of a biuret reagent provides clarification:

1. Sodium hydroxide (NaOH) to provide an alkaline medium
2. Pentahydrate copper (II) sulfate ($CuSO_4.5H_2O$) to supply Cu^{2+} ions
3. Potassium sodium tartrate ($KNaC_4H_4O_6.4H_2O$), also called Rochelle salt, to stabilize the color

Principle: The biuret reagent (blue) turns violet and pink in the presence of proteins and peptides, respectively. It requires the presence of two or more peptide bonds (e.g., tri- oligo- or poly-peptides) in a molecule for a positive reaction. The biuret reagent fails to react with amino acids because they lack peptide bonds. Therefore, there is no change in color (i.e., a negative test).

Peptide bonds (-CO-NH-) occur with approximately the same frequency per gram of the protein-containing material. Serum proteins containing peptide bonds react with an alkaline copper (II) sulfate of a biuret reagent with the formation of a violet-colored chelate:

$2H_2NCONHCONH_2 + 4NaOH + CuSO_4 \longrightarrow$

$$
\begin{array}{ccc}
& OH & OH \\
& | & | \\
CO\!-\!NH_2\!-\!\!-\!Cu\!-\!\!-\!NH_2\!-\!CO \\
\diagup & & \diagdown \\
NH & & HN \quad +Na2SO4 \\
\diagdown & & \diagup \\
CO\!-\!NH_2\!-\!Na \quad Na\!-\!NH_2\!-\!CO \\
| & | \\
OH & OH
\end{array}
$$

(I)

The intensity of the violet color produced is proportional to the number of reacting peptide bonds which, in turn, corresponds to the number of protein molecules present in a reaction system. The absorbance of the colored complex is measured spectrophotometrically at 540 nm.

2. Bradford protein assay (1976):

Principle: Coomassie Brilliant Blue G-250 binds selectively basic amino acid residues, namely arginine, lysine, and histidine in an acidic medium. As a result of binding, the color of the dye-protein complex changes from brown to blue and is measured at a wavelength of 595 nm. According to Fanglian He (2011), the interference is attributed to sodium dodecyl sulfate (SDS) even at low concentrations.

The method is easy, rapid (< 30 minutes), and extremely sensitive. The disadvantage of the method is its variability of color development with different proteins.
The method is used in the measurement of total protein in CSF.

3. Lowry's method:

The method depends upon the tryptophan and tyrosine content of an individual protein fraction. These amino acids bring about the reduction of phosphotungstic phosphomolybdic acid (Folin-Ciocalteu) reagent to develop a blue color. The intensity of the developed color is measured at 650-750 nm.
The method is unsuitable for estimating protein from urine or CSF because of its poor specificity.

4. Kjeldahl method (1883):

It is used to determine protein nitrogen in the sample. The protein nitrogen is converted to ammonium ion by acid digestion. Then, the ammonia nitrogen is measured by titration or nesslerization. Finally, ammonia nitrogen is to be multiplied by a factor 6.25 to get the protein value in the sample.
Owing to its accuracy, the method can be used as a reference method. The method is tedious, time-consuming, and inconvenient to practice in a clinical laboratory.

5. Refractometry:

It is based on refractive index measurement. The increase in the refractive index is directly proportional to the concentration of total protein (solute) in the sample. The method is quick and simple to perform.

Estimation of albumin

1. Dye-binding method:
This method was developed by Doumas et al. (1971) and modified by Spencer and Price (1977).

Principle: This one-step method uses a pH indicator dye called bromocresol green (BCG). Serum albumin binds selectively with the dye to form a blue-green colored complex. The binding occurs between an anionic dye and cationic albumin (PI 4.9)[19] at pH 4.2:

$$\text{Albumin + bromocresol green} \xrightarrow{\text{pH 4.2}} \underset{\text{yellow-green color}}{\text{albumin-BCG complex}}$$

The absorbance is measured spectrophotometrically at 620-630 nm. The intensity of the formed colored product is directly proportional to the concentration of albumin in the sample. The method is simple to perform, rapid, and cost-effective. It is performed without any pretreatment of the sample. However, it has been criticized in that the dye interacts with compounds other than albumin (e.g., serum globulins), characterizing it as a non-specific method. According to Garcia Moreira V et al. (2018), serum acute-phase proteins contribute to overestimating the concentration of albumin, especially at lower concentrations in the BCG-based method.

According to Robertson William S. (1981), factors that influence method specificity include dye concentration, reaction time, and variable protein composition of human plasma.

2. Kinetic immunoturbidimetry:
Like dye-binding methods, this technique is used in the estimation of serum albumin. It uses commercially available antisera. According to K. Spencer and C.P. Price, the technique was found to be similar to another immunological technique called radial immunodiffusion (RID). The fast assay time (30-60 seconds), cost, and sensitivity (up to 1 mg/L) makes this method suitable for the routine assay of albumin.

3. High-performance liquid chromatography (HPLC):
HPLC-based techniques are used as a reference method.

4. Electrophoresis:
The electrophoretic technique is discussed in chapter 3. Simple and satisfactory separation of serum proteins is obtained, using cellulose acetate membrane and barbiturate buffer of ionic strength 0.05 mol/liter and a pH value of 8.6. This gives well-defined bands, making an accurate quantitative study possible. The strip is to be stained by a suitable stain (e.g., Coomassie Brilliant Blue or Ponceau S). Then, bands can be eluted (Teepol 615) or the strips can be scanned. Electrophoretic patterns of serum proteins in health and disease are given in Fig. 23.1. Thus, this technique requires a very small volume of serum under examination. Furthermore, it takes no more than 1 to 2 hours.

---

[19] Isoelectric point (PI) is a pH at which the net electrical charge of a protein molecule is zero.

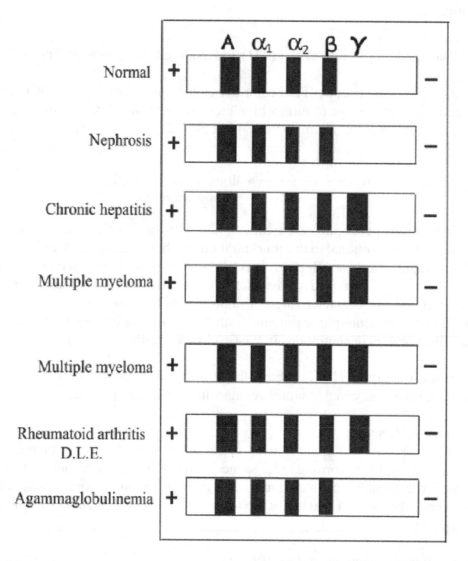

Fig. 23.1: Electrophoretic patterns of serum proteins in health and disease. At pH 8.6, all the proteins are negatively charged and migrate toward the anode (+ve electrode).

Conclusion

Currently, dye-binding methods and immunochemical methods are widely used. However, dye-binding methods and immunochemical methods are non-specific and less sensitive, respectively. Therefore, research studies are being carried out to develop better methods. Like precipitation-based old methods (i.e., salt fractionation and acid fractionation), dye-binding methods may become obsolete too.

Chapter 24

Serum Bilirubin

Formation

Bilirubin is the chief bile pigment in man. It is derived from the breakdown of hemoglobin as shown in Fig. 24.1.

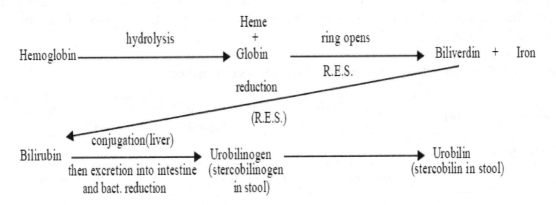

Fig. 24.1: Formation of bile pigments.

It is formed in the reticuloendothelial system (spleen, bone marrow, and Kupffer cells of the liver). In the course of the disintegration of RBCs, the protoporphyrin ring of heme derived from hemoglobin is opened to form biliverdin. The biliverdin so formed is then split off and the center of the three remaining bridges is reduced to a methene bridge to form bilirubin. It has been reported that 1 g of hemoglobin gives 35 mg of bilirubin.

Indirect bilirubin formed in the RES is not water-soluble. It is lipid-soluble and mainly associated with albumin and circulates in the blood. This insoluble bilirubin is transported to the liver (microsomes) by unknown carrier proteins called Y (ligandin) and Z. Glucuronyl transferase catalyzes the following reaction:

$$\text{Unconjugated bilirubin + glucuronic acid} \xrightarrow[\text{(microsomes)}]{\text{glucuronyl transferase}} \text{Conjugated bilirubin}$$

Unconjugated bilirubin + glucuronic acid (indirect bilirubin) → Conjugated bilirubin (direct bilirubin)

The following four fractions have been isolated from serum:

(i) Unconjugated bilirubin (α-bilirubin)
(ii) Monoconjugated bilirubin (β-bilirubin)
(iii) Diconjugated bilirubin (γ-bilirubin)
(iv) A fraction attached (irreversibly) to protein (δ-bilirubin)

Jaundice

Excessive bile pigment (bilirubin) from the blood diffuses into the tissues, turning yellow. This yellow pigmentation is called jaundice or icterus. It is easy to detect by examining the sclera (the opaque outer coat of the eyeball), skin, and mucus membranes. When the level of serum bilirubin exceeds 2 mg/dL (normal range: 0.2-1.2 mg/dL). Elevated levels of unconjugated bilirubin lead to the accumulation of bilirubin in the brain tissue. This type of pigmentation called kernicterus occurs because the unconjugated bilirubin has a high affinity for the brain tissue. Pathophysiologically, jaundice is divided into three main groups: (1) hemolytic (2) hepatocellular, and (3) obstructive. Differentiating laboratory features of these three types of jaundice are summarized in Table 24.1.

Table 24.1. Differentiating laboratory features of three types of jaundice

Laboratory feature	Hemolytic (Pre hepatic)	Hepatocellular (Hepatic)	Obstructive (Posthepatic)
Serum/Plasma			
− Color	lemon-yellow	yellow-orange	yellow-green
− Bilirubin	+ + + (unconjugated)	+ + (conjugated)	+ + + + (conjugated)
− SGPT (ALT)	N	+ +	±
− Alkaline phosphatase	N	+ +	+ + + +
Urine			
− Bilirubin	A	+ +	+ + +
− Urobilinogen	++	±	A

N = normal; A = absent

Clinical significance

Hyperbilirubinemia:
- Hemolytic jaundice
- Obstructive jaundice
- Neonatal jaundice
- Hepatitis
- Malaria

Hypobilirubinemia:
- Aplastic anemia
- Certain secondary anemias, especially those resulting from the toxic agents of carcinoma and chronic nephritis.

Sample: Samples used for bilirubin estimation need to be protected from light (artificial/ natural) because bilirubin is a photo-labile (light-sensitive) substance. Levels of bilirubin may diminish up to 50% per hour if exposed to direct sunlight. Therefore, samples are stored in dark to avoid falsely decreased results. Hemolysis-free serum or plasma is used because hemoglobin reacts with diazo reagent, causing bilirubin results to be falsely low. Lipemic samples interfere with the results too. Serum or plasma stored in the dark remains stable for one day, 7 days, and 3 months at 15°-25°C, 2°-8°C, and -20°C, respectively. Anticoagulants containing heparin and oxalate are used. Other anticoagulants should not be used.

Estimation of bilirubin *(total and direct)*

A chemical reaction between bilirubin and diazotized sulfanilic acid (diazo reagent) was described by Ehrlich (1883). This diazo reaction was named van den Bergh reaction in 1916 (i.e., the formation of azobilirubin). Based on a diazo reaction, several modified methods were developed and are classified as under:

1. Precipitation methods (e.g., McNee and Keefer, Haslewood and King, and King and Coxon)
2. Non-precipitation methods (e.g., Malloy and Evelyn, Jendrassik and Cleghorn modified by Jendrassik and Grof, Rappaport and Eichhorn, and Powell)

In precipitation methods, ethanol (a catalyst) causes precipitation of the serum proteins. This results in the loss of some azobilirubin together with the protein precipitate. Therefore, these methods are inaccurate. Non-precipitation methods use substances other than ethanol as a catalyst to avoid protein precipitation, thus increasing the sensitivity.

1. Meulengracht test (1919):
It is the simplest test to determine an increase in serum bilirubin. It is based on the assumption that all the yellow coloration is due to bile pigments, principally bilirubin. The test compares the color of blood serum with a standard (S) 1:10,000 solution of potassium dichromate and the test results are expressed in units. The normal range is 4-6 units. But, it may reach 15 units before clinical jaundice is evident. It is advisable to use hemolysis-free serum and chyle. This test can be used as a screening test for blood donors.

2. Malloy-Evelyn method:
This method was developed by Malloy and Evelyn (J. Biol. Chem., 1937, 119: 480). It is based on Van den Bergh's reaction in which azobilirubin is formed.

Principle: Bilirubin, in acidic medium, couples with diazotized sulfanilic acid with the formation of a red-purple colored complex called azobilirubin:

$$\text{Bilirubin + diazotized sulfanilic acid + 50\% methanol} \xrightarrow{\text{H}^+} \text{azobilirubin}$$
$$\text{(red-purple chromogen)}$$

Ascorbic acid stops the diazotization reaction.
The intensity of the red-purple color so developed is proportional to the concentration of the bilirubin and is measured colorimetrically or spectrophotometrically. The method is sensitive to changes in both pH and serum protein. It overestimates the direct bilirubin.

171

3. Jendrassik and Grof (1938):

Principle: This non-precipitation method uses caffeine-benzoate-acetate reagent as an accelerator. The bilirubin pigments of serum react with a diazotized sulfanilic acid reagent (coupling reaction) to produce a purple-colored complex (azobilirubin) at pH 6.5. A dissociating agent, caffeine benzoate, releases unconjugated bilirubin from albumin and makes it soluble enabling it to react with a diazo reagent. The reaction takes place at the methylene carbon atom between rings B and C. This brings about the formation of one molecule each of azobilirubin and hydroxypyromethylene-carbinol. The second molecule of azobilirubin is formed from the reaction between carbinol and diazo reagent:

(i) Sulfanilic acid + NaNO$_2$ $\xrightarrow[\text{H}_2\text{O}]{\text{2HCl 0°C; 1-2 min}}$ diazotized sulfanilic acid + 2NaCl + 2H$_2$O
    sodium salt

(ii) Bilirubin + diazotized sulfanilic acid $\xrightarrow{\text{acidic pH}}$ azobilirubin
    (purple colored)

The diazotization reaction is stopped by the addition of ascorbic acid. This also helps eliminate interference by hemoglobin.

The alkaline tartrate buffer (pH 13) is added to convert a purple-colored azobilirubin to a blue-colored complex that shows maximum absorbance at 600 nm. This helps minimize the hemoglobin-or carotene-associated absorbance. The intensity of the colored complex so developed is proportional to the concentration of the bilirubin and is measured spectrophotometrically within 30 minutes.

Direct bilirubin estimation is performed without caffeine by a direct reaction with diazotized sulfanilic acid to form azobilirubin. The absorbance is measured at 550 nm.

Indirect bilirubin can be calculated as under:

Indirect bilirubin = total bilirubin – direct bilirubin

Advantages:
1. Minimum interference by hemoglobin
2. Rapid color development
3. Measures all four fractions of bilirubin (i.e., increased sensitivity)
4. The highly precise and constant molar absorptivity of a colored azobilirubin in various protein matrices
5. Easy to standardize
6. Adaptable for neonatal bilirubin measurement

4. Bilirubin oxidase:

Bilirubin oxidase (bilirubin: oxygen oxidoreductase; EC 1.3.3.5) catalyzes the oxidation of bilirubin with the formation of an end-product called biliverdin (colorless):

$$2 \text{ Bilirubin} + O_2 \xrightarrow{\text{bilirubin oxidase}} 2 \text{ biliverdin} + 2H_2O$$

Therefore, a decrease in absorbance is measured between 405 and 460 nm and is proportional to the concentration of total bilirubin of the sample. All four fractions of bilirubin are oxidized in the presence of sodium cholate and sodium dodecyl sulfate (SDS) at pH about 8. However, the concentration of total bilirubin by this methodology is slightly lower than the diazo methods.

At pH between 3.7-4.5, the enzyme selectively catalyzes the oxidation of conjugated bilirubin and delta- bilirubin but not unconjugated bilirubin. This is how to direct bilirubin can be estimated. This method is not widely used.

5. Reflectance spectrophotometry:

Principle: Binding of bilirubin fractions causes differences in reflectance values. It uses a modified diazo reagent. The absorbance of serum bilirubin is measured at 455 nm. It needs to be correct for the hemoglobin-associated absorbance by subtracting the absorbance reading at 575 nm. The method is resistant to hemolysis. However, it is affected by the presence of lipochromes and turbidity. The method is limited to newborn infants.

6. High-performance liquid chromatography (HPLC):

Principle: Conjugated bilirubin, in an alkaline medium, is subjected to methylation while the unconjugated form remains unaffected. Later, bilirubin is extracted into chloroform and measured spectrophotometrically.

Using this highly sophisticated and extremely sensitive technique, Pieper-Bigelow C et al. (1995) reported that normal human sera contain about 0.006 mg/dL of conjugated bilirubin. The conventional laboratory methods can only detect up to 0.3 mg/dL of direct bilirubin (water-soluble) from serum/plasma samples.

Conclusion

Considering the pros and cons of available methods to date, a classical Jendrassik and Grof method (1938) ranks first as a conventional laboratory method. This method is used manually and in automated procedures worldwide.

Chapter 25

Enzymes and their Applications in Laboratory Diagnosis

Introduction

Enzymes are thermolabile organic catalysts produced by living cells. These proteinic molecules are capable of accelerating the rate of a chemical reaction without being used up. Therefore, they can be used over and over again in the process without their deterioration. The turnover number[20] of enzymes ranges between 0.5 to 600000. For example, the turnover number of lysozyme and carbonic anhydrase is 0.5 and 600000, respectively. An enzyme combines with a specific substrate to form an enzyme-substrate complex. Following an interaction between these two reactants, product(s) is produced while an enzyme remains unused at the end of a reaction:

Enzyme + Substrate $\rightleftarrows$ Enzyme-Substrate $\longrightarrow$ Product(s) + Enzyme
complex

Properties

1. Proteinic in nature and high molecular weight
2. Denaturation by heat
3. Precipitation by ethanol or high concentration of inorganic salts, e.g., ammonium sulfate
4. Non-dialyzable through semi-permeable membranes
5. The presence of cells is not necessary for their activity
6. Increase the velocity of a chemical reaction
7. Specificity, e.g., substrate specificity and group specificity
8. Reversibility (mostly catalyze reversible reactions)
9. It may be simple or conjugated

Unlike chemical reactions, enzymatic reactions are influenced by many factors.

Factors affecting enzyme activity

1. Nature and concentration of an enzyme
2. Nature and concentration of a substrate
3. Time
4. pH (minimum, optimum, maximum)
5. Temperature (minimum, optimum, maximum)
6. Ultraviolet light
7. Inhibitors (e.g., competitive and non-competitive inhibitors)
8. Activators (non-protein inorganic compounds and ions called cofactors, e.g., Mg^{++} and non-protein organic molecules called coenzymes, e.g., NAD^+)
9. Allosteric inhibitors and allosteric activators in case of allosteric enzymes
10. Ionic strength

---

[20] It is the number of substrate molecules converted to end-products by one molecule of an enzyme per second, provided the active site is saturated with the substrate.

Nomenclature and classification of enzymes

Enzymes are named and classified based on what they do rather than what they are. It is this specific property that distinguishes one enzyme from the other. A four-number system should code each enzyme. They have two names: a recommended name (formerly trivial name) and a systematic name. The recommended name is shorter and more convenient to use. In many cases, it is the name already in current use. These recommended names usually consist of three parts. They are made up of the name of the substrate, the type of a reaction catalyzed, and the "suffix -ase," e.g., alcohol dehydrogenase. Besides, a method for numbering enzymes was provided. This means that each enzyme now has an identifying classification number in addition to its recommended name and systematic name. For example, the Enzyme Commission number for alcohol dehydrogenase (a recommended name) is 1.1.1.1:

1.	oxidoreductases
1.1	acting on the CHOH group of donors
1.1.1	with NAD^+ or $NADP^+$ as an acceptor
1.1.1.1	alcohol: NAD^+ oxidoreductase (a systematic name)

The ENZYME database is a repository of information about the nomenclature of enzymes. It has become an indispensable resource because there are multiple synonyms for the same enzyme. The current version includes information on 6410 enzymes which is available through the ExPASy web (http://www.expasy.org) server. According to the recommendations of the Nomenclature Committee of the International Union of Biochemistry and Molecular biology (IUBMB), preliminary EC numbers now include an "n" as part of the fourth (serial) digit, e.g., EC 3.5.1.n3. Other cross-references, e.g., BRENDA, KEGG, IntEnz, and ExplorEnz, are also very useful in retrieving more information about enzymes.

Many enzymes occur in different structural forms but possess identical (or nearly identical) catalytic properties which have created a new problem concerning enzyme nomenclature. These enzymes are referred to as isoenzymes. The present system for enzyme nomenclature and classification makes no provision for structural diversity with similar activity.

Enzymes have been placed in seven major groups. Each group is further subdivided into different sub-groups:

  I. Oxidoreductases
  II. Transferases
  III. Hydrolases
  IV. Lyases
  V. Isomerases
  VI. Ligases (or synthetases)
  VII. Translocases (added in Aug. 2018)

I. Oxidoreductases: are enzymes that bring about simultaneous biological oxidation and reduction in a pair of compounds. In other words, the transfer of H_2 occurs from one compound to another in the presence of an oxidoreductase. For example, both NAD^+ and $NADP^+$ (coenzymes) play an important role in bringing about oxidation and reduction reactions as shown in Fig. 25.1:

$$CH_3.CHOH.COOH + NAD^+ \xrightarrow[\text{dehydrogenase}]{\text{lactate}} CH_3.CO.COOH + NADH + H^+$$

Lactate	Coenzyme		Pyruvate	Coenzyme
(Red.)	(Oxi.)		(Oxi.)	(Red.)

Fig. 25.1: LDH activity.

II. Transferases: are enzymes that bring about the transfer of a group other than hydrogen. The groups which are transferred include nitrogenous groups, phosphorus-containing groups, one-carbon groups, sulfur-containing groups, and acyl groups. The nature of transferases is exemplified in Fig. 25.2(a) and Fig. 25.2(b):

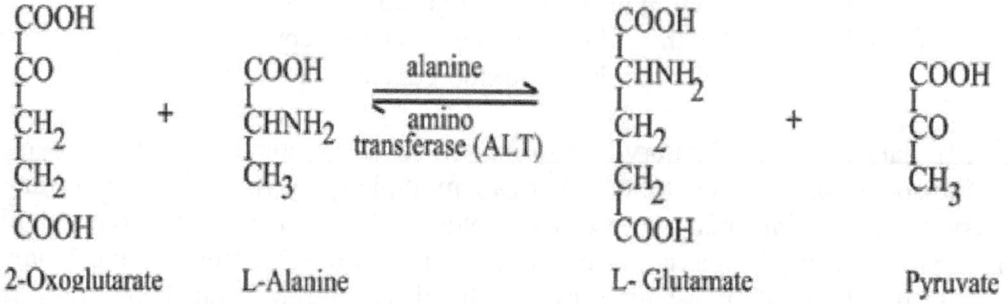

Fig. 25.2(a): Alanine transaminase (ALT) activity.

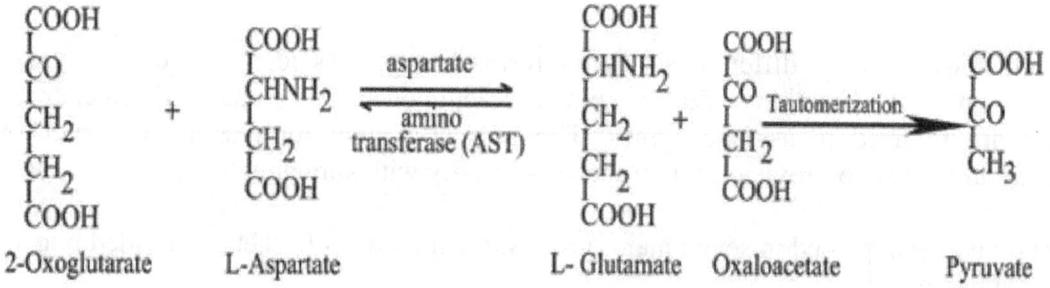

Fig. 25.2(b): Aspartate transaminase (AST) activity.

III. Hydrolases: are enzymes that bring about hydrolysis of a substrate with the formation of two products as shown in Fig. 25.3:

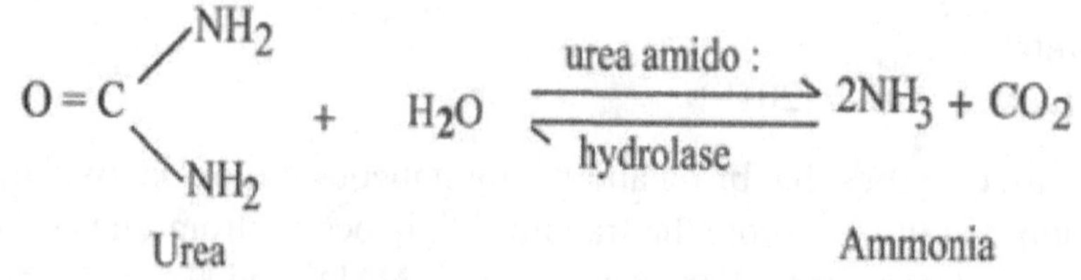

Fig. 25.3: Urea amidohydrolase activity.

176

Two phosphoric monoester hydrolases are alkaline phosphatase and acid phosphatase.

IV. Lyases: are enzymes that catalyze the addition of groups to double bonds or their formation as exemplified by carbon-oxygen lyases shown in Fig. 25.4:

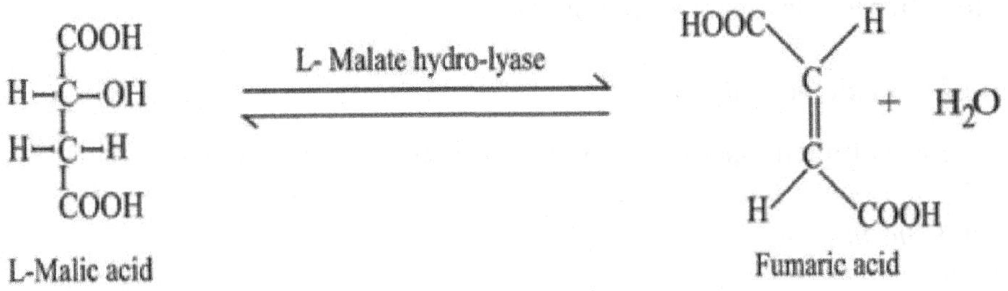

Fig. 25.4: L-Malate hydro-lyase activity.

V. Isomerases: are enzymes that bring about the interconversion between the two isomers, e.g., racemases and epimerases as shown in Fig. 25.5:

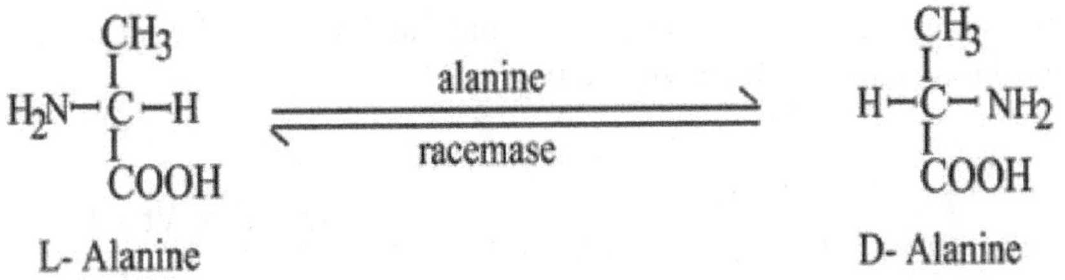

Fig. 25.5: Alanine racemase activity.

VI. Ligases or synthetases: are enzymes that bring about the linking of two compounds with the breakdown of a third energy-giving compound. This can be illustrated as shown in Fig. 25.6:

$$\underset{\text{2D-Alanine}}{2CH_3.CHNH_2COOH} + ATP \xrightleftharpoons[\text{ligase (ADP)}]{\text{D- alanine : D- alanine}}$$

$$\underset{\text{D- Alanyl- D- alanine}}{CH_3.CHNH_2.CONH.CH(CH_3).\ COOH} + H_3PO_4 + ADP$$

Fig. 25.6: D-alanine:D-alanine ligase activity.

VII. Translocases (added in Aug. 2018): are enzymes that catalyze the movement of ions or molecules across membranes or their separation within membranes:

$$\text{ATP} + H_2O + 4\,H^+ \text{ side }_1 \xrightarrow{\quad H^+\text{- transporting two-sector ATPase}\quad} \text{ADP} + \text{phosphate} + 4\,H^+ \text{ side }_2$$

The above reaction is catalyzed by H^+- transporting two-sector ATPase [ATP phosphohydrolase (H^+- transporting); EC 7.1.2.2].

Besides EC numbers there are now also, in the same style, TC numbers for the classification of transporters into different classes of transporters.

Measurement of enzyme activity

Enzyme activity measurement uses one of the following two approaches:

1. *Continuous-monitoring*
2. *Fixed-time*

A continuous-monitoring approach is a preferred one. In this method, the rate of a reaction is monitored. Therefore, coupled enzymatic reactions are adapted, allowing the measurement of the change in absorbance, e.g., changes in absorbance of NADH or NADPH during reduction at 340 nm.

The unit used to express an enzyme activity is an international unit (U). It is the enzyme activity that catalyzes one micromole of a substrate per minute under defined conditions. The following formula can be used to calculate the enzyme activity:

$$\text{Enzyme activity U/L } (\mu\,\text{mole/min/L}) = \frac{\Delta A/\text{min} \times Vt \times 10^6}{\varepsilon \times P \times Vs}$$

Where,

$\Delta A/\text{min}$ = average absorbance change per minute

Vt = total assay volume (specimen, reagent, and diluent) in mL

10^6 = factor to convert mole to micromole

ε = molar absorptivity coefficient of substrate or product, e.g., 6.22×10^3 L/mol cm of NADH at 340 nm

P = light path in cm

Vs = volume of the specimen in mL

Note: While calculating the enzyme activity using the above formula, both Vt and Vs need to be expressed in the same units.

The SI unit is katal. Therefore, $1\,U = 16.7 \times 10^9$ mol/s or 1 nkat/L = 0.06 U/L.

Michaelis-Menten curve

Various factors influence an enzymatic reaction. Importantly, the concentration of a substrate has a major impact on the velocity of a reaction. The first-order kinetics of an enzymatic reaction means the velocity is dependent on the concentration of a substrate and the concentration of an enzyme in the system. In contrast, velocity becomes zero-order kinetics in the presence of an excessive amount of a substrate and depends only on the concentration of an enzyme.

In a plot prepared by taking the substrate concentration on the X-axis and velocity of a reaction on the Y-axis (see Fig. 25.7), V_{max} represents a maximal velocity of a reaction at a substrate concentration of "c". Therefore, the concentration of the substrate would be "b" at $v = V\,max/2$ called Michaelis constant, *Km*. Thus, *Km* measures the affinity of an enzyme for its substrate. The lower the *Km* value, the greater the affinity of an enzyme for the substrate and vice versa.

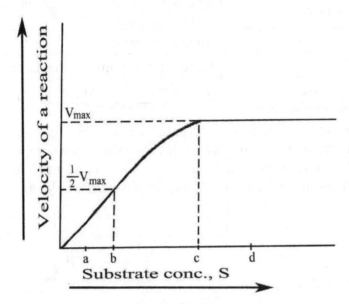

Fig. 25.7: Michaelis-Menten curve.

In developing a new enzymatic assay method, the concentration of a substrate has to be at least 10 times the *Km* ("b") to achieve the "zero-order kinetics". In other words, the substrate concentration needs to be in excess for a valid enzyme assay procedure. For practical purposes, the concentration of substrate in enzyme assay techniques is more than 20 times the *Km*.

Enzymes as analytes and reagents: Enzymes are used from two different perspectives:

   a. *Analytes*
   b. *Reagents*

a. *Analytes:* There are laboratory diagnostic tests in which enzymes are treated as analytes. Enzyme activity is measured to detect malfunctioning of an organ. In other words, some organ-specific enzymes are used as indicators of traumatic or pathological conditions as shown in Table 25.1:

Table 25.1: Relationship between enzyme activity and associated traumatic or pathologic conditions

Enzyme	Diagnostic purpose(s)
Alanine aminotransferase	liver disease
Alkaline phosphatase	bone disease, biliary obstruction
Amylase	acute pancreatitis
Aspartate aminotransferase	myocardial infarction, liver disease, muscle disease, hemolytic disease
Lipase	acute pancreatitis
Creatine kinase	muscle disease, myocardial infarction
Gamma glutamyltransferase	liver disease, alcoholism

b. Reagents: Several blood components are determined by the use of enzymes. Such determinations called enzymatic assays are highly specific. Therefore, non-specific chemical methods are replaced with enzymatic methods. Also, there is no need for pretreatment of the complex mixtures such as plasma/serum. Enzymes used as analytical reagents are listed in Table 25.2.

Table 25.2: Uses of enzymes in a clinical laboratory

Recommended name	Systematic name	Enzyme Commission number	Use
Glucose oxidase	β-D-glucose: oxygen 1-oxidoreductase	1.1.3.4	Glucose estimation (coupled with peroxidase)
Peroxidase	phenolic donor:hydrogen-peroxide oxidoreductase	1.11.1.7	Auxiliary enzyme with glucose oxidase for glucose estimation
Urease	urea: amidohydrolase	3.5.1.5	Urea estimation
Creatininase	creatinine: amidohydrolase	3.5.2.10	Estimation of creatinine
Uricase	urate: oxygen oxidoreductase	1.7.3.3	Uric acid estimation
Malate dehydrogenase	(s)-malate: NAD^+ oxidoreductase	1.1.1.37	Coupling enzyme in L-aspartate transaminase activity assay
Alcohol dehydrogenase	alcohol: NAD oxidoreductase	1.1.1.1	Ethanol estimation
DNA-directed DNA polymerase[*]	deoxynucleoside-triphosphate:DNA deoxynucleotidyl transferase (DNA-directed)	2.7.7.7	Polymerase chain reaction (PCR)
Ficin	pending	3.4.22.3	Antibody identification work-ups
Fruit bromelin	pending	3.4.22.33	Antibody identification work-ups
Papain	pending	3.4.22.2	Antibody identification work-ups

[*]Also called Taq-polymerase. It is a thermostable (optimum temperature between 75°C to 80°C) enzyme which can replicate a 1000 base pair strand of DNA in < 10 seconds at 72°C.

In many enzymatic assay methods, enzymes are immobilized on the surface of the solid support (ELISA) or paper strip.

Chapter 26

Serum Aminotransferases

Introduction

Alanine transaminase (ALT) is also commonly called alanine aminotransferase. Formerly, ALT was called serum glutamic pyruvic transaminase (sGPT). It catalyzes the reversible transfer of an amino group from L-alanine to α-ketoglutarate with the formation of L-glutamate and pyruvate [see Fig. 25.2 (a)]. ALT needs a pyridoxal-5'-phosphate (P-5'-P) to function. ALT plays an important role in cellular nitrogen metabolism, amino acid metabolism, and liver gluconeogenesis (conversion of alanine to glucose).

The distribution of ALT in different body tissues is shown in Table 26.1.

Table 26.1: The distribution of ALT in different body tissues (Wroblewski, 1958)

	Liver	Kidney	Heart	Skeletal muscle	Pancreas	Spleen	Lung
ALT*	43	19	7	4.7	2	1.2	0.7

* Values in U per 10^{-4} g wet tissue homogenates.

ALT is widely distributed in many tissues but is found predominantly in the liver and to a much lesser extent in the kidneys, heart, and brain.

Clinical significance

- Infective hepatitis
- Carbon tetrachloride poisoning

ALT is more specific than AST for liver disease. In alcoholic liver disease, AST > ALT because alcohol is a mitochondrial poison. Conversely, ALT > AST in viral hepatitis.

Sample: Hemolysis-free serum is the specimen of choice for assaying the activity of ALT and AST. Plasma (heparin or EDTA) can also be used. Serum samples can be stored for three days and long-term at 2-8°C and -20°C, respectively.

Assay of alanine transaminase (ALT) activity

1. Colorimetric method:
It was developed by Reitman and Frankel. It is a simple, economical, and reproducible method.

Principle: ALT catalyzes the transfer of an amino group from L-alanine (α-amino acid) to 2-oxoglutarate (α- keto acid) with the formation of end products, L-glutamate, and pyruvate. Pyruvate so formed, in an alkaline medium, couples with 2,4-dinitrophenylhydrazine to form a brown colored hydrazone complex.

(i) L-Alanine + 2-oxoglutarate $\xrightleftharpoons{\text{alanine transaminase}}$ L-glutamate + pyruvate

(ii) Pyruvate + 2,4-dinitrophenylhydrazine $\longrightarrow$ brown colored complex

The intensity of the brown color is proportional to the ALT activity and is measured photometrically.

2. Enzymatic assay:
This is a recommended procedure of the International Federation of Clinical Chemistry (IFCC).

Principle: Alanine transaminase (L-alanine:2-oxoglutarate aminotransferase; EC 2.6.1.2) catalyzes the reversible transfer of an amino group from L-alanine to 2-oxoglutarate with the formation of L-glutamate and pyruvate. An auxiliary enzyme, lactate dehydrogenase (lactate: NAD^+ oxidoreductase; EC 1.1.1.27) catalyzes the reduction of pyruvate to lactate with the concurrent oxidation of reduced nicotinamide adenine dinucleotide (NADH) to NAD^+:

(i) L-Alanine + 2-oxoglutarate $\xrightleftharpoons{\text{alanine transaminase}}$ L-glutamate + pyruvate

(ii) Pyruvate + NADH + H^+ $\xrightarrow{\text{lactate dehydrogenase}}$ lactate + NAD^+

The oxidation of NADH to NAD^+ is accompanied by a decrease in absorbance at 340 nm. The decrease of rate is proportional to ALT activity in the sample if the prevailing conditions are rate-limiting for ALT activity.

3. Fluorescent enzymatic assay:
This method was developed by Khampha et al. It is a sensitive and specific method.

Principle: The content of L-glutamate in the sample is amplified by bi-enzymatic reaction cycling between L-glutamate dehydrogenase [L-glutamate:NAD^+ oxidoreductase (deaminating); EC 1.4.1.2] and D-phenylglycine transaminase (D-4-hydroxyphenylglycine:2-oxoglutarate amino-transferase; EC 2.6.1.72):

(i) L-Glutamate + H_2O + NAD^+ $\xrightarrow{\text{glutamate dehydrogenase}}$ 2-oxoglutarate + NH_3 + NADH + H^+

(ii) D-4-Hydroxyphenylglycine + 2-oxoglutarate $\xrightarrow{\text{D-phenylglycine transaminase}}$ L-glutamate + 4-hydroxyphenylglyoxylate

Accumulation of NADH in the course of bi-enzymatic recycling is monitored by fluorescence ($\lambda Ex=340$ nm, $\lambda Em= 460$ nm) and used to measure L-glutamate.

Aspartate Aminotransferase

Introduction

Aspartate transaminase (AST) is also commonly named aspartate aminotransferase. Formerly, AST was called serum glutamate oxaloacetate transaminase (sGOT). Like ALT, AST catalyzes the transfer of an amino group from L-aspartate to 2-oxoglutarate to form L-glutamate and oxaloacetate [see Fig.25.2 (b)]. Like ALT, AST is also pyridoxal-5'-phosphate-dependent. The distribution of AST in different body tissues is indicated in Table 26.2:

Table 26.2: The distribution of AST in different body tissues (Wroblewski, 1958)

	Heart	Liver	Skeletal muscle	Kidney	Pancreas	Spleen	Lung
AST*	151	137	96	88	27	14	10

* Values in U per 10^{-4} g wet tissue homogenates.

Clinical significance

- Myocardial infarction
- Carbon tetrachloride poisoning
- Trauma to skeletal muscle
- Acute infectious hepatitis

Sample: similar to ALT activity assay

Assay of aspartate transaminase (AST) activity

1. Colorimetric method:
AST is also assayed by a 2,4-dinitrophenylhydrazine (2,4-DNPH) method developed by Reitman and Frankel (1957). Thus, the procedure is similar to that of ALT assay except for buffered L-aspartate-2-oxoglutarate substrate, pH 7.4.

Principle: Aspartate transaminase catalyzes the reversible bioconversion of substrates, L-aspartate, and α-ketoglutarate to yield end-products, L-glutamate, and oxaloacetate. Like a colorimetric activity assay of ALT, AST activity measurement can be performed using 2,4-dinitrophenylhydrazine:

(i) L-Aspartate + α-ketoglutarate $\xrightleftharpoons{\text{aspartate transaminase}}$ L-glutamate + oxaloacetate

Oxaloacetate $\xrightarrow{\text{tautomerization}}$ pyruvate

(ii) Pyruvate + 2,4-dinitrophenylhydrazine $\xrightarrow{\text{alkaline pH}}$ brown color complex

The intensity of the so developed brown color is measured at 505 nm and is proportional to the AST activity of the sample.

2. Enzymatic method:

Principle: Aspartate transaminase (L-aspartate:2-oxoglutarate aminotransferase; EC 2.6.1.1) catalyzes the reversible transfer of an amino group from L-aspartate to 2-oxoglutarate to form oxaloacetate and L-glutamate. An auxiliary enzyme called malate dehydrogenase ((s)-malate: NAD^+ oxidoreductase; EC 1.1.1.37) catalyzes the reduction of oxaloacetate to malate with the concomitant oxidation of NADH to NAD^+:

(i) L-Aspartate + 2-oxoglutarate $\xleftrightarrow{\text{aspartate transaminase}}$ oxaloacetate + L-glutamate

(ii) Oxaloacetate + NADH + H^+ $\xrightarrow{\text{malate dehydrogenase}}$ L-malate + NAD^+

The rate of NADH oxidation is proportional to AST activity that is measured at 340 nm.

3. Fluorescent enzymatic assay: similar to ALT method

Conclusion

Like ALT, AST is associated with liver parenchymal cells. AST is routinely tested as a part of liver function tests. When AST is higher than ALT, one should consider a muscle source of both enzymes, e.g., muscle inflammation due to dermatomyositis. Therefore, both ALT and AST are not good indicators of liver function because they do not reliably reflect only the liver source but also other sources, e.g., muscle. Since ALT is a non-specific test for hepatocellular injury, ancillary clinical chemistry and/or histopathology tests are often used to interpret ALT values.

In human clinical trials, it is a recommended practice to interpret a higher than three times the elevation of ALT above the upper limit of normal combined with a total bilirubin (TBILI) elevation higher than two times above the upper limit of normal as suggestive of severe injury with/without any other evidence. This medicine practice is called Hy's Law.

Chapter 27

Serum Lactate Dehydrogenase

Introduction

Lactate dehydrogenase (LD) is present in most tissues. It has a molecular weight of about 140,000 daltons. It is a tetramer molecule (four subunits). In other words, it consists of four polypeptide chains of the following two types:

1. H (heart muscle)
2. M (skeletal muscle)

Thus, five different combinations are possible: H_4, H_3M, H_2M_2, HM_3, and M_4, and these correspond to LD_1, LD_2, LD_3, LD_4, and LD_5. LD_1 and LD_2 are much more inhibited by oxalate than LD_4 and LD_5. But, the effect of urea is the reverse. Distribution of LD isoenzymes in different body tissues is listed in Table 27.1.

Table 27.1: The distribution of LD isoenzymes in different body tissues

Isoenzyme	Sources	Serum concentration, % (in adults)
LD_1	heart and erythrocytes	17-27
LD_2	heart and erythrocytes	27-37
LD_3	lymph tissue, lungs, platelets, and pancreas	18-25
LD_4	liver and skeletal muscle	3-8
LD_5	liver and skeletal muscle	0-5

Normal ratios are:

$LD_1 < LD_2$
$LD_5 < LD_4$

Usually, LD_2 is a major isoenzyme in the serum. When LD_1 is greater than LD_2 ("flipped LD), it could mean a heart attack in the past. But, the LD test is no longer requested in cardiac disorders and is largely replaced by a troponin test (i.e., troponin T and troponin I). The results of a troponin test are directly proportional to the degree of damage to the heart muscles e.g., heart attack.

When LD_5 is higher than LD_4, it could indicate liver damage.

Clinical significance

Elevated levels

- Myocardial infarction
- Liver diseases
- Various malignant diseases
- Leukemias
- Pancreatitis

- Secondary hepatocellular diseases
- Megaloblastic anemia
- Hemolytic anemia
- Muscular dystrophy

Sample: Hemolysis-free serum is the preferred sample for assaying lactate dehydrogenase (LD) activity. Erythrocytes contain large amounts of LD. Therefore, any degree of hemolysis will yield abnormally high results.

If plasma must be used as the source of the specimen, the sample must be centrifuged to obtain a platelet-free plasma. Various anticoagulants, namely oxalate, and fluoride are inhibitory to LD. Heparin was found erratic (Batsakis and Henry).

Serum samples for LD isoenzymes' measurement can be stored at room temperature for 3 days without substantial loss of activity. To protect cold-labile LD_4 and LD_5 forms, samples are stored at room temperature.

For long-term storage, samples are frozen with glutathione added.

Assay of lactate dehydrogenase activity

1. Colorimetric method:
This chemical method was developed by King. J. and modified by himself. The principle is the same as in cases of AST and ALT. It is a highly economical, highly reproducible, simple, and quick procedure.

Principle: L-Lactate dehydrogenase [(S)-lactate: NAD^+ oxidoreductase; EC 1.1.1.27] catalyzes the reversible reaction (L $\longrightarrow$ P[21]) with the formation of pyruvate and reduced form of nicotina-mide adenine dinucleotide (NADH):

$$\text{L-Lactate} + NAD^+ \xrightarrow[\text{pH 8.8-9.8}]{\text{lactate dehydrogenase}} \text{pyruvate} + NADH + H^+$$

The reaction is monitored by measuring the increase in NADH at 340 nm and is proportional to the LD activity in the sample. The main factors, namely temperature, pH, hemolyzed samples, and use of a poor quality NAD^+ (as a reagent) influence the test results.

---

[21] Also, a reversible reaction P $\longrightarrow$ L can be used at pH 7.4 to 7.8.

Alternatively, the reduction of NAD can be coupled to the reduction of 2-*p*-iodophenyl-3-*p*-nitrophenyl-5-phenyl tetrazolium chloride (INT) with phenazine methosulfate acting as an electron carrier. The molar absorptivity of the formazan[22] is 19.3×10^3 at 503 nm. This is how a three-fold increase in sensitivity over the UV (340 nm) kinetic assay can be obtained.

Advantages of L $\longrightarrow$ *P assay:*

1. Lower substrate inhibition by lactate as compared to pyruvate
2. The lower content of endogenous LD inhibitors present in NAD^+ preparations used in the assay
3. Highly extended reaction linearity

Note:

L $\longrightarrow$ P assay is preferred to P $\longrightarrow$ L assay.

2. Electrophoretic technique:
Electrophoretic technique on various support media is very popular.

Principle: Isoenzymes, namely LD_1 to LD_4 migrate towards the anode and LD_5 moves towards the cathode on the agarose film at a pH value of 8.6 at 20°C. The isoenzymes are then detected after a short incubation with a liquid overlay containing L-lactate and NAD^+. The reaction generates NADH which fluoresces at alkaline pH following excitation by light at approximately 360 nm. The isoenzymes are measured by the relative proportion of fluorescence produced by each isoenzyme band. The technique is accurate and precise.

Other methods, namely column chromatography and rapid immunological techniques can be used for the assay of LD_1 alone.

---

[22] Are chromogenic products of the reduction of tetrazolium salts mediated by dehydrogenases and reductases.

Chapter 28

Serum Phosphatases

Introduction

Phosphatases are group-specific enzymes. Therefore, they catalyze the splitting of phosphoric acid from monophosphoric esters. The major sources of alkaline phosphatases are the liver, bone, intestine, placenta, and kidney.

Alkaline Phosphatase

Alkaline phosphatase is a glycoprotein with a molecular weight of 140,000 daltons. It is a dimer of two very similar or identical subunits. Each subunit contains a tightly bound zinc atom contributing towards the structural integrity of the polypeptide and a loosely bound zinc atom that is required for catalysis. Similarly, each subunit has a different binding site for magnesium ions associated with a stimulatory effect. The effect of physical and chemical agents on alkaline phosphatase isoenzymes is shown in Table 28.1.

Table 28.1: Effect of physical and chemical agents on alkaline phosphatase isoenzymes

Isoenzyme	Heat	Urea	L-Phenylalanine
Bone	sensitive	sensitive	resistant
Liver	resistant	intermediate stability	resistant
Intestinal	resistant	resistant	resistant

Clinical significance

Elevated levels:
- Obstructive jaundice
- Hepatic jaundice
- Paget's disease
- Carcinomatous metastases in the bone
- Osteomalacia
- Rickets
- Hyperparathyroidism
- In the healing stage of fractures
- Pregnancy (third trimester)

It becomes necessary to do a differential diagnosis, especially in cases of the liver- and bone-related disorders. The gamma-glutamyl transferase (GGT) measurement serves this purpose. In liver-associated conditions (e.g., acute hepatitis and primary liver tumor), both serum alkaline phosphatase and gamma-glutamyl transferase are elevated. In bone-related disorders, gamma-glutamyl transferase value stays normal.

Low levels:
- Wilson disease
- Chronic myeloid leukemia (CML)
- Hypothyroidism
- Post-menopause

Sample: Hemolysis-free serum/heparinized plasma is used in the measurement of alkaline phosphatase activity. Samples need to be frozen for storage because values falsely increase in samples stored at either room temperature or refrigerator temperature (2-8°C).

The alkaline phosphatases are not sensitive to fluoride ions but are inhibited by divalent-chelating agents, e.g., EDTA (disodium salt).

Assay of alkaline phosphatase activity

1. Colorimetric method:

This method was developed by Kind and King. It is a popular, simple, and economical method.

Principle: Alkaline phosphatase [phosphate-monoester phosphohydrolase (alkaline optimum); EC 3.1.3.1] catalyzes the hydrolysis of the colorless substrate, *p-nitrophenyl phosphate* (*p*-NPP), to produce *p*-nitrophenol (yellow color) and inorganic phosphate at alkaline pH:

$$p\text{-nitrophenyl phosphate} + H_2O \xrightarrow[\text{pH 10; Mg}^{2+}]{\text{alkaline phosphatase}} p\text{-nitrophenol} + Pi \;\; (\text{yellow})$$

The reaction is terminated by the addition of NaOH.

The rate of formation of the *p*-nitrophenolate anion (yellow) is monitored at 405 nm and is directly proportional to the alkaline phosphatase activity.

Phenol so formed is allowed to react with 4-aminoantipyrine in the presence of an alkaline oxidizing agent, potassium ferricyanide, to form an orange-colored complex. The intensity of the color is measured at 510 nm and is proportional to the enzyme activity in the sample.

Factors that influence the enzyme activity

1. *pH:* The activity keeps increasing with increasing pH in the range from 7.0 to 9.0.
2. *Magnesium (Mg²⁺):* The velocity of the reaction increases two-fold by increasing the Mg^{2+} concentration up to the nominal value of 5 mM.
3. *Zinc ions (Zn²⁺):* The effects of various concentrations of zinc are complex. Low concentrations (0.5-1 mM) are slightly stimulatory in the initial velocity whereas higher concentrations (>3 mM) are inhibitory.
4. *p-Nitrophenol:* a competitive inhibitor of alkaline phosphatase activity
5. *Inorganic phosphate:* a competitive inhibitor of alkaline phosphatase activity
6. *L-Phenylalanine:* a non-competitive inhibitor of alkaline phosphatase activity

2. Electrophoretic method:

Several electrophoretic techniques are employed to separate and distinguish the isoenzymes of these alkaline phosphatases. Usually, polyacrylamide gel is used as a supporting medium.

Acid Phosphatase

Introduction

The major sources of acid phosphatase include prostate, liver, erythrocytes, and bone-marrow. A total of three active acid phosphatase forms in serum have been separated utilizing the electrophoretic technique. These forms can be inhibited as shown in Table 28.2.

Table 28.2: Inhibition of acid phosphatase isoenzymes

Isoenzyme	Inhibitory agent
erythrocytes*	formaldehyde
serum	fluoride ions
prostrate	tartrate (20 mM)
bone	resistant to tartrate

* Resistant to tartrate.

Clinical significance

Acid phosphatase:
- Thrombocytosis
- Gaucher's disease
- Ulcerative colitis
- Benign hypertrophy of the prostate
- Thrombocytopenic purpura
- Medicolegal work (vaginal discharges)

Acid phosphatase measurement was used as a screening test for prostate cancer. It is used to distinguish B cell acute lymphoblastic leukemia (negative) from T cell acute lymphoblastic leukemia (positive).

Sample: Hemolysis-free serum is the specimen of choice. The serum is separated from erythrocytes. Acidification (pH <6.5) of the sample followed by freezing is a satisfactory method of storage. It is to be reminded that improper storage methods yield falsely decreased results. Acid phosphatase is an extremely heat-labile enzyme. Its activity decreases in storage at room temperature or even at 2°-8°C. The acid phosphatases are inhibited by fluoride ions but not by divalent cation-chelating agents.

Assay of acid phosphatase activity

1. Colorimetric method:

This method was also developed by Kind and King. Thus, the procedure remains the same as in the case of serum alkaline phosphatase except pH 4.9 and the incubation time.

Principle: Acid phosphatase [phosphate-monoester phosphohydrolase (acid optimum); EC 3.1.3.2] catalyzes the hydrolysis of the colorless substrate, *p*-nitrophenyl phosphate (*p*-NPP), to form *p*-nitrophenol (yellow color) and inorganic phosphate at acidic pH:

$$p\text{-nitrophenyl phosphate} + H_2O \xrightarrow[\text{pH 4.9}]{\text{acid phosphatase}} p\text{-nitrophenol} + Pi$$
$$\text{(yellow)}$$

The substrate phenolphthalein monophosphate is suitable for automation whereas α-naphthyl phosphate is substrate specific for prostatic acid phosphatase.

2. Electrophoretic technique:
Several electrophoretic techniques are employed to separate and distinguish the isoenzymes of these acid phosphatases. Usually, polyacrylamide gel is used as a supporting medium.

3. Radioimmunoassay:
This immunological technique is reliable in the measurement of prostatic acid phosphatase activity.

Other Clinically Significant Enzymes (see Table 28.3)

Table 28.3: Other clinically significant enzymes

Enzyme	Source(s)	Clinical significance	Comment(s)
Amylase	Pancreas, salivary glands	-Acute pancreatitis	-Hydrolysis of starch produces free glucose molecules -Measurement of increase in absorbance of NADH at 340 nm
Lipase	Pancreas	-Acute pancreatitis	-Splits triglycerides into glycerol and fatty acids -Turbidimetric assay
Aldolase	Skeletal muscle	-Muscle necrosis	-Rarely tested
Gamma-glutamyl transferase(GGT)	Liver, kidneys	-Alcoholic cirrhosis -Metastatic carcinoma	-Uses gamma-glutamyl-3-carboxy-4-nitroanilide

Table 28.3 (cont.): Other clinically significant enzymes

Enzyme	Source(s)	Clinical significance	Comment(s)
Creatine kinase (CK)	Brain, heart skeletal muscle	-Myocardial infarction -Muscular dystrophy	-Assayed by monitoring an increase in NADPH
Pseudocholinesterase(PCHE)	Liver, brain	-Decreased levels in insecticide poisoning	-Spectrophotometric assay of thiocholine
Glucose-6-phosphate dehydrogenase	RBCs	-Hemolytic anemia following the use of oxidant drugs, e.g., primaquine	-Assayed from hemolysate of whole blood

Chapter 29

Endocrine System

Introduction

Endocrinology deals with endocrine glands and tissues that secrete hormones. Unlike exocrine glands (e.g., salivary and mammary glands), endocrine glands lack ducts. In other words, hormones secreted by endocrine glands diffuse into the bloodstream via the interstitial fluid instead. Hormones are chemical signals that influence their respective target tissues, thus maintaining homeostasis. Chemically, hormones may be proteins or steroids. Examples of each chemical class are:

1. *Protein hormones*: adrenocorticotropic hormone (ACTH), thyroid-stimulating hormone (TSH), follicle-stimulating hormone (FSH), prolactin (PRL), human chorionic gonadotropin (HCG), antidiuretic hormone (ADH), oxytocin, growth hormone (GH), insulin, and glucagon
2. *Steroid hormones*: C_{21} corticosteroids and progestins, C_{19} androgens and C_{18} estrogens, cortisol, and aldosterone

The locations of major endocrine glands in a human body are highlighted in Fig. 29.1.

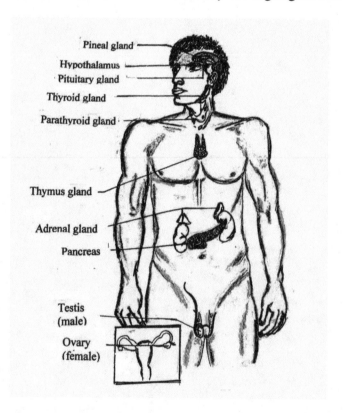

Fig. 29.1: The locations of major endocrine glands in a human body.
(Drawing by Heli Mistry).

194

1. *Hypothalamus:* is a region of the brain associated with homeostasis. It regulates sleep, appetite, body temperature, water balance, and blood pressure. It acts as a link between the endocrine system and the nervous system. It secretes five releasing factors that stimulate the anterior pituitary lobe to secrete the corresponding hormones:

a. *thyrotropin-releasing hormone* (TRH)
   - stimulates the anterior pituitary to secrete thyroid-stimulating hormone (TSH)
b. *corticotropin-releasing hormone* (CRH)
   - stimulates the anterior pituitary to secrete adrenocorticotropic hormone (ACTH)
c. *gonadotropin-releasing hormone* (GnRH)
   - stimulates the anterior pituitary to secrete follicle-stimulating hormone (FSH) and luteinizing hormone (LH)
d. *growth hormone-releasing hormone* (GHRH)
   - stimulates the anterior pituitary to secrete growth hormone (GH)

2. Anterior pituitary gland
a. *thyroid-stimulating hormone* (TSH)
b. *adrenocorticotropic hormone* (ACTH)
c. *follicle-stimulating hormone* (FSH) *and luteinizing hormone* (LH)
d. *prolactin* (PRL)
   - also called luteotropin
   - secreted during pregnancy and after childbirth
   - stimulates mammary glands to produce milk
   - plays a role in fat and carbohydrate metabolism

e. *melanocyte-stimulating hormone* (MSH)
   - associated with skin color changes, e.g., amphibians
   - very low in humans
f. *growth hormone* (GH)
   - also called somatotropin
   - promotes the growth of cartilage, bone, and many soft tissues
   - hyposecretion and hypersecretion during childhood cause pituitary dwarfism and gigantism, respectively
   - hypersecretion in adults causes acromegaly

3. Posterior pituitary gland
a. *antidiuretic hormone* (ADH)
   - also called vasopressin
   - produced in the hypothalamus and stored in the posterior lobe of the pituitary gland
   - promotes the reabsorption of water in distal renal tubules
   - deficiency leads to diabetes insipidus and polyuria
b. *oxytocin*
   - produced in the hypothalamus and stored in the posterior lobe of the pituitary gland
   - regulates uterine muscle contractions during childbirth
   - causes the ejection of milk from mammary glands

4. *Thyroid gland* (butterfly-shaped structure)
a. thyroxine (T_4)
- ten times more T_4 than T_3 produced
- most of the T_4 converted to T_3 by the liver

b. triiodothyronine (T_3)

Biosynthesis of T_4 and T_3 depends on the availability of iodine. The thyroid gland contains approximately 25 times more iodine than the blood. This explains why iodized table salt is used in the kitchen. Both hormones accelerate metabolism.

Hypothyroidism causes cretinism (congenital hypothyroidism) and myxedema in children and middle-aged adults, respectively. Hashimoto thyroiditis (an autoimmune disorder) and a simple goiter are also disorders of hypothyroidism. Conversely, hyperthyroidism results in Graves' disease.

Expected laboratory results in thyroid disorders are summarized in Table 29.1.

Table 29.1: Expected laboratory results in thyroid disorders

Disorder	T4	T3	THBR	FTI	FT4	TSH
Primary hypothyroidism	↓	↓	↓	↓	↓	↑
Secondary hypothyroidism*	↓	↓	↓	↓	↓	↓
Hyperthyroidism	↑	↑	↑	↑	↑	↓

* Secondary hypothyroidism due to pituitary insufficiency.

c. calcitonin
- helps regulate blood calcium (Ca^{2+}) level

5. *Parathyroid gland*
a. parathyroid hormone (PTH)
- regulates calcium and phosphorus levels in the blood

Parathyroid hormone (PTH) is synthesized by four parathyroid glands present in the neck. These glands secrete PTH when the calcium level is low. Conversely, the secretion of PTH is stopped if the calcium level becomes high. The major target cells of PTH are bone and kidney. Parathyroid hormone controls the blood calcium level by influencing the following three target tissues:

(i) *Bone*: the liberation of calcium to blood by stimulated osteoclasts
(ii) *Kidney*: reabsorption of calcium by kidney tubules, thus preventing the loss of calcium
(iii) *Small intestine*: indirect enhancement of calcium absorption from the small intestine

The effects of PTH on calcium and phosphorus are reciprocal as shown in Table 29.2.

Table 29.2: Regulation of calcium and phosphorus by PTH

Disorder	PTH	Calcium	Phosphorus
Primary hyperthyroidism	↑	↑	↓
Primary hypothyroidism	↓	↓	↑

6. Adrenal medulla
   a. epinephrine
   b. norepinephrine

Both hormones are classified as catecholamines. Dopamine, a precursor, is converted to norepinephrine and later to epinephrine by dopamine β hydroxylase and phenylethanolamine *N*-methyltransferase, respectively. Hypersecretion of catecholamines occurs in cases of pheochromocytoma and neuroblastoma. Symptoms of pheochromocytoma include hypertension with episodic palpitations, excessive sweating, anxiety, and headache.

7. Adrenal cortex
   a. aldosterone (principal mineralocorticoid)
   - regulated by the renin-angiotensin system
   - promotes sodium (Na^+) reabsorption and potassium (K^+) loss in the renal tubules
   b. cortisol (principal glucocorticoid)
   - a significant role in carbohydrate, protein, and lipid metabolism
   - exhibits diurnal variation (peak level at 8 am; the low level at 8 pm)
   - elevated levels cause Cushing's syndrome
   - adrenal gland insufficiency causes Addison disease
   c. sex hormones

8. Testes
testosterone (androgen) secreted by Leydig cells
   - stimulates and maintains secondary sex characteristics in males
   - circulates by sex hormone-binding globulin

9. Ovaries
   a. estradiol (E_2)
   - primary estrogen
   - secreted by non-pregnant females
   - causes the breast to enlarge via the accumulation of adipose tissue
   - regulates the menstrual cycle and maintains the pregnancy as well
   b. estriol (E_3)
   - secreted by pregnant females (synthesized by the placenta)
   - aids in the evaluation of fetoplacental integrity
   c. estrone (E_1)
   - secreted after menopause
   d. relaxin

- secreted before childbirth

e. *inhibin*
- inhibits the secretion of the follicle-stimulating hormone by the anterior pituitary gland

10. Placenta

a. *estriol*
- a minor hormone that is almost undetectable

b. *Progesterone*
- prepares the uterus for pregnancy and maintains pregnancy

c. *Human chorionic gonadotropin* (HCG)
- a glycopeptide hormone produced by corpus luteum during early pregnancy
- is used to detect pregnancy
- is also used in the diagnosis of gestational trophoblastic disease, testicular tumor, and other HCG-producing tumors

d. *Human placental lactogen* (HPL)
- participates in the development of mammary glands
- is used to assess placental function

11. Pancreas

a. *insulin*
- produced by the *beta cells* of the islets of Langerhans in the pancreas
- promotes the uptake of glucose by target tissue cells, e.g., liver cells, muscle cells, and fat cells

b. *glucagon*
- produced by the *alpha cells* of the islets of Langerhans in the pancreas
- increases the plasma glucose level
- elevated levels found in diabetes mellitus, glucagonoma, and pancreatitis
- excessive secretion leads to metabolic acidosis

c. *somatostatin*
- produced by the *delta cells* of the islets of Langerhans in the pancreas
- inhibits the release of the growth hormone (anterior pituitary) and many digestive hormones, e.g., glucagon

12. Gastrointestinal tract

a. *gastrin*
- regulates the secretion of HCl by parietal cells of the stomach
- elevated levels found in Zollinger-Ellison syndrome

b. *secretin*
- helps regulate the pH of the duodenum

13. Pineal gland

a. *melatonin*
- suppresses the secretion of growth hormone and gonadotropin
- regulates circadian and circannual rhythms

b. *serotonin*
- stimulates or inhibits different types of smooth muscles and nerves

14. Thymus gland: located behind the sternum and between lungs. It remains active until puberty. After puberty, it undergoes a gradual shrinkage and is replaced by fat.

thymosin
- promotes the development and maturation of T lymphocytes. Some lymphocytes (in lymph nodes or thymus) may develop into tumors, e.g., Hodgkin disease and non-Hodgkin lymphomas

15. Kidney

a. erythropoietin (EPO)
- controls the production of erythrocytes by bone marrow
- produced by cells close to the proximal renal tubule
- also produced (small quantity) by macrophages and hepatic Kupffer's cells
- levels can increase 100-fold due to hypoxemia (e.g., high altitudes and emphysema)
- binding of EPO to erythroid progenitor cell stimulates proliferation and maturation

b. 1,25-(OH)$_2$ vitamin D
- facilitates absorption of calcium and phosphorus in the gastrointestinal tract

Regulation of hormone secretion

A. Negative feedback: is the most common means of controlling the secretion of hormones. There are three levels of control as listed below:

a. *Target gland* (primary): is the one that secretes a specific hormone and acts on a respective body tissue
b. *Pituitary* (secondary): is engaged in secreting trophic hormones to further stimulate the target glands at a distance to secrete their specific hormones
c. *Hypothalamus* (tertiary): is the one that secretes releasing factors which, in turn, stimulate the pituitary to secrete its hormones

B. Positive feedback: increased accumulation of an end-product enhances the activity of a hormone, resulting in the higher yield of the product itself, e.g., stimulation of luteinizing hormone by estradiol before ovulation

Assay of hormones

Specimens: The requirement of a sample depends upon the analyte in question. It can be either

a. serum/plasma
b. 24-hour urine

In some measurements, the collection time is critical because of diurnal variation. There are several antigen-antibody based techniques available to measure the hormones. They include:

1. Radioimmunoassay (RIA)
2. Enzyme multiplied immunoassay technique (EMIT)
3. Enzyme-linked immunosorbent assay (ELISA)
4. Particle counting immunoassay (PACIA)
5. Chemiluminescence assay (CLIA)

Chapter 30

Blood Gases, pH, and Electrolytes

Introduction

Ideally, the pH of blood is between 7.35-7.45. The body manages to maintain blood pH within a reference range. Components that contribute to regulating pH are given in Table 30.1.

Table 30.1: Normal ranges of pH-determining components

Component	Normal range
PO_2, mm Hg	80-100
PCO_2, mm Hg	35-45
HCO_3^-, mEq/L	22-26

The following two systems play a major role:

1. *Respiratory system* (lungs): involves a gaseous exchange of CO_2 for O_2 in alveoli called ventilation. This is how blood is oxygenated. The oxygenated blood is pumped from the heart to tissues through a systemic vein. Tissues, in turn, produce CO_2 as a waste product that is exhaled through the lungs. The respiratory system attempts to compensate much faster (minutes) than the renal system.
2. *Renal system* (kidneys): involves retention or excretion of bicarbonate ions to maintain normal pH. Unlike the respiratory system, the renal system takes hours to days to correct the pH.

In addition to the main buffer system of carbonic acid and bicarbonate, deoxyhemoglobin, plasma albumin, and monohydrogen phosphate also contribute to normalizing the blood pH.

Henderson-Hasselbalch equation

This equation explains the relationship among pH, PCO_2, and HCO_3^-:

$$pH = pK' + \log \frac{cHCO_3^-}{cdCO_2}$$

Where,
pH = negative logarithm of H^+ activity
pK' = dissociation constant for dissolved CO_2 in plasma (i.e., 6.1)

HCO_3^- = concentration of bicarbonate ions
$cdCO_2$ = concentration of dissolved CO_2 (PCO_2 x 0.030[23])

The ratio of the concentration of HCO_3^- (bicarbonate ions) to the concentration of dissolved CO_2 ($cdCO_2$) in plasma is 20:1.

---

[23] 0.030 = solubility coefficient at 37°C.

Substituting values in the above equation,

$$pH = 6.1 + log\ \frac{20}{1}$$

pH = 6.1 + 1.3
pH = 7.4

Specimen: It is very important to collect a representative arterial blood sample. For the collection of an arterial blood specimen, the anticoagulant of choice is lithium heparin (100 U/mL blood). The specimen is collected anaerobically without a tourniquet. Exposure of specimens to air results in a decrease of PCO_2 and an increase of both pH and PO_2.

Once an arterial blood specimen is collected, glycolysis and other oxidative processes are inhibited by placing the syringe into ice water (valid up to 1 hour). Failure to do so, PCO_2 increases whereas both pH and PO_2 decrease. Oxalate, citrate, and EDTA are not used because they absorb CO_2, decreasing the values in the specimen.

Physiological acid-base imbalance

Some diseases or conditions may lead to alkalosis (pH > 7.45) or acidosis (pH < 7.35). They are classified as under:

1. *Respiratory acidosis:* is associated with an increase in blood PCO_2 (>45 mm Hg). Causes include airway obstruction, pulmonary emphysema, respiratory distress syndrome (RDS), pulmonary fibrosis, and trauma. The kidneys respond by reabsorption of bicarbonate ions(proximal tubules), and increased exchange rate of Na^+ for H^+ with the excretion of H^+ (distal tubules) to compensate. Also, the elimination of CO_2 can be triggered due to a higher concentration of PCO_2 in the blood, causing hyperventilation.

2. *Respiratory alkalosis:* is associated with a decrease in the concentration of PCO_2 (< 35 mm Hg). Causes include hypoxia, hysteria, and fever. The kidneys respond by the elimination of bicarbonate ions and a low exchange rate of $Na^+ - H^+$ with the retention of H^+ to compensate.

3. *Metabolic acidosis:* is linked with a decrease in bicarbonate ions level (< 22 mEq/L). Causes include diabetic ketoacidosis, renal failure, lactic acidosis, and severe diarrhea. The lungs attempt to compensate by decreasing the concentration of PCO_2 (hyperventilation).

4. *Metabolic alkalosis:* is linked with an increase in bicarbonate ions level (>26 mEq/L). Causes include vomiting and excess consumption of alkali. The lungs try to compensate by increasing the concentration of PCO_2 (hypoventilation)

Clinical case scenarios: Presentation of clinical case scenarios can be helpful for a better understanding of acid-base imbalance as shown in Table 30.2.

Table 30.2: Clinical case scenarios of acid-base imbalance

Disorder	pH	PCO$_2$ (mm Hg)	HCO$_3^-$ (mEq/L)	Compensation
Respiratory acidosis	7.15	55	29	Partial
Respiratory alkalosis	7.6	25	18	Partial
Metabolic acidosis	7.15	25	15	Partial
Metabolic alkalosis	7.7	50	30	Partial

Electrolytes

Introduction

Though electrolytes are required in trace quantities, they play a key role in metabolism. Electrolytes maintain osmotic pressure and water distribution in the various body fluid compartments. Also, they regulate the proper function of the heart and other muscles. Therefore, abnormal levels of electrolytes can lead to many disorders. Thus, it is important to determine their concentrations (levels). Electrolytes can be anions or cations. In other words, they can have a negative or positive electrical charge. The dietary requirements for electrolytes are different because some of them are consumed in small quantities or at rare intervals and are retained. On the other hand, calcium, potassium, and phosphorus are excreted regularly and must be obtained regularly to prevent deficiencies. The key electrolytes are calcium, potassium, sodium, magnesium, chloride, bicarbonate, phosphate, and sulfate.

1. Sodium (Na$^+$)

Sodium is the major extracellular cation, representing approximately 90% of inorganic cations per liter of plasma water. Sodium accounts for approximately half the osmolality of the plasma. It plays a key role in maintaining the normal distribution of water and the osmotic pressure in the extracellular fluid compartment. The daily requirement of sodium is only 1-2 mmol/day. The level of sodium is regulated by aldosterone in the distal tubules. The renal threshold[24] of sodium is 110-130 mmol/L. Thus, it determines the amount of sodium excreted in the urine. The sodium concentration in urine ranges between 40-220 mmol/day.

Measurement
Hemolysis-free serum/plasma (Lithium or ammonium salt of heparin) is used as a specimen. The specimen is frozen for long-term storage. Urine is collected without a preservative. Erythrocytes contain one-tenth of the sodium present in plasma. Therefore, slight hemolysis does not make a significant decrease in sodium values. Other specimens for sodium determinations include sweat, feces, and gastrointestinal fluid. Whole blood may be used. Sodium is measured by flame-emission-spectrophotometry and ion-selective electrodes.

---

[24] The renal threshold of a substance is the plasma concentration at which the rate of glomerular filtration of the substance begins to exceed the rate at which the tubules can reabsorb it.

Clinical significance

Hypernatremia
- Excessive intake
- Hyperaldosteronism
- Decreased ADH
- Hyperadrenocorticism (Cushing's syndrome)
- Diabetes insipidus
- Metabolic acidosis
- Burns

Hyponatremia
- Decreased intake
- Aldosterone deficiency
- Diuretic therapy
- Dilutional (water retention)
- Depletion (sodium loss exceeds water loss)
- Addison's disease
- Renal failure

2. Potassium (K$^+$)

Potassium is the major intracellular cation. Potassium is secreted in the distal tubules of the kidney. Potassium is essential for neuromuscular function. The concentration of potassium is approximately 23 times greater inside the cells compared to that of extracellular fluid. The potassium level is controlled by aldosterone that promotes potassium excretion.

Measurement
Hemolysis-free serum/plasma (heparin) is the specimen of choice. Plasma is separated from RBCs to avoid falsely elevated levels and stored at 2-8°C. For long-term storage, the specimen needs to be frozen. Urine and sweat specimens are also tested for potassium levels. It is measured by flame-photometry and ion-selective electrodes with a membrane containing valinomycin. Falsely elevated potassium results may be attributed to one or more factors of the collection and processing of the blood specimen, e.g., squeezing site of capillary puncture, pumping fist during venipuncture, prolonged tourniquet time, IV fluid contamination, hemolysis, and delay in separating serum/plasma.

Clinical significance
Hyperkalemia
- Dehydration
- Renal failure
- Diabetic ketoacidosis
- Aldosterone deficiency

Hypokalemia
- Alkalosis
- Decreased intake
- Insulin administration
- Loss of fluid containing potassium
- Aldosteronism

Note: Both hyperkalemia and hypokalemia can result in cardiac arrest.

3. Chloride (Cl⁻)

Chloride is one of the major extracellular anions. It controls body water distribution and osmotic pressure. Also, chloride maintains electrical neutrality. When bicarbonate leaves the red blood cells, chloride enters into the cells to maintain an overall electrical neutral charge (chloride shift).

Measurement
Hemolysis-free serum/plasma is required for chloride determination. It is required to collect the specimen anaerobically because CO_2 loss changes the concentration in the sample. Sometimes, urine and sweat specimens are also tested for chloride values. Urinary chloride can be useful in the differential diagnosis of persistent metabolic alkalosis. The colorimetric method using mercury thiocyanate and ion-selective electrode method can be used for measurement. Falsely elevated results can be encountered while using a titration method because other halogens (Br, Fl, etc.) also participate in the reaction.

Clinical significance
Hyperchloremia[25]
- Dehydration
- Renal failure
- Excessive intake
- Primary hyperparathyroidism

Hypochloremia
- Prolonged vomiting
- Defective reabsorption
- Addisonian crisis

4. Carbon dioxide (CO₂)

Carbon dioxide exists largely as HCO_3^- in solution. Total carbon dioxide (tCO_2) consists of:
1. Dissolved gas
2. Carbon dioxide bound to protein (hemoglobin)
3. Carbonic acid
4. Bicarbonate (HCO_3^-)

---

[25] Elevated sweat chloride values, along with other symptoms, may be indicative of a diagnosis of cystic fibrosis.

Measurement
Serum/plasma (heparinized) is the specimen of choice for HCO_3^- estimation. It is required that the specimen is collected and processed anaerobically because exposure to air decreases the result. The ion-selective electrode method and enzymatic method can be used for HCO_3^- determination. Also, it can be calculated using measured pH and pCO2 results. The measurement of bicarbonate is useful to evaluate acid-base balance.

Clinical significance
Elevated levels
- Metabolic alkalosis
- Compensated respiratory acidosis

Decreased levels
- Metabolic acidosis
- Compensated respiratory alkalosis

5. Calcium (Ca^{2+})

Calcium is important in the structure of bones and teeth. Over 99% of total body calcium is in the bone. Uptake of calcium (intestine) is mediated by vitamin D. Loss of calcium is 'fine-tuned' by the distal tubules of the kidneys under the control of parathyroid hormone (PTH). PTH increases the reabsorption of calcium. Calcitonin decreases the concentration of calcium in the serum. The concentration of calcium is also influenced by pH and the amount of bone resorption. Also, calcium is important for neuromuscular activity and blood coagulation. There are three forms of calcium:

1. Ionized calcium: the physiologically active entity
2. 40% of total calcium is bound to albumin and other proteins
3. Complexed: usually with phosphate and bicarbonate

Calcium is regulated by parathyroid hormone (PTH), calcitonin, vitamin D, pH, and protein concentration.

Measurement
Whole blood (heparinized) is the specimen of choice for ionized calcium. It is also required to collect specimens under anaerobic conditions. Total calcium determination requires hemolysis-free serum/plasma (heparinized). Ionized calcium is determined using an ion-selective electrode. Total calcium can be determined by the atomic absorption spectrophotometry method (reference method) or colorimetric method.

Clinical significance
Hypercalcemia
- Primary hyperparathyroidism
- Malignancy
- Vitamin D excess
- Chronic renal failure

Hypocalcemia: Vitamin D affects the level of calcium and helps absorb calcium.
- Hypoparathyroidism
- Malabsorption
- Vitamin D deficiency
- Rickets

6. Phosphorus (PO_4^{3-})

Phosphorus is present intracellularly as well as extracellularly. It is present as phosphate in the body. About 85% of the total phosphorus is present in bones and teeth. It plays an important role in the bone structure, regulation of pH, cell membrane transport, and energy storage and transfer.

Measurement
Hemolysis-free serum/plasma (heparinized) is the specimen of choice. It is advisable to collect a fasting specimen because the results are low following a meal. The colorimetric method using ammonium molybdate reagents can be used to determine inorganic phosphate. Urine must be acidified to pH 6 to prevent precipitation of phosphates. The reference range for phosphorus is higher in growing children compared to that of adults.

Clinical significance
Hyperphosphatemia
- Hypoparathyroidism
- Excess intake
- Chronic renal failure
- Excessive vitamin D

Hypophosphatemia
- Rickets
- Decreased vitamin D
- Malabsorption

7. Magnesium (Mg^{2+})

Magnesium is essential as a cofactor in many enzymatic reactions, e.g., alkaline phosphatase and muscle contraction. It is usually present in muscle, bone, and plasma.

Measurement
Hemolysis-free serum/plasma (heparinized) separated from RBCs and urine are used for the measurement of Mg^{2+}. Atomic absorption (reference method) is not routinely used but gives accurate results and a colorimetric method that uses methylthymol blue reagent.

Clinical significance
Hypermagnesemia
- Excess intake
- Dehydration
- Chronic renal failure
- Diabetic ketoacidosis (DKA)

Hypomagnesemia
- Malabsorption
- Alcoholism
- Diuretics
- Hyperaldosteronism
- Tetany

Anion gap

Anion gap can be used as a quality control tool to detect problems with the measurement of Na^+, Cl^-, and tCO_2 (HCO_3^-). Estimation of unmeasured cations and anions based on the measurements of serum sodium (Na^+), potassium (K^+), chloride (Cl^-), and carbon dioxide (CO_2) is possible too.

Formulae

$(Na^+ + K^+) - (Cl^- + CO_2)$: reference range = 10-20

$Na^+ - (Cl^- + CO_2)$: reference range = 8-16

Clinical significance
Elevated values
- Metabolic acidosis
- Decrease in cations
- Elevated albumin levels
- Renal failure
- Toxic ingestion

Decreased values
- A decrease in anions
- A decrease in albumin levels
- Abnormal proteins

REVIEW QUESTIONS

1. Which instrument is used to measure the optical density (OD) of colored solutions?
2. Who developed electrophoresis?
3. Which S. I. (Systeme Internationale) unit is used to report glucose concentrations?
4. Which compound is present in the liver and muscle to store an excess of glucose?
5. Which term is used to denote the formation of glucose from non-carbohydrate sources?
6. How long does the plasma glucose level take to return to the control value in a standard glucose tolerance curve?
7. What is the strength of concentrated sulfuric acid?
8. Which compound forms the bulk of the non-protein-nitrogen fractions in serum?
9. Which factor is used in the multiplication of urea nitrogen value to obtain urea concentration?
10. What is the end-product of purine catabolism in men?
11. What is the chemical compound that is deposited in the joints in gout?
12. What source is used in the preparation of uricase?
13. Which key compound is used in most non-enzymatic uric acid assay methods?
14. Which reaction forms the basis for most creatinine assay methods?
15. Which test is routinely used to assess the glomerular filtration rate?
16. Which particles cause the lipemic (turbid) appearance of serum?
17. Which chemical reagents in the Salkowski reaction react with cholesterol to develop a green color?
18. Which enzyme is used to bring about hydrolysis of triglycerides in the enzymatic assay of serum triglycerides?
19. What is the synonym for conjugated bilirubin?
20. What is the name of the reaction that forms the basis for the estimation of bilirubin?
21. Which chemical solution is used as an artificial standard while assaying serum bilirubin?
22. What term is used to describe the yellow pigmentation of certain body areas (e.g., sclera and skin) due to the excessive accumulation of bilirubin in the blood?
23. What is the site for the formation of albumin?
24. Which dye is used in the determination of serum albumin?
25. Which of the following two proteins is water-soluble: albumin and globulin?
26. What is the electrical charge carried by protein molecules at pH 8.6?
27. What is the nature of enzymes?
28. What is the optimum pH of alkaline phosphatase?
29. Which enzymatic assay is performed in the diagnosis of metastatic prostatic carcinoma?
30. How many isoenzymes of lactate dehydrogenase are known?
31. Which type of diabetes is prone to ketoacidosis and diabetic complications?
32. Which test is performed to assess the average plasma glucose level over the past 2-3 months period?
33. What anticoagulant inhibits urease that is used as part of the reagent system in some urea assay methods?
34. Why must the pH of the urine sample for uric acid determination be adjusted to 7.5-8?
35. Which lipoprotein transports most cholesterol?
36. What is the relationship between HDL cholesterol and the risk of CAD?
37. Which bilirubin fraction is elevated in HDN?

38. What is the normal A:G ratio?

39. What causes elevated albumin?

40. What causes decreased gamma globulin?

41. Which protein fraction is the fastest moving in electrophoresis at pH 8.6?

42. What stain is used in serum protein electrophoresis?

43. What instrument is used to quantitate protein fractions following serum protein electrophoresis?

44. Which protein fraction contains copper?

45. What is the major clinical significance of elevated alkaline phosphatase?

46. Which enzymes are elevated in acute pancreatitis?

47. Which enzyme is an indicator of alcoholism?

48. Which cardiac enzyme is most specific?

49. Which clinical condition occurs in the highest levels of LD?

50. What are the major electrolytes?

51. What is the major extracellular cation?

52. How are the sodium and potassium usually assayed?

53. What clinical condition results from very high *or* very low potassium levels?

54. Which disease is characterized by a high concentration of sodium and chloride?

55. What pretreatment of urine is required before performing a urine phosphorus analysis?

56. What happens to CO_2 if the specimen is exposed to air?

57. Which hormone is tested to detect pregnancy?

58. What type of method is used for most hormone assays?

59. Where is the growth hormone produced?

60. Where is aldosterone produced?

61. What substances can cause a *false* positive VMA?

62. What is the precursor in the biosynthesis of all steroid hormones?

63. What is Addison's disease?

64. Which is the physiologically active form of T_4?

65. What is the name of an autoimmune disease, the most common type of hyperthyroidism in the U.S.?

Answers

1. Photoelectric colorimeter
2. Arne Wilhelm Kaurin Tiselius
3. mmol/L
4. Glycogen
5. Gluconeogenesis
6. 120 minutes
7. 34 N
8. Urea
9. 2.14
10. Uric acid
11. Uric acid
12. Jack bean meal
13. Alkaline phosphotungstate
14. Jaffe reaction (1886)
15. Creatinine clearance test
16. Chylomicrons
17. Ferric chloride in acetic acid and concentrated sulfuric acid
18. Lipase
19. Direct bilirubin
20. Van den Bergh reaction
21. Methyl red solution at pH 4.6 to 4.7
22. Jaundice (icterus)
23. Liver
24. Bromocresol green (BCG)
25. Albumin
26. Negative
27. Proteinic
28. 10
29. Acid phosphatase
30. Five
31. Type I (juvenile-onset diabetes or IDDM)
32. Glycated hemoglobin (hemoglobin A1c)
33. Sodium fluoride
34. To prevent precipitation of uric acid
35. Low-density lipoprotein (LDL)
36. Inverse
37. Indirect bilirubin
38. 1-1.8
39. Dehydration
40. Hypogammaglobulinemia
41. Albumin
42. Coomassie Brilliant Blue
43. Densitometer
44. Ceruloplasmin

45. Liver and bone disorders
46. Lipase and amylase
47. Gamma-glutamyl transpeptidase (GGT)
48. CK-2
49. Pernicious anemia
50. Sodium, potassium, chloride, and bicarbonate
51. Sodium
52. Ion-selective electrode
53. Cardiac arrhythmias
54. Cystic fibrosis
55. Acidified to pH 6
56. Decreases
57. Human chorionic gonadotropin (hCG)
58. Radioimmunoassay (RIA)
59. Anterior pituitary
60. Adrenal cortex
61. Banana, vanilla, and some drugs
62. Cholesterol
63. Adrenal insufficiency
64. Free T$_4$
65. Graves' disease

Section III: Immunology/Serology

Chapter 31

Antigens

Introduction

Those substances which, upon introduction into a foreign animal species, induce the biosynthesis of immunoglobulins and specifically react with these immunoglobulins are called antigens.

Many diagnostic laboratory tests are based on antigen-antibody reactions. Serological reactions are simple, rapid, and specific. Their test results are reliable and reproducible. Therefore, it is necessary to understand:

1. *What are these substances?*
2. *Where are they found?*
3. *How are they biosynthesized?*

Properties

1. Although most of the complete antigens are proteins, some of them may be polysaccharides, polypeptides, lipids, or nucleic acids. Some complex substances are unable to stimulate the biosynthesis of antibodies by themselves and require a protein molecule are defined as haptens or partial antigens. Capsular polysaccharide materials of pneumococci and capsular glutamyl polypeptide of *B. anthracis* and penicillin are good examples of haptens.
2. Most antigens are macromolecules with high molecular weight (>10,000 daltons). For example, the molecular weight of hemocyanins is 6.75 million daltons.
3. Antigens should have an aromatic radical, e.g., gelatin is a non-antigenic substance as it lacks aromatic radical, tyrosine.
4. Antigens are 'foreign' or 'non-self' to an animal.
5. Antigens are susceptible to tissue enzymes. Polystyrene latex particles are not antigenic due to the insusceptibility of tissue enzymes. In other words, antigens are soluble in the tissues.
6. Antigens exhibit marked specificity. However, antigenic specificity is not absolute. Portions of antigen molecules that determine the specificity of antigen-antibody reactions are called antigenic determinants (epitopes). The size of the determinant group may be quite small to the size of the whole antigen molecule, e.g., 5-7 amino acid residues.

Types of antigens based on their origin

a. Exogenous antigens: Those antigens that enter the body from outside and circulate in the body fluids are called exogenous antigens. Such foreign antigens are held by antigen-presenting cells (APCs), e.g., macrophages and dendritic cells through phagocytosis. Bacteria, viruses, and fungi are categorized under exogenous antigens.

b. Endogenous antigens: Agents that may be the body's cells, fragments, chemical substances, or products capable of producing antibodies are called endogenous antigens. Cytotoxic T cells accept them only after the processing of these antigens by macrophages. Endogenous antigens can be autologous, homologous, or heterologous. Blood group antigens and histocompatibility leukocyte antigens (HLA) are examples of endogenous antigens.

c. Autoantigens: Normally, some individual's simple proteins (e.g., thyroglobulins) or conjugated proteins (e.g., nucleoproteins) do not stimulate the immune system in a healthy person. But, the immune system may be stimulated by these molecules in patients suffering from a specific autoimmune disease. This occurs due to the altered genetic and environmental conditions, thus losing the normal immunological tolerance to such molecules (autoantigens).

Antigenic substances

There are many substances capable of stimulating the formation of antibodies. Some important antigenic substances are:

1. Blood corpuscles, e.g., RBCs
2. Viruses, e.g., influenza virus
3. Rickettsiae, e.g., *R. prowazeki*

Bacteria, e.g., *Salmonella typhi,* possess three main antigens as shown in Table 31.1.

Table 31.1: Antigens of *Salmonella typhi*

	"H" or flagellar Ag*	"O" or somatic Ag**	"Vi" or "K" Ag
a. Treatment by:			
heat	destroyed over 70°-75°C	resists a temperature of 100°C	destroyed at 60°C for 1 hour
absolute alcohol	sensitive	resistant	resistant
weak acids	sensitive	resistant	sensitive
formalin	resistant	sensitive	resistant (0.2%)
b. Diphasic variation	present	absent	absent

*"H" Ag is proteinaceous, highly immunogenic, and capable of inducing an antibody with high titers.
**"O" Ag is a polysaccharide by nature, less immunogenic, and capable of inducing an antibody with low titers.

4. Bacterial toxins, e.g., exotoxins of *Cl. botulinum* and *C. diphtheriae* and endotoxins of *V. cholerae* and *P. pestis*
5. Vegetable toxins, e.g., ricin and abrin
6. Serum, e.g., globulin

The antigenic structure of a bacterial cell is not simple. This multiplicity of bacterial antigens has been likened to a mosaic. Raffel has suggested that we should 'look upon a microbe as a bag of distinct antigens' (see Fig. 31.1). Moreover, different bacterial species may possess some common antigens which are responsible for cross-reactions.

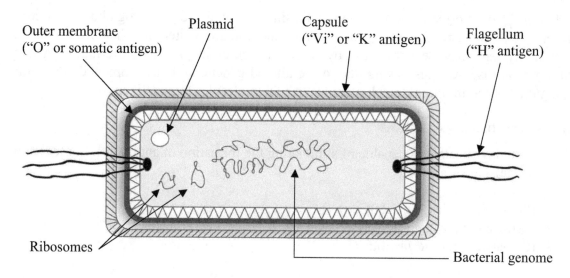

Outer membrane ("O" or somatic antigen) Plasmid Capsule ("Vi" or "K" antigen) Flagellum ("H" antigen)

Ribosomes Bacterial genome

Fig. 31.1: Antigenic structure of *Salmonella typhi*.

The heterophile antigen is defined as an antigen that occurs in different biological species, classes, and kingdoms, e.g., Forssman antigen (a lipid carbohydrate complex) found in man, animals, plants, birds, and bacteria.

Vaccines

Dr. Edward Jenner (1796) successfully developed an immune response in an eight-year-old boy against a deadly infection, smallpox. Since he had used the cow-pox virus (less virulent to humans) to develop an acquired immunity, it tempted him to coin the term "vaccine" (Latin *vacca* = cow). Louis Pasteur (1885), a French chemist, developed the rabies vaccine as a second revolutionary immunization technique. He succeeded to save the life of Joseph Meister, a nine-year-old boy, who had been bitten by a rabid dog. Vaccines are categorized according to the nature of the material used to trigger the immune response:

(i) Live (attenuated or weakened) vaccines: They develop a long-lasting immunity require a low dose. Some of these vaccines may revert to the pathogenic form. Examples include measles/mumps/rubella (MMR), chickenpox, yellow fever, and rotavirus.

(ii) Dead (killed or inactivated) vaccines: They require a higher dose as well as booster immunizations. Though dead vaccines develop a shorter-lasting immunity, they are safer and stable. The agents used to kill microbes include heat, radiation, or chemicals. Vaccines namely, polio (Salk vaccine), rabies, cholera, flu, hepatitis A, and plague are good examples of inactivated vaccines.

(iii) Toxoids: Purified exotoxins are treated to selectively destroy the toxicity while preserving the antigenicity. This can be accomplished by inactivating a toxin with heat or chemical (e.g., formalin) treatment. It may need booster shots to provide ongoing protection. Examples include tetanus and diphtheria toxoids (Tdap vaccine).

(iv) Subunit vaccines: A specific part of a microorganism, e.g., protein or polysaccharide, is used instead of a whole microorganism to serve the purpose. Examples include hepatitis B and acellular pertussis.

(v) Conjugate vaccines: It is self-explanatory because antigens are fused with polysaccharides. These vaccines are more effective for immature immune system of infants, e.g., *H. influenzae* type b (Hib)

(vi) Messenger RNA (mRNA)-based vaccines: This innovative vaccine contains mRNA encased in lipid nanoparticles LNPs). mRNA directs the biosynthesis of a spike-specific protein (antigen) which, in turn, modulates the immune system to produce a specific antibody. The LNPs play a promising role as a vaccine delivery system:

    (i) Protect the mRNA against the degradation
    (ii) Facilitate endosomal escape
    (iii) Enable to target to the desired cell type
    (iv) Can be co-delivered with adjuvants if needed

mRNA-based vaccines have inherent instability. For example, Moderna's mRNA-1273 vaccine needs a temperature of -20°C for 6 months storage, and thawed vaccine remains stable at 2°-8°C for up to 30 days. The Pfizer/BioNtech's mRNA vaccine is to be stored at -75°C and the thawed vaccine is good for 5 days at 2°-8°C.

The claimed efficacy of about 95% by the manufacturers remains controversial.

DNA-based vaccination is also a novel approach in building up the acquired immunity. The research is underway.

Chapter 32

Immune System

Introduction

The host defense mechanism involves a complex immune system as outlined in Fig. 32.1.

    A. Innate immunity
    B. Adaptive immunity

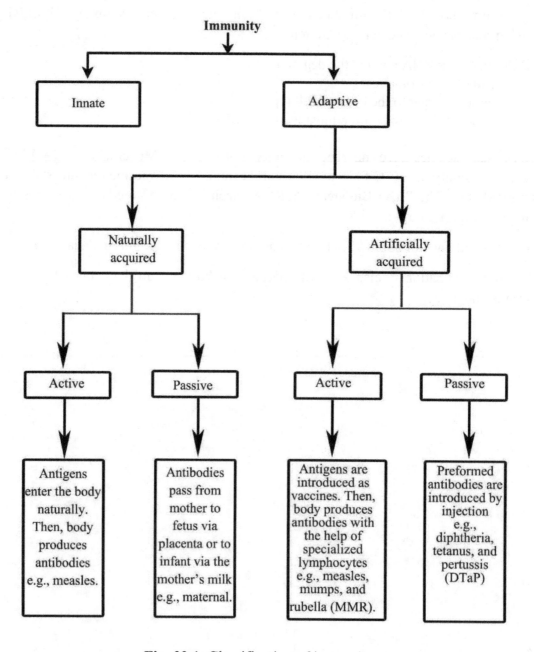

Fig. 32.1: Classification of immunity.

A. Innate immunity

Innate immunity is inherited from parents to their offspring. It involves physical barriers (skin and mucous membranes), phagocytic leukocytes (macrophages), body secretions (bile, saliva, and tears), inflammatory response (mast cells), and complement.

Since innate immunity is non-specific, the system is engaged in the removal of any kind of invading agents, e.g., bacteria, viruses. This is mainly accomplished by:

(i) *Inflammatory response*: Inflammatory response activates the mast cells to release histamine. Such chemical mediators have an inflammatory cascade effect, involving the increased cell trafficking at the site of damaged tissue.

Following an infection, traumatic injury, or a burn on external surfaces, it is readily noticeable with the following typical signs and symptoms in a sequence listed below:

- redness
- heat
- swelling
- pain

(ii) *Phagocytosis*: Macrophages not only invade the pathogens at the site of an infection but also release chemical mediators (cytokines) to attract more cells to the area of damaged tissue. The mechanism of phagocytosis is depicted in Fig. 32.2.

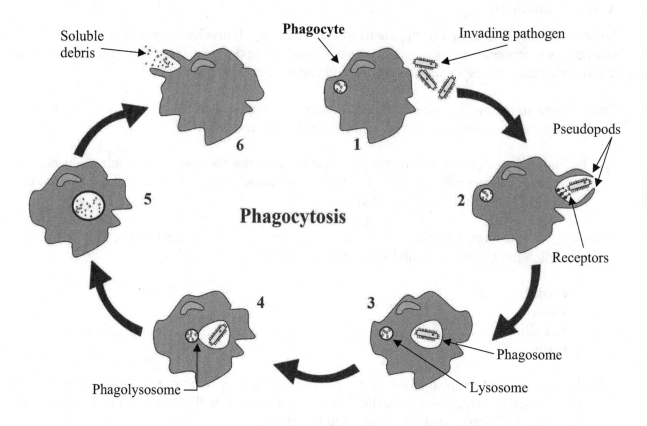

Fig. 32.2: Steps of phagocytosis, a type of innate immunity.

1. Chemotaxis
2. Entrapment
3. Ingestion (engulfment)
4. Formation of phagolysosome
5. Destruction and digestion
6. Exocytosis (elimination of soluble debris)

Dendritic cells (DCs) are bone-marrow-derived phagocytes and roam around in the blood, lymph, and tissue. They capture and process antigens followed by their union with major histocompatibility complex (MHC) II molecules before the presentation. Additionally, they secrete a cytokine called interleukin-1 (IL-1) that stimulates helper T cells to release a growth factor, interleukin-2 (IL-2). Thus, they play a major role as antigen-presenting cells (APCs) while activating the T_H (CD4) cells of the adaptive immunity.

(iii) *Natural killer (NK) cells:* they are capable of killing many potentially harmful foreign materials with the help of their enzymes. Like cytotoxic T cells, NK cells use a similar mechanism called apoptosis for killing the target cells.

(iv) *Protective proteins:*
   1. Interferon
   2. Complement

1. Interferon: There are three major classes of interferon produced following the exposure to antigens, e.g., viruses and RNA. They are classified as interferon alpha, interferon beta, and interferon-gamma. They participate in intercommunication, thus performing a regulatory role in the immune system. Besides, the inhibitory effect of interferon against many viruses, they also play other roles, e.g., activation of natural killer cells and inhibition of cancer cells by interferon-alpha and interferon-gamma, respectively.

2. Complement: Complement cascade is engaged in the destruction and removal of pathogens. There are more than 30 serum proteins in a complement system that are activated to facilitate this task. To accomplish this, the following pathways are triggered as depicted in Fig. 32.3.

   a. Classical pathway: is activated in the presence of antigen-antibody complex
   b. Lectin pathway: is activated in the presence of mannose-binding lectin (MBL)
   c. Alternative pathway: is activated in the presence of bacterial endotoxin

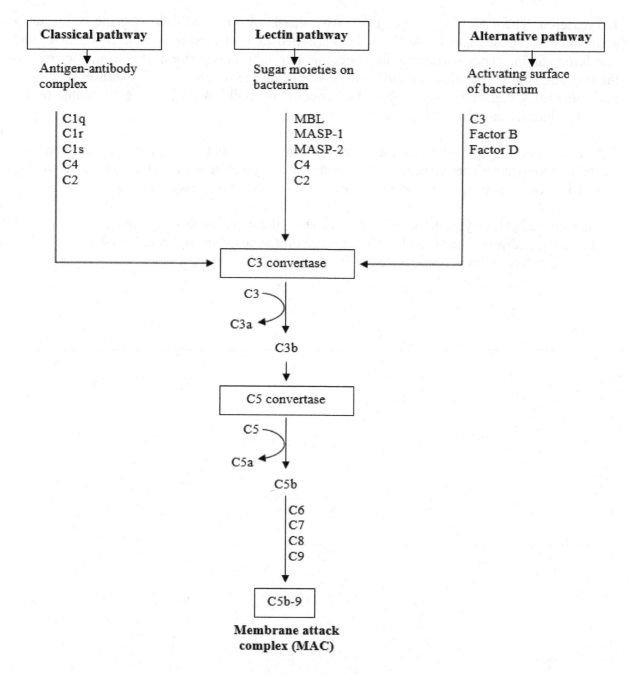

Fig. 32.3: Complement cascade.

In all three pathways, the formation of homologous variants of the protease called C3 convertase takes place. The resulting ring-shaped complex molecule called a membrane attack complex (MAC) makes holes in the surface layers of bacteria and enveloped viruses. Later, such damaged bacterial cells and viral particles fail to survive. The overall effect of the activated complement cascade is to enhance inflammation, facilitate phagocytosis, and lysis of pathogens.

B. Adaptive immunity

  a. *Antibody-mediated immunity*
  b. *Cell-mediated immunity*

a. Antibody-mediated immunity: B cells and T cells

It seems necessary to understand the steps involved in the formation of plasma cells (see Fig. 6.1). Following exposure to antigens, B cells are activated and then undergo differentiation into two types of B cells, namely long-lived memory B cells and plasma cells. Plasma cells, in turn, secrete antibodies into circulation (i.e., humoral immunity).

The cells engaged directly or indirectly in adaptive immunity are B cells and T cells. These cells originate and undergo maturation in primary lymphoid organs, namely red bone marrow and thymus. Distinctive features B cells and T cells are listed in Table 32.1.

Table 32.1: Brief overview of the differences between B cells and T cells

Characteristic	B cells	T cells
Origin	Bone marrow	Thymus
Location	Outside of lymph node	Inside of lymph node
Life span	Short	Long
Surface antibodies	Present	Absent
Secretion	Immunoglobulins(antibodies)	Lymphokines
Blood	20% of lymphocytes	80% of lymphocytes
Formation of cells	Plasma and memory cells	Killer, helper, and suppressor cells
Type of immune system	Antibody-mediated	Cell-mediated
Inhibition of immune system	No	Yes (suppressor cells)
Response to transplants and cancer cells	No	Yes
Migration to the site of infection	No	Yes(lymphoblasts)
Defensive against?	Bacteria and viruses	Protists and fungi
Tissue distribution	Spleen, gut, respiratory tract, and germinal centers of lymph nodes	Parafollicular parts of cortex and periarteriolar of the spleen

Biosynthesis of immunoglobulins

Biosynthesis of immunoglobulins begins with the phagocytosis of antigen by macrophages. Macrophages, in turn, present antigen in their active form to B lymphocytes to stimulate them. These stimulated B lymphocytes then undergo proliferation, maturation, and differentiation into plasma cells-large lymphocytes. In this way, the actual biosynthesis of immunoglobulins largely occurs in the plasma cells. Some large lymphocytes can probably revert to small B lymphocytes (memory cells).

In some instances, the biosynthesis of immunoglobulins against certain large antigenic polymers (e.g., *Pneumococcus* polysaccharide) involves only B cells. Antigens, with a smaller number of determinants and requiring a carrier, need T cell co-operation for the biosynthesis of immunoglobulins. Unlike B cells, T cells do not undergo differentiation into immunoglobulin-producing cells.

Antibodies are immunoglobulins that appear in the blood and tissue fluids as a result of the entrance into the tissues of antigens, and which can react specifically with the corresponding antigen.

Immunoglobulins comprise about 20% of total serum proteins. Depending on the nature of the antigen-antibody reaction, they are named variously as agglutinins, precipitins, antitoxins, and so on. On the other hand, antibodies may be designated by the name of antigen with the prefix 'anti-' e.g., anti-hCG, anti-A, anti-DNA.

Factors affecting the formation of immunoglobulins (antibody):

1. Nature of antigen
2. Dosage of antigenic material and number of doses (anamnestic reaction)
3. Age, nutritional status, and nature of animal species used
4. Routes of administration
5. Adjuvants, e.g., aluminium hydroxide (alum), Freund's adjuvant
6. Immunosuppressive agents, e.g., X-irradiation, antimetabolites
7. Genetic factors: Some substances can be antigenic in one species but not in another. Also, it is true for members belonging to the same species.

The rate of antibody formation following the initial injection of antigen and 'booster' injection is illustrated in Fig. 32.4. The secondary response produces a high titer of antibodies in a short period in comparison with the primary response. This phenomenon is called 'anamnestic reaction'.

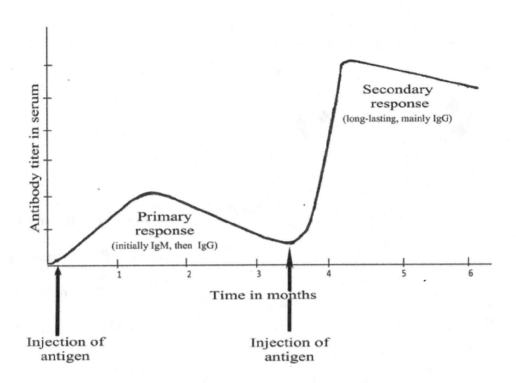

Fig. 32.4: Rate of antibody formation following 'initial' injection of antigen and 'booster' injection (anamnestic response).

Structure of immunoglobulins

Many immunoglobulins are produced in response to a single pure antigen. But, they are not homogenous as they are developed by different clones of cells. These molecules have been studied in detail. Chemically, they are glycoproteins. They possess similar structural patterns. They consist of two pairs of polypeptide chains of different sizes (i.e., heavy and light). Furthermore, these chains are held together by disulfide (S-S) linkages. There is the presence of a constant carboxyl-terminal portion, as well as a variable amino-terminal portion in each chain.

Light (L) chains of all classes of immunoglobulins show similarity. They have molecular weights of approximately 25,000 daltons. There are two types of chains:

(i) K (Kappa) - Originally described by Korngold
(ii) λ (Lambda) - Originally described by Lapari
    Only one type of chain is found in immunoglobulin.

Heavy (H) chains have molecular weights of 50,000-70,000 daltons. Each of the 5 immuno-globulins has an antigenically distinct set of H chains (i.e., λ, α, μ, δ, and ε). There may be 1 to 5 disulfide (S-S) bonds to hold two heavy chains together. Splitting of immunoglobulin by papain forms three fragments in all, namely two Fab and one Fc. Similar fractions can be obtained by the action of pepsin. The flexible hinge region is present in the C region of the H chain. The joining (J) chain is found in polymeric structures of IgA and IgM. Structures of IgG, IgA, and IgM are depicted in Fig. 32.5 (a), (b), (c).

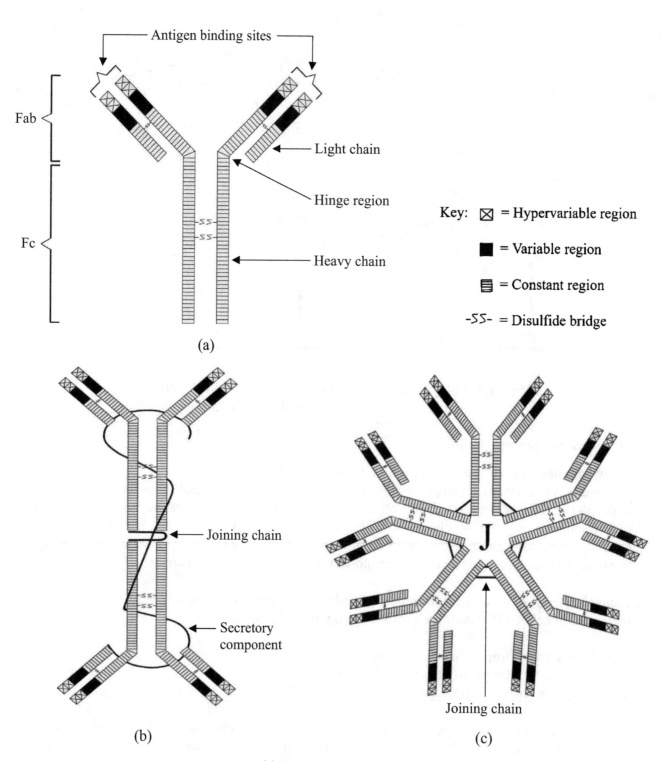

(a) Immunoglobulin G (monomer)
(b) Immunoglobulin A (dimer)
(c) Immunoglobulin M (pentamer)

Fig. 32.5: Structure of immunoglobulins.

Characteristics of immunoglobulins (see Table 32.2):

Tiselius (1937) fractionated serum proteins into albumin, alpha, beta, and gamma globulins. He used electrophoresis (see chapter 3) to do so. From anode towards the cathode, albumin travels the shortest distance, alpha, and beta globulins a little farther, and gamma globulins faster and farther than the other fractions. Tiselius and Kabat (1938) equated the gamma globulin fraction with the antibody activity. Later, many antibodies were reported to migrate as alpha or beta globulins. Antibody activity resides in any one of three fractions of globulin. As it offers immunity, it is called 'immunoglobulin'.

Immunoglobulins have been studied and characterized by many workers. They are classified into five classes, namely IgG, IgA, IgM, IgD, and IgE. Each of the five immunoglobulin classes has a distinct set of chains. The five heavy chain types are designated by the Greek alphabet letter as under:

IgG	γ (gamma)
IgA	α (alpha)
IgM	μ (mu)
IgD	δ (delta)
IgE	ε (epsilon)

Thus, each class is named by Ig (immunoglobulin) followed by the first alphabet of the Greek letter, indicating the type of heavy chain. The immunoglobulins of IgG class have been divided into four subclasses viz., IgG_1, IgG_2, IgG_3, and IgG_4. Each subclass possesses a distinct type of gamma chain. The occurrence of these four subclasses in human serum is in the approximate proportions of 65%, 23%, 8%, and 4%, respectively.

Table 32.2: Characteristics of immunoglobulins

Characteristic	IgG	IgA	IgM	IgD	IgE
Structure	monomer	dimer(with secretory component)	pentamer	monomer	monomer
Location	blood,lymph, intestine	secretions (tears,saliva, mucus, intestine,milk), blood,lymph	blood,lymph, B cell surface (as monomer)	B cell surface, blood,lymph	bound to mast and basophil cells throughout body,blood
Sedimentation coefficient, S	7	7 or 11*	19	7	8
Molecular weight, g·mol^{-1}	150	170 or 400	900	180	190
Heavy chain symbol	γ	α	μ	δ	ε
Normal serum conc.,%	80	10-15	5-10	0.2	0.002
Half life, days	23	6	5	3	2.5
Daily formation, mg./ kg.	34	24	3.3	0.4	0.0023
Intravascular distribution,%	45	42	80	75	50
Carbohydrate,%	4	10	15	18	18
Heat stability, 56°C.	+	+	+	+	-
Presence in milk	+	+	-	-	-
Complement fixation	+	-	+	-	-
Crosses placenta	+	-	-	-	-
Prominent in external secretions	-	++	-	-	+

*7S, mol.wt. 170 g·mol^{-1} IgA in serum;11S, mol. wt. 400 g·mol^{-1} IgA in external secretions, e.g., saliva milk, and tears.

b. Cell-mediated immunity
- *helper T cells:* express the CD2 (E rosette), CD3 (mature T cell), and CD4 (helper) markers. They help cytotoxic T cells and B cells through the substances they produce.
- *cytotoxic T cells:* express CD8 and act against invaders, namely virus-infected cells and tumor cells.
- *suppressor (regulatory) T cells:* express CD3, CD4, and CD25 markers. They control the activity of B cells and T cells, thus preventing them to overreact and cause harmful effects to healthy tissues.

The distinctive features of innate and adaptive immunity are outlined in Table 32.3.

Table 32.3: Brief outline between innate and adaptive immunity

Characteristic	Innate immunity	Adaptive immunity
Composition	Phagocytic leukocytes, dendritic cells, natural killer cells, plasma proteins, and physicochemical barriers	B cells and T cells
Specificity	Non-specific	Specific
Response	Fast	Slow
Potency	Low	High
Inheritance	Yes	No
Allergic reaction	No	Immediate and delayed hypersensitivity
Memory	No	Yes
Speed of response	Fast	Slow
Complement system activation	Alternative and lectin pathways	Classical pathway
Physiological and anatomical barriers	Skin and mucous membranes	Lymph nodes and spleen
Defensive against?	Any foreign invader	Only specific infection
Distribution	Vertebrates and invertebrates	Vertebrates

Irregularities of the immune system

a. Hypersensitivity reactions

Adverse responses by a normal immune system to cause damage rather than protection. They are classified as under:

1. *Type I-Immediate hypersensitivity*: IgE-mediated response which may manifest as systemic anaphylaxis and localized anaphylaxis, e.g., Bee stings, asthma, and hay fever.
2. *Type II-Antibody-dependent cytotoxic hypersensitivity*: binding of immunoglobulin (IgG or IgM) to the antigen on cells followed by cell destruction via complement activation, e.g., hemolytic transfusion reaction (HTR) and hemolytic disease of the fetus and newborn (HDFN).
3. *Type III-Immune complex-mediated hypersensitivity*: Formation and deposition of antigen-antibody complexes in organs or tissues. Complexes so formed induce complement activation and the subsequent inflammatory response mediated via massive infiltration of neutrophils, e.g., Arthus reaction (localized) and serum sickness (generalized).

4. *Type IV-Delayed hypersensitivity*: Antigen-sensitized T cells (T$_H$1) response, causing them to release lymphokines that activate macrophages or T cytotoxic cells (T$_C$) that mediate direct cellular damage, e.g., graft rejection, contact dermatitis, and poison ivy.

b. Autoimmune diseases

Disorders are implicated with the malfunctioning of the immune system where the immune system attacks the body's tissues or molecules. This is due to a failure of the immune system to discriminate between "self" and "non-self". Examples of autoimmune diseases are:

- Rheumatoid arthritis (RA)
- The systemic lupus erythematosus (SLE)
- Inflammatory bowel diseases, e.g., ulcerative colitis and Crohn's disease
- Idiopathic thrombocytopenic purpura (ITP)
- Type 1 diabetes mellitus
- Guillain-Barre syndrome
- Psoriasis
- Graves' disease
- Hashimoto's thyroiditis
- Myasthenia gravis
- Multiple sclerosis
- Vasculitis

c. Immunodeficiency diseases

These disorders are caused due to B cell deficiencies or T cell deficiencies and sometimes both. Individuals with immunodeficiency diseases are susceptible to opportunistic infections, e.g., *Candida albicans* infections. Immunodeficiency diseases are subdivided into two categories:

1. Primary (congenital): are usually inherited in which components of an immune system are either absent or adversely affected:

- B cell deficiencies, e.g., agammaglobulinemia
- T cell deficiencies, e.g., DiGeorge syndrome (thymic hypoplasia)
- Combined B cell and T cell deficiencies, e.g., Severe combined immunodeficiency syndrome (SCIDS)

2. Secondary (acquired): associated with the underlying diseases or conditions:

- Human immunodeficiency virus (HIV) infection
- Multiple myeloma
- Malignancy, e.g., ALL, AML
- Immunosuppressive medications, e.g., corticosteroids

Chapter 33

Agglutination and Precipitation

Introduction

Antigen-antibody reactions, *in vitro*, are also called "serological reactions". They are highly specific reactions. They help:

1. To identify infectious agents (e.g., members of typhoid and dysentery groups isolated from stool) and non-infectious agents (e.g., enzymes).
2. To know the presence of specific antibodies in the patient's serum (e.g., typhoid).
3. To determine antibody titer (e.g., epidemiological surveys). Some important antigen-antibody reactions are listed in Table 33.1.

Table 33.1: Antigen-antibody reactions

Reaction	Antigenic substance	Antigen	Antibody
Agglutination or clumping	Bacteria	Agglutinogen	Agglutinin
Precipitation or flocculation	'Soluble' carbohydrate or protein	Precipitinogen	Precipitin
Complement-fixation	Bacteria, protein	-	Complement fixing Ab
Neutralization	Toxin	Toxin	Antitoxin

Agglutination (Clumping)

Agglutination was described by Gruber and Durham (1896). It was applied shortly afterwards by Widal (1896) to the laboratory diagnosis of enteric fever. It is probably the most extensively applied reaction of serological reactions and is performed either by slide or tube method. It is more sensitive than precipitation.

Factors governing agglutination reactions

1. Nature of an agglutinogen:
The participating agglutinogen is particulate. It consists of suspensions of bacteria, cells (e.g., RBCs), or uniform particles (e.g., polystyrene latex and bentonite) onto which agglutinogen is coated. This is the reason why agglutinogen is not subjected to serial dilutions.

2. Agglutinin:
An antiserum should contain a corresponding agglutinin. Serial dilutions of the serum containing the agglutinin may be prepared to determine the agglutinin titer[26]. Agglutinin belongs to the IgM class of immunoglobulins.

---

[26] The 'titer' of the agglutinin in serum is the highest dilution with clearly visible agglutination.

3. The concentration of reactants:

Sometimes, agglutination occurs only at a higher dilution instead. It occurs owing to the presence of a blocking antibody and such phenomenon is termed zoning or the prozone phenomenon, e.g., *Br. abortus*.

4. Menstruum:

Agglutination occurs in the presence of an electrolyte. On the other hand, agglutination of bacteria may occur by electrolytes alone, e.g., acid agglutination. Thus, the nature and concentration of the electrolytes used are of great importance. The physiological or normal saline provides a very satisfactory menstruum.

5. Temperature:

Although the elevated temperatures (37°C - 56°C) accelerate the agglutination reaction, extremely high temperatures (60°C and over) may damage the agglutinins.

6. Agitation:

The velocity of the agglutination increases by agitation (e.g., stirring, shaking, or centrifuging).

Applications
1. Identification of an isolated species
2. Study of the antigenic structure of bacteria
3. Laboratory diagnosis of typhoid fever (Widal test), typhus fever (Weil-Felix test), infectious mononucleosis (Paul-Bunnell test), and other infections
4. Determination of human blood groups (hemagglutination)
5. Anti-globulin (Coombs) test

Laboratory diagnostic tests

1. Widal (tube) test

Fever caused by *S. typhi* and *S. paratyphi* is called 'enteric fever'. Either of the following two ways, one can carry out laboratory diagnosis of enteric fever:

1. Isolation and identification of bacteria from blood, feces, or urine
2. Agglutination (Widal) test developed by Widal (1896)

Principle
Agglutinins against 'O' (somatic) and 'H' (flagellar) agglutinogens of *Salmonella* group of bacteria is detected quantitatively, using killed and stained smooth suspension of appropriate bacteria.

Specimen
0.4mL of serum is required. In case of any delay in testing, it is stored at 2°-8°C.

Procedure (see Fig. 33.1)
a. Master dilution: Prepare a master dilution serially
b. Assay

1. Arrange four rows of 6 tubes (3" x 3/8") each in a rack
2. Transfer the diluted serum (from master dilutions) in vertical rows
3. Transfer the bacterial antigens in horizontal rows
4. Mix well and incubate overnight at 37°C

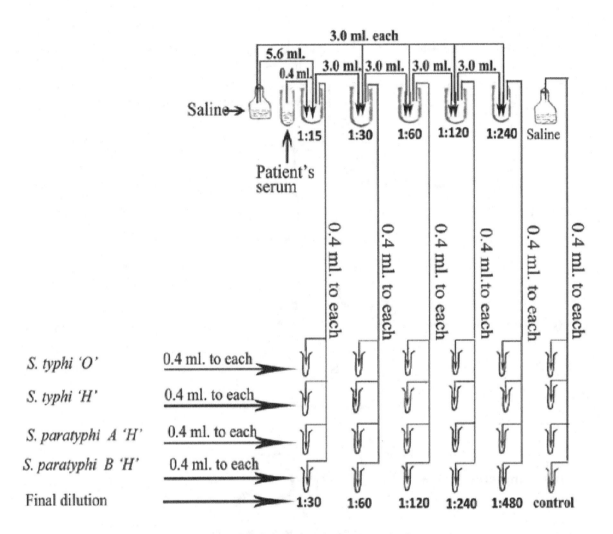

Fig. 33.1: Widal (tube) test for enteric fever.

Interpretation

Agglutination titers of 1:120 and more are clinically significant. A rise in the titers on the repetition of the test after 5-7 days will confirm the diagnosis of enteric fever.

2. Enzyme-linked immunosorbent assay (ELISA)

ELISA (also called enzyme immunoassay) technique is relatively inexpensive and simple to perform. It is used for qualitative and quantitative studies of either antigen or antibody in the serum specimen. There are four types of ELISA techniques as shown in Fig. 33.2.

a. *Direct*
b. *Indirect*
c. *Sandwich*
d. *Competitive*

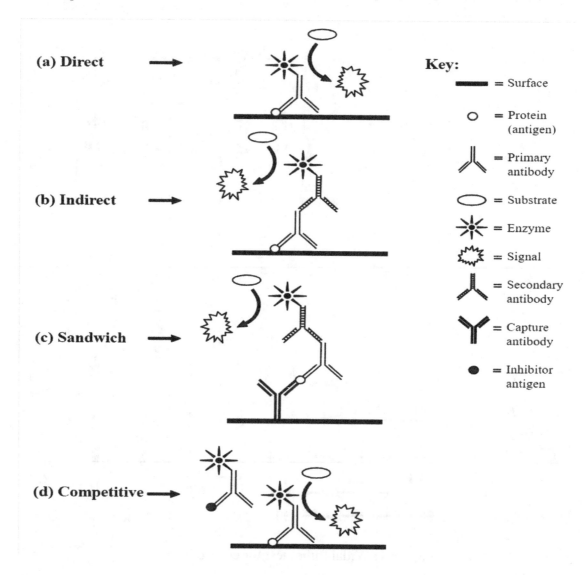

Fig. 33.2: Different formats of ELISA.

Enzymes used for enzyme labeling include horseradish peroxidase, alkaline phosphatase, glucose-6-phosphate dehydrogenase, and β-galactosidase. Generally, the ELISA technique involves the following four key steps:

1. Trapping of an antigen or antibody from a specimen by a corresponding specific antibody or antigen coated on the surface of solid-phase support (a polystyrene microtiter plate).
2. Washing with a mild detergent helps remove any antibodies or other proteins that are non-specifically attached.

234

3. Developing a plate by adding an enzyme-substrate. The formed complex reacts with substrate in proportion to the quantity of antigen or antibody first bound by the antibody or antigen coating.

4. Recording a color change (signal), using a variety of methods, e.g., absorbance, fluorescence, or electrochemical. Thus, an analyte (antigen or antibody) from a liquid specimen can be detected and quantitated. ELISA technique is used extensively in the detection of antibodies to viruses and parasites. Also, ELISA finds its application in a toxicology laboratory in screening some drugs.

Enzyme-linked immunosorbent assay (ELISA) is a specific and sensitive technique. It is a widely used technique and amenable to automation.

ELISA has the following applications:

a. Estimation of tumor markers, e.g., prostate-specific antigen (PSA)
b. Estimation of hormones, e.g., human chorionic gonadotropin (hCG) in urine (pregnancy test)
c. Screening of viral infections, e.g., Covid-19 and human immunodeficiency virus (HIV)
d. Detection and/or quantification of antibodies in blood/tissue, e.g., antinuclear antibody (ANA) and autoantibodies

3. Western blot technique

Originally, the technique was developed for assaying DNA by Sir Edwin Mellor Southern. Afterwards, Northern and Western blotting techniques were named for RNA and protein macromolecules, respectively. Western blotting (immunoblotting) helps detect the protein of interest from a mixture of proteins, e.g., cell lysate and blood plasma. The basic steps are outlined in Fig. 33.3.

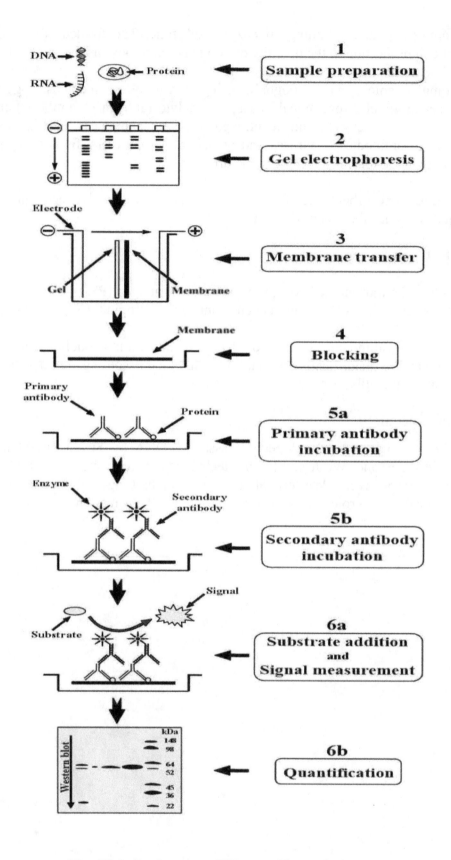

Fig. 33.3: Basic steps of Western blot technique.

1. *Sample preparation*: An extract of microbial cells, e.g., viruses, bacteria, or fungi, is prepared. This lytic process makes use of a mixture that comprises a cold cell lysis buffer and a fresh protease inhibitor.

2. *Gel electrophoresis*: It uses sodium dodecyl sulfate-polyacrylamide gel electrophoresis (SDS-PAGE) to separate protein macromolecules based on their molecular weight. Interestingly, all protein macromolecules carry a negative electrical charge, enabling them to migrate towards a positive electrode (anode).

3. *Membrane transfer*: Since membrane has affinity for proteins, they can easily be transferred onto a membrane, e.g., nitrocellulose and polyvinylidene difluoride. This step involves packing the membrane up to make a sandwich. The component materials are assembled and pressed (removal of air bubbles) to form a sandwich as shown in Fig. 33.4.

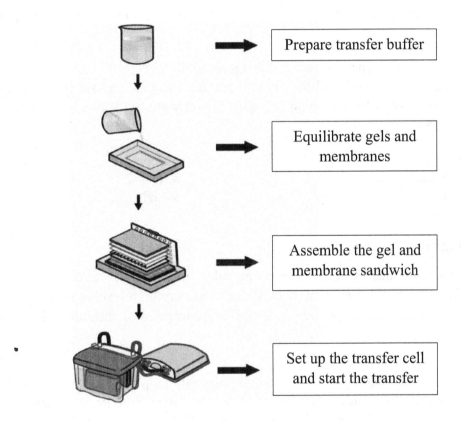

Fig. 33.4: General workflow for electrophoresis transfer.
(Reproduced with permission from Creative Proteomics, Shirley, New York)

The transfer sandwich is placed in a transfer chamber and fully covered with a transfer buffer and a coolant-filled bag. The electrophoretic unit is connected to a power supply and allows it to run for optimal power and time as recommended by the manufacturer.

4. *Blocking*: A blocking protein such as 5% non-fat milk or bovine serum albumin can be used to block sites other than the protein of interest on the membrane. This reduces the

non-specific binding of antibodies (primary and secondary) that are proteins too. Such a blocking minimizes the background signals.

5. *Incubation with antibodies*: A membrane is incubated overnight at 4°C (or one hour at room temperature) with a diluted primary antibody (monoclonal mouse) specific to the target protein (5a). The membrane is washed with Tris-buffered saline Tween 20 (TRIS) three times for five minutes each before and after incubation with a labeled secondary antibody[27] (5b). Both the incubation and washing steps are performed in the tray that is placed on a shaker.

6. *Detection*: For the purpose of detection, the added substrate (e.g., luminol) reacts with the enzyme (e.g., horseradish peroxidase) with chemiluminescence (6a):

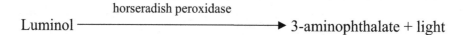

$$\text{Luminol} \xrightarrow{\text{horseradish peroxidase}} \text{3-aminophthalate} + \text{light}$$

The emitted light (i.e., signal) is captured using an X-ray film (6b). Alternatively, a fluorescent-tagged antibody can be used and the subsequent detection by an instrument that captures the fluorescent signal. Since the technique is highly specific and sensitive, it is used to confirm the following diseases:

- AIDS
- Lyme disease
- Peptic ulcer
- Hepatitis B
- HSV-2
- Alzheimer disease

4. Urine pregnancy test

The pregnancy hormone, a human chorionic gonadotropin (hCG), is released into the body by the placenta when a woman is pregnant. It is produced at very high levels in the first 3-4 months of pregnancy. It is advisable to wait 12-14 days after conception to accurately detect hCG in urine samples.

Principle
The test is based on the agglutination inhibition test. In pregnancy, the anti-hCG serum is neutralized by urine-hCG and fails to agglutinate the polystyrene latex particles antigen. In the absence of pregnancy, hCG free urine fails to neutralize anti-hCG serum, which in turn, reacts with latex antigen-forming agglutinate.

Specimen
The first morning urine sample is collected and stored at 2°-8°C until tested. The patient should be instructed to restrict fluid intake during nighttime. Samples that are heavily contaminated with pus, bacteria, or blood should be avoided.

---

[27] Rabbit anti-mouse.

5. Weil-Felix test

The Weil-Felix reaction (1916), a non-specific agglutination test, was first described in the laboratory diagnosis of rickettsial infections. It has largely been replaced with indirect immunofluorescence tests. However, the Weil-Felix test continues to hold its importance in resource-limited areas. For more details, the reader is requested to refer to chapter 41.

Precipitation (Flocculation)

Introduction

Precipitation was first described by Kraus (1897). He mixed bacteria-free filtrates of broth cultures of the typhoid bacillus, the cholera bacilli, and other bacteria with the antisera prepared against the homologous organism. As a result of this, he observed a macroscopic insoluble precipitate.

The phenomenon of precipitation is considered to be analogous to agglutination. But, the precipitinogen (antigen) is in an extremely fine colloidal solution. Therefore, the precipitate is formed largely by the precipitin (antibody). Flocculation involves non-specific antigens, e.g., cardiolipin antigen in venereal disease research laboratory (VDRL) test.

Factors controlling precipitation

1. Nature of precipitinogen
2. Nature of precipitin
3. The concentration of reactants
4. Temperature[28] (optimum:37°C)
5. Nature and concentration of an electrolyte
6. pH (optimum: 6.6-8.2)
7. Time (several hours at 37°C)
8. Agitation

Applications

The precipitation test may be performed qualitatively as well as quantitatively. In the case of a quantitative test, the antigen is diluted and the antiserum is kept constant. It is carried out in various ways:

1. Ring test, e.g., C-reactive protein test for serotyping of pneumococci and grouping of streptococci
2. Tube test, e.g., Kahn test for syphilis
3. Agar gel diffusion test (Ouchterlony), e.g., Elek test for detecting toxigenic strains of *C. diphtheriae*
4. Slide test, e.g., VDRL test (flocculation) for syphilis, detection of the origin of bloodstains in medico-legal work (forensic medicine)
5. Ascoli's test (Postmortem diagnosis of anthrax from the tissue of a dead or decomposed animal)

---

[28] The maximum amount of precipitate is formed at very low temperatures. On the other hand, a temperature of 55°C or higher may cause a precipitate to dissolve.

6. Determination of the kind of animal a mosquito has recently fed on

Rapid plasma reagin (RPR) test

The RPR test is a screening test for detecting reagin (serum antibody) in syphilitic cases. It is a non-treponemal test. It is a simple, rapid, economical, and reliable test with a high degree of reproducibility. The immunoglobulin belongs to the IgE class.

Principle
Under the standard set of test conditions, serum-containing reagin brings about co-agglutination of the carbon particles of the RPR antigen (appearing as black clumps against a white background). The RPR antigen is simply a carbon-containing cardiolipin antigen. Oppositely, reagin-free serum fails to form black aggregates of the RPR antigenic carbon particles (appearing as an even light gray color).

In the case of a positive RPR test, a quantitative test is performed to know the reagin titer. This is accomplished by diluting serum with 0.85% NaCl solution to give serial dilutions as shown in Fig. 33.5.

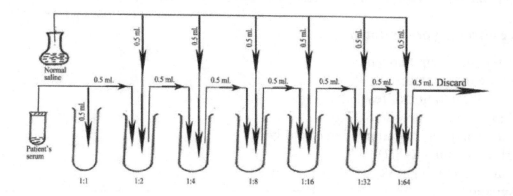

Fig. 33.5: Serial dilutions of serum.

Repeat the qualitative test, taking a drop (0.05 mL) of each serial dilution (i.e., from 1:2 to 1:32) on a separate card.

Results
The reagin titer is that titer indicated by the tube carrying the highest dilution with any degree of visible clumping.

Limitations
1. As the test is a screening test, one should confirm positive specimens with other methods, e.g., Treponema pallidum particle agglutination assay (TPPAA) and Treponema pallidum hemagglutination assay (TPHA).
2. The result may be falsely positive in certain diseases (e.g., malaria, leprosy, and infectious mononucleosis) and in specimens that are highly contaminated with bacteria.

Chapter 34

Complement-Fixation and Toxin-Antitoxin Neutralization

Complement-Fixation

The complement-fixation test was introduced by Bordet and Gengou (1901). It is a very versatile and sensitive test. But, it is a complex procedure that involves two systems:

1. Complement-fixing or bacteriolytic system
2. An indicator system

The test requires five reactants and only one is unknown. Therefore, the remaining four must be accurately standardized before the test. The reactants are (1) antigen (2) patient's serum (3) complement (4) sheep erythrocytes and (5) anti-sheep hemolysin. Saline containing calcium and magnesium ions are used as electrolytes.

Principle
The test is based on the fact that if the complement is fixed by reacting with antigen and its homologous antibody, lysis of sheep erythrocytes does not take place even in the presence of antibodies against the sheep erythrocytes.

Procedure {see Fig. 34.1 (a), (b)}
1. Mix the bacterial suspension or other antigen preparation with the test serum and complement
2. Incubate for 1 hour at 37°C to allow the reactants to react
3. Add sheep RBCs sensitized by homologous hemolysin (an indicator system)
4. Reincubate at 37°C for 1 hour
5. Keep in a refrigerator for 24 hours
6. Record the results

Results
(a) NO LYSIS: indicates the presence of homologous antibodies in the serum.
(b) LYSIS: suggests the absence of homologous antibodies in the serum.

(a) Positive :

Specific antigen(X) + Homologous antibody (anti-X) in serum (heated)

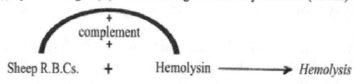

+
complement
+

Sheep R.B.Cs.   +   Hemolysin ————————→ *No hemolysis*

(b) Negative :

(i) Specific antigen (X) + No homologous antibody in serum (heated)

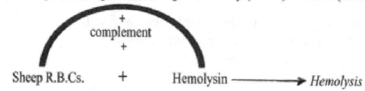

+
complement
+

Sheep R.B.Cs.   +   Hemolysin ————————→ *Hemolysis*

Or (ii) No specific antigen + Homologous antibody (anti-X) in serum (heated)

+
complement
+

Sheep R.B.Cs.   +   Hemolysin ————————→ *Hemolysis*

Fig. 34.1 (a), (b): Diagrammatic presentation of 'Complement-Fixation Test' (CFT).

Applications
Complement-fixation reaction is widely used as a diagnostic laboratory test for the following infectious diseases:

a. Viral diseases: yellow fever, dengue fever, and lymphogranuloma venereum
b. Rickettsial diseases: typhus fever
c. Bacterial diseases: syphilis (Wassermann test), yaws, pinta, chronic gonorrhea, and brucellosis
d. Protozoal diseases: kala-azar, malaria, and Chagas disease

One of the best-known applications of this reaction is the Wassermann test. The test procedure is general and is similar to that of the Wassermann test, the main difference being the antigen. A positive reaction may be expected from 5 to 7 weeks from the date of infection.

There are many modifications to the test after Wassermann developed the technique. The reagents required in the test are summarized below:

1. Antigen
It is a non-specific antigen. It is an ether-alcoholic extract of beef-heart powder called cardiolipin (complex phospholipid). Specificity and sensitivity of this antigen are increased by the addition of

cholesterol and lecithin. It is tested for anti-complementary activity as it frequently absorbs a certain amount of complement non-specifically.

2. Patient's serum

It is heated at 56°C for 30 minutes or at 60°C for 4 minutes to destroy any complement that may be pre-existing. It should be free from hemoglobin. It is diluted in a definite proportion (1:5).

3. Complement

It is obtained from guinea pigs as it combines with most antigen-antibody complexes. It is always necessary to titrate guinea pig serum for complement activity. One unit or 1 minimal hemolytic dose (MHD) of complement is defined as the highest dilution of the guinea pig serum which will bring about complete lysis of one-unit volume of washed sheep RBCs in 1 hour at 37°C in the presence of an excess of hemolysin. In practice, 2, 3, or 4 MHD of complement are usually used. It must be fresh as it deteriorates by preservation.

4. Sheep RBCs

They are recovered from defibrinated jugular venous blood. 5 or 10% of washed red cell suspension is used. It can be stored for about 3 days at 0°C. It is to be standardized before the actual test.

5. Anti-sheep hemolysin (amboceptor)

It is prepared by injecting rabbits with sheep RBCs. It is titrated similarly to complement and should be over 1:10,000. It is heat stable and is preserved by adding an equal volume of glycerol to it.

Procedure

Steps involved in the complement-fixation test are listed in Table 34.1.

Table 34.1: Complement-fixation test

	Tube 1*	Tube 2	Tube 3	Tube 4
Serum (inactivated), mL	0.5 (1/2)	0.5 (1/2)	0.5 (1/8)	0.5 (1/32)
Complement (3 MHD), mL	0.5	0.5	0.5	0.5
Antigen (1/15), mL	-	0.5	0.5	0.5
Saline, mL	0.5	-	-	-
	Incubate at 37°C for 1 hour			
Hemolysin (3 MHD), mL	0.5	0.5	0.5	0.5
Corpuscles (5 percent), mL	0.5	0.5	0.5	0.5
	Incubate at 37°C for 1 hour and then leave overnight at 0°- 4°C			

* Serum control: It should show complete hemolysis.

Results
  (i)   Absence of hemolysis = Positive
  (ii) Complete hemolysis = Negative
  (iii) Incomplete hemolysis = ±

Note: The test proper is performed along with the known negative control, the known positive control, and the antigen control.

Limitations
The test may give false-positive results in the presence of diseases, such as leprosy, malaria, malignancy, and other febrile conditions and after vaccination. Biologically false-positive results may be found in some normal individuals.

Toxin-Antitoxin Neutralization

Introduction

Bacterial exotoxins, on injection into the tissues of laboratory animals (e.g., horse), stimulate the formation of homologous neutralizing antibodies called antitoxins. Exotoxins of *Cl. tetani* and *C. diphtheriae* are converted to toxoids (anatoxins) by treatment with formalin. The importance of antitoxins in increasing the resistance offered to infection with the homologous toxigenic bacteria was first shown by Behring and Kitasato (1890).

Toxin-antitoxin neutralization can be demonstrated *in vivo* and *in vitro*. *In vivo* experiments, appropriate mixtures of toxin and antitoxin (after keeping *in vitro* for definite periods) are injected into an experimental animal (e.g., guinea pig, or mouse). A similar mixture where saline is substituted for the serum is used as a control. The test animal remains unaffected, provided serum contains an adequate quantity of antitoxin. On the other hand, the control animal shows characteristic signs of toxemia. This toxin-antitoxin neutralization was considered to be analogous to the reaction between strong acids and alkalis by Ehrlich. It is a reversible reaction. So, dissociation occurs by various physical and chemical processes, e.g., dilution, heating, freezing, and treatment with weak acids. The union becomes more stable by increasing the time of contact in vitro.

Danysz (1902) established an important fact that the amount of toxin neutralized by a fixed amount of antitoxin varied according to the way toxin was added. He showed that the bulk addition of toxin was more promising than the addition of separate fractions.

Applications
  1. To differentiate between virulent and avirulent strains, e.g., *C. diphtheriae* and various members of clostridia producing gas-gangrene.
  2. Intracutaneous diagnostic tests, e.g., Schick test for diphtheria and Dick test for scarlet fever.
  3. To determine the potency of both toxin and antitoxin. Units used during the standardization of reactants are:

MLD (minimal lethal dose) = the smallest amount of toxin killing a 250 g guinea pig in 4 days after subcutaneous injection.

Antitoxin unit = the smallest amount of antitoxin neutralizing 100 MLD of the toxin.

L0 (*Limes nul*) dose = the largest amount of toxin which is just neutralized by 1 unit of antitoxin.

L+ (*Limes tod*) dose = the smallest amount of toxin killing a 250 g guinea pig in 4 days when mixed and injected with 1 unit of antitoxin.

Neutralizing antibodies are also produced by viruses and enzymes.

Review questions

1. Which term is applied for a substance that increases the formation and persistence of antibody(ies) upon the injection of an animal with the antigen?
2. Which term is used for a substance that becomes antigenic after combining with body protein and can react specifically with the formed antibody?
3. What is the name of the protein that lacks aromatic radical, making it non-antigenic?
4. Which class of immunoglobulins have a pentameric structure?
5. Which class of immunoglobulins are present in the highest concentration in normal adults?
6. Which class of immunoglobulins routinely cross the placenta?
7. Which class of immunoglobulins are easily detectable serologically in rheumatoid arthritis (RA)?
8. Which substance of urine is detected serologically in pregnancy tests?
9. What is the nature of a serological reaction employed in a C-reactive protein (CRP) test?
10. What is the nature of a serological reaction used in a Venereal Disease Research Laboratory (VDRL) test for syphilis?
11. Which serological test is performed in the diagnosis of a Rocky Mountain spotted fever?
12. Which serological test is commonly used to detect recent infection caused by β hemolytic streptococci, Lancefield Group A?
13. Which serological test is used to differentiate between hepatitis A and hepatitis B?
14. Which non-specific antigen is used in both the VDRL and Kolmer complement-fixation tests?
15. What is the source of erythrocytes used in the indicator system of the complement-fixation test?
16. Which skin test is carried out in the detection of infection with *Mycobacterium tuberculosis*?
17. What is the name of the substance that is capable of rendering immunity without harming the patient?
18. Which class of immunoglobulins are most frequently seen in agglutination reactions?
19. Which antibody leads to the occurrence of the prozone phenomenon?
20. Which type of serological reaction finds its application in medico-legal work (forensic medicine)?
21. Which class of immunoglobulins can mediate atopic allergies?
22. Which cell is the principal source of Interleukin 2 (IL-2)?
23. Which complement protein is present in the highest concentration in human serum?
24. Which ion is essential as a cofactor in the complement cascade?
25. How are monoclonal antibodies produced?
26. Which rickettsial organism gives a characteristic pattern OX-19: +ve; OX-2: +ve; OX-K: 0 on a Weil-Felix test?
27. Which is a B cell surface marker engaged in T and B cell cooperation?

Answers

1. Adjuvant
2. Hapten (partial antigen)
3. Gelatin
4. IgM
5. IgG
6. IgG
7. IgG
8. Human chorionic gonadotropin (hCG)
9. Precipitation
10. Flocculation reaction
11. Weil-Felix test
12. Antistreptolysin O (ASO) test of Rantz and Randall
13. HbsAg (Australia antigen) test
14. Cardiolipin-lecithin
15. Sheep
16. Mantoux test
17. Toxoid (anatoxin)
18. IgM
19. Blocking antibody
20. Precipitation
21. IgE
22. T cell
23. C3
24. Mg^{++}
25. Hybridomas
26. Rocky Mountain spotted fever
27. MHC class II antigens

Section IV: Clinical Microbiology

Chapter 35

Sterilization

Introduction

Sterilization is a process that completely removes or kills all living microorganisms present in a given object or a given area. Sterilization methods may be grouped as under:

1. Physical
2. Chemical
3. Mechanical

1. Physical

Physical agents commonly used are heat and radiation. Heat is used in two forms:

a. Dry heat
b. Moist heat

a. Dry heat
Dry heat has a relatively low power of penetration. The destructive effect of dry heat is due to the coagulation of the cell protein. Vegetative forms of bacteria are destroyed after 1 1/2 to 2 hours of exposure at 100°C. But, bacterial endospores are destroyed after 3 hours of exposure at 140°C or 1 hour of exposure at 160°C. Important applications of dry heat are discussed below:

(i) Incineration
Incineration is a process of burning disposable and contaminated materials. The actual burning of material destroys microorganisms. Incineration is used for the destruction of carcasses, infected laboratory animals, and other infected materials to be disposed of.

(ii) Flaming
The naked flame is used to sterilize platinum wire loops, needles, glass slides, coverslips, or other non-flammable objects.

(iii) Hot air:
Satisfactory sterilization in a hot air oven requires 160°C for 1 hour, provided the door of the oven is not opened during this period. Glassware (Petri dishes, pipettes, flasks, bottles, test tubes), needles, syringes, powders, gauze dressings, petroleum, and other oily materials are sterilized by a hot air oven. Precautions to be taken during its operation are:

1. The glassware should be completely dry.
2. The oven must be at room temperature while keeping the glassware. Thereafter, the oven is put on and the temperature is adjusted according to the requirement.
3. It is advisable to let the oven cool before taking out the glassware.

This practice avoids cracking of the glass.

b. Moist heat

Robert Koch demonstrated and applied the marked bactericidal action of moist heat. Moist heat destroys both vegetative and spore forms at much lower temperatures than those required by dry heat because:

1. It has more power of penetration.
2. It denatures the protein more easily.
3. It has better heat conductivity.

Important applications of moist heat are discussed below:

(i) Boiling

Boiling is the easiest method. It is a common method for sterilizing syringes and blunt instruments. It readily destroys vegetative microorganisms (bacteria, fungi, and viruses) in a few minutes. For example, *Neisseria gonorrhoeae* can be destroyed at 50°C in 3 minutes. Some spores are destroyed in 30 minutes. But, certain spores are not destroyed even after exposing them for 24 hours or longer. Two percent sodium carbonate solution may be added in boiling water to speed up the destruction of spores. Moreover, it helps prevent rusting of instruments. Precautions to be taken during boiling are:

1. Instruments to be sterilized by this method should be cleaned thoroughly.
2. The time of sterilization is considered only after reaching the temperature of boiling water to 100°C.
3. No instrument should be added or removed from the boiling water bath during the process.
4. The boiling water bath should be covered with a lid.
5. The boiling period for rubber articles should not exceed 5 minutes. After five minutes, they should immediately be removed from the water bath.
6. Boiling time should be 5 minutes more for every 1000 feet above sea level because the boiling temperature of water decreases at higher altitudes.

Limitation:

Boiling is not a very safe sterilization method.

(ii) Pasteurization:

Pasteurization is a common method in the dairy industry. Milk is heated at 62°C for 30 minutes. In the process, all non-spore-forming pathogens (e.g., *Mycobacterium tuberculosis* and *Brucella abortus*) and other microorganisms are destroyed without affecting the chemical composition of milk.

(iii) Tyndallization:

Tyndallization is also called fractional or intermittent sterilization. In this method, the material is exposed to free-flowing steam at atmospheric pressure (100°C) for 30 minutes for three successive days. All vegetative forms present in the culture medium are killed at the first heating stage. But, spores remain alive during this first stage. Therefore, the culture medium is incubated after the first heating stage to allow the spores to germinate (i.e., heat resistant spores are converted into heat-sensitive vegetative cells). These newly formed vegetative cells are destroyed at the second heating stage. Finally, the third heating stage ensures complete sterilization.

Culture media (e.g., gelatin and egg-albumin containing media) that cannot withstand autoclaving temperature are subject to sterilization by tyndallization.
Vaccines and sera are sterilized at 55°-60°C for 1 hour for 5 or 6 successive days since these materials cannot withstand 100°C.

(iv) Autoclaving (see Fig. 35.1):
An autoclave is a basic equipment for any microbiological laboratory. Generally, though not always, the 2 is operated at a pressure of approximately 15 lbs/in^2 (121°C) for 15-20 minutes. It varies somewhat depending upon the nature and quality of the material to be autoclaved. Precautions to be taken during autoclaving are:

1. Materials to be sterilized by autoclaving are loosely packed and the bundles are small and kept separately in a closed chamber.
2. All the air in the closed chamber is to be displaced by the incoming steam.
3. The thermometer should measure 121°C without decreasing for 20 minutes.
4. In the case of autoclaving of liquids, the pressure should fall gradually while shutting off the autoclave, because the sudden release of pressure causes the liquids to boil in the containers, wetting the cotton plugs, and blowing them out.
5. If the articles are damaged by prolonged heating or evaporation, allow them to cool promptly before removing them from the chamber.

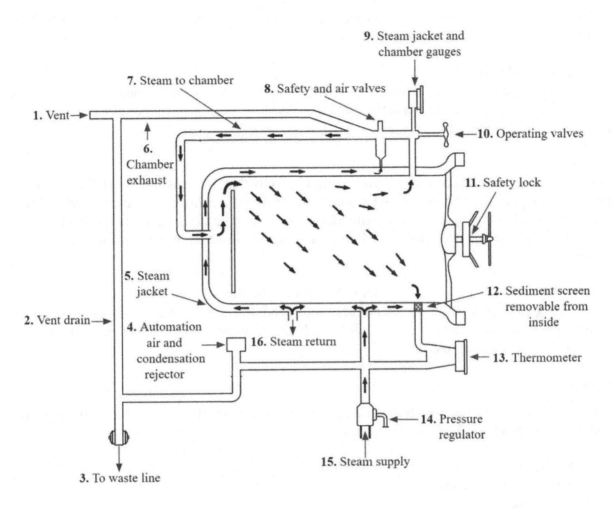

9. Steam jacket and chamber gauges

7. Steam to chamber

8. Safety and air valves

1. Vent

6. Chamber exhaust

10. Operating valves

11. Safety lock

5. Steam jacket

2. Vent drain

4. Automation air and condensation rejector

16. Steam return

12. Sediment screen removable from inside

13. Thermometer

14. Pressure regulator

15. Steam supply

3. To waste line

Fig. 35.1: Autoclave - a basic instrument for microbiological laboratory.

The information regarding time, pressure, and temperature needed for different materials to satisfactorily sterilize is provided in Table 35.1.

Table 35.1: The information regarding time, pressure, and temperature needed for different materials for satisfactory sterilization

Article	Time (mins)	Pressure (lbs/in^2)	Temperature (°C)
Instruments	30-40	22	121
Syringes	15-20	18-20	115-118
Gloves, catheters, and rubber articles	15	15	115-118
Culture media	20	20	116-118
Empty bottles and injections	15	15	115-117

Note: It is not possible to sterilize mineral oil or petroleum products by autoclaving since steam does not penetrate them.

Factors affecting autoclaving include temperature, moisture, pressure, time, entrapped air, and the nature of the load.

(v) High vacuum sterilizer
This sterilizer is a new type of sterilizer in which compressed steam under vacuum is used. Thus, this method has shortened the sterilizing time. It is used for sterilizing rubber gloves and clothes at 33 lbs/in^2 for 5-7 minutes.

Radiation
Irradiation is the best alternative for sterilizing materials that are sensitive to heat or chemical agents. It is a type of cold sterilization because it sterilizes without heating. There are two types of radiation, namely ionizing and nonionizing. Ionizing radiation includes gamma rays and X-rays. Gamma radiation is the most popular form of radiation sterilization in medicine and healthcare-related fields.

Nonionizing radiation such as ultraviolet (UV) rays can be successfully used to disinfect surgical rooms, tissues for grafting, drugs, meat, nuts, etc. It should be noted that UV radiation is not as penetrating as ionizing radiation. Ultraviolet radiation causes massive dimerization (e.g., T-T dimer) that is detrimental to cells.

2. Chemical

Chemical agents are used for sterilization purposes. The type of chemical agent required for sterilization depends on the following factors:

1. Nature and concentration of the chemical agent
2. Microorganism involved
3. Temperature
4. Time
5. Menstruum in which reaction occurs

Most of the chemical agents have bactericidal as well as bacteriostatic action, depending upon the concentration used. For example, phenol acts as a bactericidal agent (1:20) as well as a bacteriostatic agent (1:80).

(i) Acids:
Acids exercise a disinfecting effect that is dependent on the degree of electrolytic dissociation (i.e., on the concentration of the H ions). Generally, inorganic acids are more active than organic acids. Thus, inorganic acids (HNO_3, HC1, and H_2SO_4) are powerful bactericidal agents.

Glassware (e.g., bottles, pipettes, and test tubes) can quickly be sterilized by immersing them in a strong mineral acid and then thoroughly washing them with boiling water. Chromic acid (a mixture of $K_2Cr_2O_7$ and H_2SO_4) is routinely used for cleaning glassware. Moreover, it removes the greasy matter, protein, pus, and similar materials associated with the glassware.

(ii) Alkalis:

Alkalis have a disinfecting effect in proportion to the degree of electrolytic dissociation (i.e., to the concentration of the OH⁻ ions). Generally, H^+ ions exert a more disinfecting effect than OH ions.

KOH and NaOH are powerful disinfectants. Thus, alkalis are used in the manufacture of soaps. Caustic action of alkali is prohibited in the treatment of wounds.

(iii) Oxidizing agents:

Some chemical compounds readily give up nascent oxygen and are called oxidizing agents. This nascent oxygen has a strong disinfecting action. Oxidizing agents are not effective in the presence of organic matter (e.g., blood, pus, or lymph) since nascent oxygen combines indiscriminately with any associated organic compounds. Thus, hydrogen peroxide, potassium permanganate, and sodium perborate are used as oxidizing agents.

(iv) Halogens:

Halogens are strong disinfectants. They are difficult to apply in practice since they disintegrate rapidly in the presence of water. The disinfecting effect of halogens tends to be inversely proportional to their atomic weights. So, the order of their bactericidal action is chlorine, bromine, and iodine.

a. *Chlorine and its derivatives*

Chlorine gas is a highly effective disinfectant. It is used extensively for the disinfection of drinking and swimming-pool water in a free state. The content of Cl_2 gas in water should be in the range of 0.5-1.0 parts per million parts of water.

Calcium hypochlorite ($CaClO_2$) or bleaching powder exerts its disinfecting action due to the breakdown of calcium hypochlorite to hypochlorous acids. It is mostly used for the disinfection of excreta. For this purpose, a 5 percent solution of $CaClO_2$ is mixed with an equal amount of feces or urine and left for one hour before disposing it into the sewer. Typhoid bacilli can be destroyed by a 1:100,000 $CaClO_2$ solution in 24 hours.

Sodium hypochlorite ($NaClO_2$) solution (5-25%) is sold in the market as a laundry bleach. A mixture of bleaching powder and boric acid, called Eusol, is used for disinfecting wounds.

b. *Iodine and its derivatives*

Iodine is a strong disinfectant among the halogens. It is used extensively as a tincture (alcoholic solution of iodine) or iodoform (dry form). The tincture is used for sterilizing the skin. A promising development has been the combination of a compound of iodine and a non-ionic detergent. The resulting product is called iodophor. Iodophors are water-soluble, less staining action, and increased disinfecting activity.

(v) Alcohols and ether:

The bactericidal action of absolute alcohol is limited. The bactericidal action of alcohol becomes more effective after dilution with water. For example, absolute alcohol has no killing effect on staphylococci even after the treatment of several days. But, 50% or 70% of alcohol can destroy them in about 1 hour. Methylated spirit is used to disinfect the skin before hypodermic injections.

Formaldehyde, prepared from methyl alcohol, has wide applications as formalin (40% aqueous solution of formaldehyde) and also in the gaseous state for fumigation of rooms. Some surgical instruments cannot be sterilized by heat and they are sterilized by formalin vapor. An atmosphere saturated with formalin vapor for 24 hours is needed for satisfactory sterilization. It should be noted that absolute alcohol loses the bactericidal action of most disinfectants while using alcohol as a solvent. Ether is a weak bactericidal agent.

(vi) Dyes:
Organic dyes (e.g., crystal violet, gentian violet, and brilliant green) are useful as bactericidal agents. For example, gentian violet (1:100,000) exercises strong bactericidal action against Gram-positive microorganisms but has little effect on Gram-negative bacteria. 1% gentian violet is used for boils and burn cases. Certain selective culture media make use of dyes. For example, brilliant green is used as an inhibitory agent for the isolation of typhoid bacilli.

(vii) The carbolic acid family:
Members of this family are coal-tar products. Except for phenol, they are almost insoluble in water and form colloidal suspensions. Phenol is poisonous and corrosive. Its odor is objectionable. The concentration of phenol determines whether it is bacteriostatic or bactericidal. Phenol is fairly effective against vegetative bacteria, tubercle bacilli, and certain fungi. But, it cannot destroy spores and viruses. Phenol is an excellent disinfectant for blood, pus, sputum, feces, and albuminous materials. 0.5 to 1.0% of phenol can safely be used for disinfection of skin, since a stronger solution may kill the tissue. Five percent of carbolic lotion is used for carbolization of theaters and to disinfect contaminated linens and clothes by soaking them for 24 hours.

Cresol is also corrosive to living tissues. It is a stronger disinfectant than phenol and it is less poisonous. 1% of cresol lotion can be used for floor disinfection. Lysol® is a solution of cresol with soap. It is used to disinfect furniture, instruments, table surfaces, floors, walls, rubber articles, rectal thermometers, and contaminated materials. Lysol® lotion is used for disinfecting articles contaminated by tuberculous patients since Lysol® is fairly effective against tubercle bacilli. For this purpose, contaminated articles are soaked in 1 to 2% Lysol® lotion for 24 hours. Pure Lysol® is used for sterilizing sharp instruments. It should be noted that Lysol®-treated sharp instruments must be rinsed with boiled or distilled water before using them to avoid its irritating effect and tissue injury on the skin.

Dettol is prepared from cresol and chlorine. It is less toxic and, therefore, can be used on wounds. Dettol is used for dressing wounds (1:80) and in obstetric (1:40).

(viii) Salts of heavy metals:
Salts of certain heavy metals (mercury, silver, copper, and zinc) exert a detrimental effect upon microorganisms. The use of the concentration of heavy metal salt is important since the concentrations of such salts have stimulating, inhibitory, and destructive effects on bacteria. Gram-positive bacteria are more susceptible to the action of metallic salts than Gram-negative bacteria. Some important metallic salts are included in Table 35.2.

Table 35.2: Some important metallic salts

Heavy metal	Salt(s)	Use(s)
Mercury	Merthiolate	– As a skin disinfectant – As a preservative in some vaccines
	Mercurochrome	– As a skin antiseptic
Silver	Argyrol	– 20% aqueous solution in the treatment of infections of the mucous membrane of the eyes, nose, and urethra
Copper	Copper sulfate	– To control algal growth in open water reservoirs – As a fungicidal agent in garden sprays

(ix) Ethylene oxide (C_2H_4O):

Heat- or moisture-sensitive materials (e.g., medical devices and disposable plastic syringes) are sterilized by using ethylene oxide gas (gaseous sterilization). It causes the alkylation of proteins and nucleic acids, thus interfering with the normal metabolism and replication of microbes.

3. Mechanical

Certain materials (e.g., blood, serum, and certain sugars) are heat-sensitive. Therefore, they cannot be sterilized by heat. Under such circumstances, mechanical methods can be used for sterilizing purposes.

Filtration is a mechanical means for sterilizing certain liquids that cannot be heated up to sterilizing temperature. This is accomplished by passing liquid material through a bacteria-proof filter. Bacteria are removed while filtering liquid in two ways:

1. Bacteria are held back due to a smaller pore size than bacterial size.
2. The electrical charge between the filter and the bacterial surface is different. This leads to the adsorption of bacteria on the inner surface of the filter. The main types of bacterial filters include membrane filter, diatomaceous earth filter, Chamberland filter, and Seitz filter.

Unfortunately, soluble substances (e.g., toxins) cannot be removed from the material in question.

Also, airborne contaminants can be removed by filtration. Usually, high-efficiency particulate air (HEPA) filters are extensively used to supply contaminant-free air to hospital rooms and biosafety cabinets.

Conclusion

Autoclaving is a gold standard method of sterilization for a wide variety of materials. However, the chemical agents are the only choice in certain circumstances, e.g., disinfection of working surfaces. Most of the chemical agents only reduce the microbial load to safe levels. Ideal antiseptics and disinfectants kill microbes in the shortest possible time without harming the living tissues and inanimate objects, respectively.

Chapter 36

Staining Techniques

Introduction

Many microorganisms are omnipresent. They are found not only in the environment (e.g., soil, air, and water) but also in various parts of the human body. Some of them are pathogenic bacteria that may harm the body. On the other hand, some bacteria are part of the normal flora of the body, e.g., *Escherichia coli*, a commensal of the digestive tract. Morphologically, they may be round (coccus), rod-shaped (bacillus), or coiled forms (spirochete). In some bacterial species, cells remain together and form a particular type of arrangement (e.g., pairs, chains, and irregular clusters) following the process of cell-division as shown in Fig. 36.1.

Group	Appearance	Figure		
		(i)	(ii)	(iii)
Cocci	Spheres	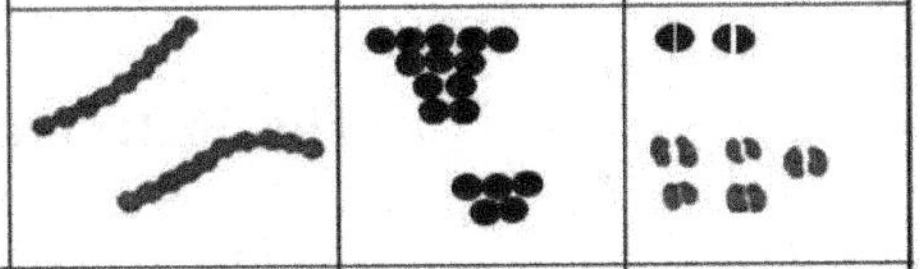		
Bacilli	Rods	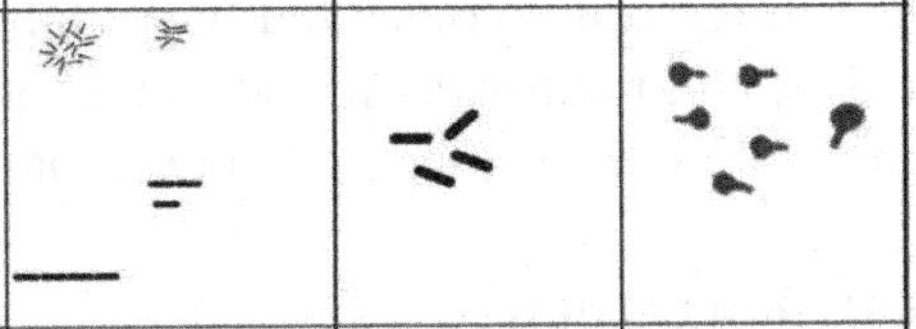		
Spirochetes	Coiled forms	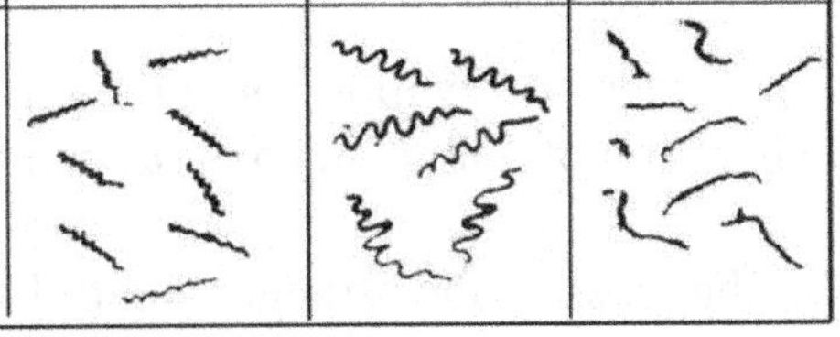		

Fig. 36.1: Morphology of bacteria.

Bacteria are unicellular prokaryotic microorganisms. They possess various types of cellular structures, namely endospores, flagella, pili, capsules, and metachromatic granules as shown in Fig. 36.2.

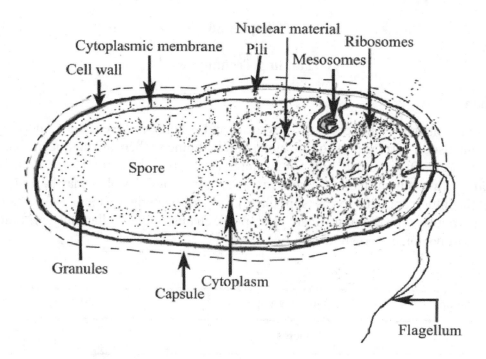

Fig. 36.2: Structure of a bacterial cell.

These structures can be observed by suitable staining techniques. Staining techniques are quick, inexpensive, and relatively simple to perform. For example, *Clostridium tetani* can be identified by demonstrating the presence of a terminal endospore in a Gram-positive bacillus.

Why is staining required?

Staining provides information about the physiology and primary criteria used in the identification and classification of unknown bacterial cultures:

1. The shape, size, and arrangement of bacterial cells can be studied.
2. The presence or absence of cellular parts can be known, e.g., endospores, flagella, and metachromatic granules.
3. The chemical nature of various cellular components can be understood, e.g., acidic, basic, or neutral.
4. Bacterial cells and their structures too thin to be seen under the ordinary microscope can be made visible. This is accomplished by impregnation of silver on the surface, increasing the thickness.
5. The permeability property of cells can be studied by vital staining.
6. Stained smears can be preserved as a permanent record for future study.

Factors affecting the staining procedure

1. The glass slide should be clean, dry, grease-free, and without scratches.
2. The thin and uniform smear should be prepared in the limited area marked with the help of a marker.
3. The smear is fixed by a physical agent (e.g., heat) or a chemical agent (e.g., formalin and mercuric chloride), depending upon the nature of cells and their parts to be demonstrated.

260

4. Nature and concentration of stain used in the staining technique.
5. Use of a mordant.
6. Time of stain reaction: Weak stains allowed to react for a long period yields better results than strong stains allowed to react for a short period.
7. Decolorization of smear in differential staining procedures.

Staining techniques may be divided into three categories:

A. **Simple stains:** use only one stain
B. **Differential stains:** help in the differentiation of two different groups of cells or structures within a cell
C. **Special stains:** aid to accentuate a specific structure of a cell

A. Simple (monochrome) stains

The monochrome staining technique is relatively simple to perform because it involves the use of only one stain during the method. It is very useful for studying the morphology (i.e., size, shape, and arrangement) of bacteria, yeasts, and related microorganisms.

Principle
Since the electrical charge on the surface of bacteria is negative (i.e., acidic), it is easy to color them using a positively charged stain called a basic stain e.g., methylene blue, crystal violet, and safranin). In other words, there is an attraction between the two oppositely charged molecules.

Test organism
Corynebacterium diphtheriae

Procedure
1. Cover the fixed film with methylene blue for 3 minutes.
2. Wash off with tap water.
3. Allow it to air-dry by keeping the slide vertical on a draining rack.
4. Examine it under an oil-immersion lens.

Results
Blue-colored cells in different forms, namely club-, needle-, or sperm-shaped seen.

B. Differential stains

1. Gram stain

The Gram staining technique was developed by Hans Christian Gram (1884). This is a differential staining technique because it enables to classify bacteria into two large groups:

1.Gram-positive (stained dark purple)
2.Gram-negative (stained pink)

Test organisms
(i) Staphylococcus aureus

(ii) Escherichia coli

Procedure
1. Fix the smear by passing the slide over the flame.
2. Cover the slide completely with the violet stain and allow it to react for 1 minute.
3. Replace the stain with Gram's iodine for 1 minute.
4. Drain off the solution and rinse it with tap water.
5. Wash off with 95% alcohol and continue until no more color comes off the smear.
6. Wash the smear with water.
7. Flood the smear with safranin for 2 minutes.
8. Wash off with water.
9. Drain and allow it to air-dry.

Results

Cells of *S. aureus* and *E. coli* stain purple (Gram-positive) and pink (Gram-negative), respectively.

Recognition of the common bacterial morphotypes is listed in Table 36.1.

Table 36.1: Gram reaction and common bacterial morphotypes

Morphotype/ Gram reaction	Description	Group(s)
Gram-positive:		
cocci	– chains	– *Streptococcus, Peptostreptococcus*
	– pairs, short chains, clusters	– *Staphylococcus, Peptococcus*
	– pairs, lancet-shaped forms	– *Pneumococcus*
bacilli	– large, broad, square-ended	– *Bacillus, Clostridium*
	– small – may occur in palisades	– *Corynebacterium, Listeria*
	– long, slender in chains, branching	– *Lactobacillus, Actinomyces, Nocardia*

Table 36.1 (cont.): Gram reaction and common bacterial morphotypes

Morphotype/ Gram reaction	Description	Group(s)
Gram-negative:		
diplococci	– long, slender in chains, branching	– *Lactobacillus, Actinomyces,* and *Nocardia*
	– Coffee-bean, intracellular	– *Neisseria, Branhamella,* and *Veillonella*
coccobacilli	– Small, single or pairs extracellular	– *Acinetobacter, Moraxella,* and *Haemophilus*
	– Large, plump, bipolar staining comma-shaped slender	– Enteric bacteria, *Campylobacter, Vibrio,* and *Pseudomonas*
bacilli	– Elongated, occur as end-to-end pairs, intensely stained. Pleomorphic, coccobacillary pointed end filaments	– *Bacteroides* – *Fusobacterium*

Applications

Gram staining results are valuable in the rapid presumptive diagnosis of many diseases as listed below:

(i) Cerebrospinal fluid (CSF)
Diagnosis: Meningitis
- Gram-negative, kidney-shaped diplococci: *N. meningitidis*
- Pleomorphic, Gram-negative coccobacilli: *H. influenzae*
- Gram-positive, lancet-shaped diplococci: *Strep. pneumoniae*
- Gram-positive cocci in pairs and short chains: Lancefield's group B streptococci
- Small Gram-positive rods: *L. monocytogenes*
- Spherical Gram-variable encapsulated budding yeasts: *Crypt. neoformans*

(ii) Skin lesions
Diagnosis: Pyoderma
- Gram-positive cocci in pairs and chains: Group A β-hemolytic streptococci, *Staph. aureus* or both
- Large Gram-positive rods with blunt ends, single, and short chains: *B. anthracis*

(iii) Stool
Diagnosis: Acute enteritis
- Numerous PMNs with comma-shaped pleomorphic Gram-negative rods: *Campy. jejuni*

(iv) Urethral exudate
Diagnosis: Urethritis

- Gram-negative diplococci inside PMNs: *N. gonorrhoeae*

It should be noted that the gonococcus may be indistinguishable on the smear from *Acinetobacter* (Mima-Herellea) and *Moraxella*.

(v) Urine
Diagnosis: Cystitis
  - Plump Gram-negative rods 2-3μ in length: *E. coli*

(vi) Vaginal secretions
Diagnosis: Bacterial vaginosis
  - Numerous clue cells covered by small Gram-variable rods: *G. vaginalis*

(vii) Pus
Diagnosis: Brain abscess
  - The typical presence of proteinaceous debris in the center of which is a cluster of short Gram-negative rods: *Bacteroides*
  - Many brain abscesses are the result of a mixture of microorganisms, one of which is usually an anaerobe.

(viii) Peritoneal fluid
Diagnosis: Peritonitis
  - Much proteinaceous material, occasional pus cells, and Gram-positive cocci in pairs and chains: enterococci

(ix) Purulent discharge
Diagnosis: Infected incision of the eye
  - Many pus cells and Gram-positive cocci in pairs and chains: Group A β-hemolytic streptococci

(x) Sputum
Diagnosis: Pneumonia
  - Many PMNs and Gram-positive lancet- or helmet-shaped diplococci: *Strep. pneumoniae*
  - Gram-positive cocci in pairs, tetrads, and clusters commonly within PMNs: *Staph. aureus*
  - PMNs and encapsulated Gram-negative rods: *Klebsiella pneumoniae*

(xi) Bone aspirate or pus
Diagnosis: Osteomyelitis
  - Many PMNs and Gram-positive cocci: *Staph. aureus*

(xii) Abscess
Diagnosis: Gas gangrene
  - Cellular debris, degenerating cells, and large darkly-staining Gram-positive rods: typical of clostridia

One seldom sees spores in clinical material with *Clostridium perfringens*.

(xiii) Swab (from advancing margin)
Diagnosis: Cellulitis
- Many PMNs and Gram-positive cocci in clusters: *Staph. aureus*

2. Acid-fast (Ziehl-Neelsen) stain

Ziehl-Neelsen or acid-fast staining method is useful for the laboratory diagnosis of tuberculosis and leprosy (Hansen's disease).

This is also a differential staining method since it divides microorganisms into two groups:
1. Acid-fast organisms (stained red)
2. Non-acid-fast organisms (stained blue)

Principle
Acid-fast organisms are not decolorized by acid alcohol once they have been stained since they have a high content of fatty substances (mycolic acid).

Test organism
Mycobacterium tuberculosis

Procedure
1. Cover the fixed smear with carbol fuchsin, and heat it until the steam rises.
2. Allow it to stain for 5 minutes, applying heat intermittently.
3. Wash off gently with tap water.
4. Decolorize with 20% H_2SO_4 and 90% alcohol for 5 minutes and 2 minutes, respectively. (Use 5% H_2SO_4 while decolorizing smear of *M. leprae*).
5. Wash with tap water and drain.
6. Cover the smear with methylene blue or malachite green for 30 seconds.
7. Wash well with tap water and allow it to dry in the air.

Results
Acid-fast organisms stain bright pink against blue or green background (see Fig. 36.3).

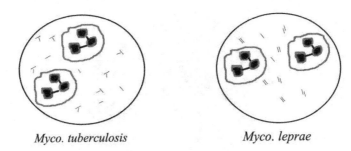

Myco. tuberculosis   *Myco. leprae*

Fig. 36.3: Acid-fast bacilli.

Fluorochrome stains (e.g., auramine O) are relatively more sensitive than conventional carbol-fuchsin stains, namely Ziehl-Neelsen and Kinyoun (a cold stain).

3. Endospore stain (Schaeffer-Fulton method)

Endospores (spores) are heat-resistant structures that are formed by some genera of bacteria, e.g., *Bacillus* and *Clostridium*. They germinate to form vegetative cells when environmental conditions become favorable. Stains cannot penetrate the spore coat in cold conditions. Based on the presence or absence of spores, bacteria are divided into two categories:

1. Spore formers
2. Non-spore formers

Principle
Bacterial endospores once stained by malachite green (primary stain) in hot condition retain green color as opposed to the vegetative cells that take up safranin (secondary stain) and appear pink.

Test organism
Bacillus megaterium

Procedure
1. Place the heat-fixed slide over a screened water bath and then add malachite green.
2. Keep the slide over the steaming water bath for 5 minutes. Be sure to add more stain to avoid drying out of the stain.
3. Remove the slide from the steaming water bath and rinse the slide with a gentle flow of tap water. Do not forget to wash off any stain leftover on the bottom of the slide.
4. Cover the smear with safranin and allow it to react for 30-60 seconds.
5. Wash off the stain with tap water and blot dry.
6. Examine the smear using an oil-immersion lens and record the results.

Results
Endospores appear green against the pink-colored vegetative cells (see Fig. 36.4)

Alternatively, bacterial endospores can be demonstrated using carbol fuchsin (primary stain) and methylene blue (secondary or counterstain). Endospores appear as oval red structures against the blue-colored vegetative cells.

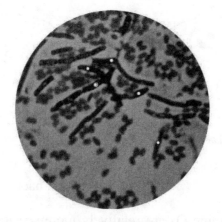

Fig. 36.4: Endospore of *B. megaterium*.

C. Special stains

1. Capsule stain

Some bacteria and yeasts form a thick layer of a capsular substance surrounding the cell wall. It is made up of polysaccharides or polypeptides that offer resistance against phagocytosis. It is neither an acidic nor a basic structure.

Principle
The India ink, being an acidic (anionic) stain, fails to stain cells and capsules but the background. However, counterstaining with a basic (cationic) stain can color the negatively charged cells.

Test organism
Klebsiella pneumoniae (> 5 days old culture)

Procedure
1. Place a drop of India ink on a clean microscope slide (close to the frosted edge).
2. Using a sterile technique, apply a loopful of cells and mix with a drop of stain. Avoid clumps of cells to make an ideal smear.
3. Using another clean microscope slide at an angle of 45°, spread the contents of a drop gently to make a thin film.
4. Allow the film to air-dry. Do not heat or blot dry.
5. Apply crystal violet and allow it to react for 1 minute.
6. Rinse the smear gently with tap water.
7. Allow the smear to air-dry.
8. Examine the smear under an oil-immersion lens.

Results
Capsules appear clear (halo-like) areas surrounding purple-colored cells against the dark background (see Fig. 36.5).

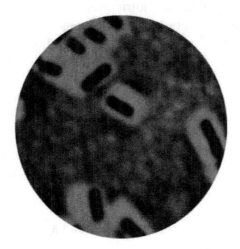

Fig. 36.5: *Klebsiella pneumoniae* and its capsule.

2. Negative stain

The negative staining technique is superior to other staining techniques to study cellular morphology because cells remain unstained without distortion of their features.

Principle
The nigrosin, an acidic (anionic) stain, is repelled by a negatively charged surface of cells, leaving them unstained against the dark background. Alternatively, India ink may be used as an acidic stain.

Test organism
Spirillum volutans

Procedure
1. Place a drop of nigrosin (10%) on a clean microscope slide (adjacent to the frosted edge).
2. Using an aseptic technique, transfer a loopful of bacterial cells and mix with a drop of nigrosin. Avoid clumps of cells to make a satisfactory smear.
3. Using another clean microscope slide at an angle of 45°, spread the contents of a drop to make a thin smear.
4. Allow the smear to air-dry.
5. Examine the smear using an oil-immersion lens.

Results
Colorless (unstained) spirochetes against the dark background seen.

3. Flagella (Leifson) stain

Flagella are thin and fragile appendages present in some bacteria. They cannot be visualized under a compound light microscope unless artificially thickened. Based on their presence, number, and arrangement, bacteria are grouped as under:

1. Absence of flagella: atrichous
2. Presence of a single polar flagellum: monotrichous
3. Presence of tufts of flagella at each pole: lophotrichous
4. Presence of one or more flagella at both poles: amphitrichous
5. Presence of flagella all over the cell surface: peritrichous

Therefore, these traits aid in the phenotypic characterization and classification of bacteria.

Principle
The mordant (e.g., tannic acid) gets deposited on the surface of flagella, thus thickening them to visualize within the limits of resolving power of a compound light microscope.

Test organism
Proteus vulgaris (18-48 hours old culture grown on a blood agar medium)

Procedure
a. Preparation of smear
1. Using a wax pencil, mark a rectangular area around a clear part of a microscope slide.
2. Place a drop of distilled water approximately 1 cm far from the frosted edge.
3. Using a sterile technique, charge the sterile wire loop by a gentle touching of a colony followed by a light touching of the charged wire loop to only the drop of water. Avoid mixing.
4. Allow the drop to flow toward the other end of the slide.
5. Allow the film to air-dry. Avoid heat-fixation.

b. Staining procedure
1. Flood the smear with flagella stain (pararosaniline acetate or basic fuchsin) and allow it to remain on the bacterial film for approximately 15 minutes until a precipitate appears. The reaction time is influenced by some variables, e.g., the age of the stain and the room temperature.
2. Rinse the smear by keeping the slide on a staining rack and let the water run over the surface of the slide.
3. Following the rinsing step, put the slide in a tilted position to allow water to run off the slide.
4. Allow the smear to air-dry.
5. Examine the smear using an oil-immersion lens and record the results.

Results
Flagella, including the bacterial cells, stain red.

4. Fontana's stain

Spirochetes are thin-walled, flexible, and spiral-shaped Gram-negative bacteria. They are measured in their length and width. They use axial filaments for their motility.

Principle
Artificial thickening under silver oxide precipitates formed following heat treatment to ammoniacal silver nitrate (Fontana's stain) enables one to visualize under a compound light microscope.

Test organism
Treponema pallidum

Procedure
1. Prepare a thin smear on a clean microscope slide and allow it to air-dry.
2. Treat the smear three times at an interval of 1 minute, for 30 seconds each time, with Fontana's fixative.
3. Wash off the fixative with absolute alcohol, allowing it to react for 3 minutes.
4. Drain off the excess alcohol and dry the smear by burning off the residue.
5. Cover the smear with Fontana's mordant, heating it till steam rises, then let the mordant remain on the smear for 30 seconds.
6. Wash well with distilled water and again dry the slide.

7. Cover the smear with the ammoniacal silver nitrate solution, heating it till the steam rises, then let the solution remain on the smear for 30 seconds. The film turns brown.
8. Wash well with distilled water and keep the slide on its end in a draining rack for drying.

Results
The spirochetes appear brownish-black against a brownish-yellow background.

5. Feulgen stain

Feulgen stain is a valuable stain in histology to detect chromosomal material or DNA.

Some clinical isolates can easily be identified by staining techniques alone as shown in Table 36.2.

Table 36.2: Identification of bacteria by staining techniques

Bacterial species	Staining technique	Description	Disease caused
Mycobacterium leprae	ZNCF	pink slender rods occurring singly in parallel bundles or globular masses	leprosy
M. tuberculosis	ZNCF	pink slender rods occurring singly or angularly	tuberculosis
Neisseria gonorrhoeae	Gram	Gram-negative bean-shaped diplococci are seen inside of neutrophils	gonorrhea
N. meningitidis	Gram	Gram-negative diplococci with flat sides inside and found inside neutrophils	meningitis
Clostridium tetani	Gram	Gram-positive pointed rods with terminal spore, giving the appearance of a 'drum-stick'	tetanus (lock-jaw)
Treponema pallidum	Fontana	brownish-black slender spirals against a brownish-yellow background	Syphilis
Corynebacterium diphtheriae	Neisser	yellow rods with blue metachromatic granules, giving a 'club' appearance	diphtheria
Yersinia pestis	Wayson	Gram-negative rods show a bipolar appearance, resembling safety pins	plague

Chapter 37

Specimens, Growth Media, and Anaerobiosis

Introduction

Laboratory diagnosis is crucial in the management of the patient. For many diseases, it is necessary to confirm the clinical diagnosis for successful treatment. Despite the accuracy of clinical diagnosis, the etiological agent for a bacterial infection is to be recovered as a pure culture for the susceptibility test. Therefore, it is important to understand the basics of a disease process, e.g., epidemiology and tissue tropism. There are various means of transmission of bacterial diseases:

1. Foods and drinks, e.g., bacillary dysentery, typhoid, and cholera
2. Air (droplet infection), e.g., tuberculosis
3. Direct contact, e.g., gonorrhea and syphilis
4. Insects, e.g., bubonic plague by the rat flea
5. Inanimate objects, e.g., diphtheria

Koch's Postulates

The relationship between a disease and a pathogen can clearly be understood from four postulates assumed by Robert Koch:

1. The pathogen must be present either alive or dead in the diseased host.
2. It must be possible to isolate the pathogen in pure culture in the laboratory.
3. When such a pure culture is introduced into a susceptible laboratory animal, typical signs and symptoms of disease must develop after an appropriate incubation period.
4. Re-isolation of a pathogen in a pure form from such an artificially developed disease must be possible.

Etiology

One has to keep in mind that simple entry of an organism into the body does not necessarily lead to the development of a disease. There are mainly three infection-determining factors:

1. Number of invading bacteria
2. Virulence of bacteria
3. The resistance offered by the host

These controlling factors are related to the development of disease as under:

$$\text{Disease} = \frac{\text{Number of bacteria x Virulence of invading bacteria}}{\text{Resistance offered by the host}}$$

Also, a definite length of the period is required before the disease becomes evident. This is called the incubation period of the disease. It may be a few days or several weeks, depending on the bacterial species involved in the infective process.

Laboratory diagnosis

Some bacterial pathogens are easily identified with the help of staining techniques. They are dealt with in chapter 36. In some cases, information about colony characteristics, presence or absence of a specific enzyme is very useful in the identification of an isolate.

Collection and care of clinical microbiology specimens

A variety of clinical specimens for routine microbiological examination are requested by health care providers. They may be bacterial (aerobic and anaerobic), fungal, parasitic (ova and cysts), or viral specimens. Unlike specimens for chemistry, hematology, immunohematology, and immunology, this draws special attention in terms of contamination with normal flora (e.g., skin and mucous membranes) and system for transport of microbiologic specimens to preserve their integrity. Some general precautions to be exercised are:

1. Collect a sufficient quantity of a representative specimen
2. Avoid contamination with indigenous flora by using only sterile equipment under aseptic conditions
3. Secure meaningful specimens before treatment
4. Label the specimen container with full details: patient's name, medical record number, date of birth, gender, date, and time of collection
5. Place the specimen container in a biohazard bag and bring the specimen to the laboratory for examination without any delay (e.g., pneumatic tube transport or a runner)
6. Use disposable rubber gloves and mask as safety measures

1. *Urine cultures:* addressed in chapter 38.

2. *Blood cultures:* Blood culture is the most widely used laboratory diagnostic test to establish the etiology of bloodstream infections, e.g., acute infective endocarditis. Typically, two blood culture bottles, namely aerobic (gray cap) and anaerobic (purple cap) are used for the detection of bacteremia or septicemia. The skin area should be well disinfected with 70% isopropyl alcohol followed by a 2% tincture of iodine swipe in concentric circles. For optimum aseptic blood collection, iodine should be allowed to remain on the skin for at least 1 minute. The septa of culture bottles are disinfected by using chlorhexidine swipes (15 seconds) before collection as well.

Usually, the nutrient broth media employed for blood cultures are supplemented with 0.025% of sodium polyanethol sulfonate (SPS) because of the following properties:

- anticoagulant
- antiphagocytic
- anticomplementary

- anti-Lysozyme
- neutralization of potential antimicrobial agents, e.g., aminoglycoside antibiotics

However, SPS may be inhibitory to some *Neisseria* spp. and *Peptostreptococcus* spp. This adverse effect can be overcome by adding 1.2% gelatin. Approximately, 5-10 mL of venous whole blood (adults) is inoculated into 50 mL each of blood culture broth, i.e., aerobic (1st) and anaerobic (2nd) bottles. In the case of children, 1-2 mL of blood is used to inoculate 20 mL of blood culture broth (pink cap). Thus, the blood-to-broth ratio is maintained between 1:5 to 1:10 to improve the recovery of true pathogens.

Guidelines recommend that the initial 2-3 paired sets of blood culture should be collected at one time or over a brief time interval from multiple anatomic sites. Additional 2-3 paired sets of blood culture may be needed if the first 2-3 blood culture results turn out negative after 24-48 hours of incubation, e.g., severe infection.

Inoculated culture bottles are swirled several times for mixing and transported immediately to a microbiology laboratory. They are then incubated at 35°C for 5 days with continuous-monitoring (24/7) blood culture instruments, e.g., BD BACTEC™ FX40. During incubation, the CO_2 based built-in fluorescence-detector system indicates positive cultures (flagged) which are then subjected to Gram stain, subculturing onto suitable media and the antimicrobial susceptibility test as per the institution's protocol.

If delayed transport of inoculated culture bottles to a microbiology laboratory is anticipated, the bottles are incubated at 35°C in a 5% CO_2 atmosphere until their transport to a microbiology laboratory.

Immediate performance of the Gram stain on all positive blood cultures and the submission of a preliminary report (presumptive diagnosis) is very helpful to the physician (Barenfanger, et al.). Following the Gram stain, subculturing is carried out on appropriate culture media as under:

1. Positive aerobic cultures: blood agar, chocolate agar, and MacConkey's agar
2. Positive anaerobic cultures: blood agar, chocolate agar, MacConkey's agar, and CDC/ PEA

The most common isolates recovered from blood cultures are:

- *Staphylococcus aureus*
- *Escherichia coli*
- other coliforms
- *Streptococcus pneumoniae*
- *Enterococcus* spp., e.g., *Enterococcus faecalis*
- *Pseudomonas aeruginosa*
- *Candida albicans*

3. Stool cultures: Stool culture may be requested by a healthcare provider in one of the following indications:

- bloody diarrhea
- tenesmus (continual feeling of the need to empty the bowel accompanied with cramping rectal pain)
- high fever
- persistent or severe signs and symptoms
- recent travel to a third world country
- known exposure to a bacterial agent
- presence of leukocytes in a fecal specimen

The fresh stool is collected in a clean, dry bedpan or a similar wide-mouth container, avoiding contamination from toilet water or urine. A portion of stool (5 g), preferably tainted with mucus, pus, or blood, is transferred to a clean leak-proof dry plastic container followed by lid replacement and transportation to a laboratory within one hour. To increase the probability to recover pathogenic bacterial agent(s), it is highly desirable to submit 2-3 stool specimens collected on separate days.

For children, a rectal swab is usually used to recover intestinal pathogens, if any.
Intestinal parasites (e.g., *Giardia lamblia*) are detected by direct microscopy in physiological saline preparation.

4. Cerebrospinal fluid (CSF): An invasive procedure called a lumbar puncture (spinal tap) is performed by experienced personnel to collect the CSF. It is collected with strict aseptic precautions. The specimen of CSF for bacteriological examination is collected second in a row while collecting multiple tubes for other tests, e.g., chemistry tests, to avoid potential skin normal flora.

It is highly recommended that the CSF specimen should be treated as STAT (urgent) and hand-delivered. Ideally, a CSF specimen received in less than one hour is centrifuged at 1000 x g for 10-15 minutes to recover sediment. The sediment is then used to perform Gram stain as well as plating on chocolate and blood agar media. If delayed processing is expected, specimens need to be inoculated to Trans-Isolate (T-I) media and incubated overnight in 3-7% CO_2 at 35°C. Specimens are never stored at 2°-8°C because the common causative agents of meningitis, namely *Haemophilus influenzae* and *Neisseria meningitidis* are susceptible to refrigeration.

5. Sputum: It includes three early mornings deeply coughed up sputum samples collected on three consecutive days. Avoidance of contamination with saliva is highly desirable during coughing.
Before acid-fast stain and plating, sputum for TB is processed as under:

1. Digestion: *N*-acetyl-L-cysteine
2. Decontamination: sodium hydroxide (NaOH)
3. Neutralization: buffer or H_2O
4. Centrifugation: 5000 rpm

Precautions must be taken during the handling of a specimen of sputum. Thus, the formation of infectious aerosols can be avoided by a careful treatment of sputum while dispatching, opening, closing, shaking, and centrifuging sputum containing vial. This explains why laboratories that process specimens supposedly loaded with pathogenic *Mycobacterium* spp. meet biosafety level 3 requirements.

6. Swabs: A swab is a simple tool used to collect microbiology specimens from different sites of the body. It is convenient to collect a representative specimen, especially from some awkward sites. For example, a flexible calcium alginate nasopharyngeal swab is used to collect a specimen from the posterior nares and pharynx.
The swabbing technique is used in cases of many infections to recover potential pathogens, e.g., eye, ear, nose, and genital.
It is recommended that two swabs should be collected: (1) for the culture (2) Gram stain.

7. Tissue: A sterile screw-cap container or anaerobic collection jar is used for collecting small pieces of tissue. A few drops of sterile saline are added to keep the specimen moist. It should be transported to a microbiology laboratory in less than 15 minutes.

8. Abscess: Using a sterile syringe and needle, a purulent material is collected after decontaminating the surface of an undrained abscess. Once the specimen is aspirated, the needle is detached followed by capping of the syringe and prompt transportation to a laboratory.
Alternatively, 5-10 mL of the aspirated material can be transferred to an evacuated anaerobic gel transport container.

9. Wound: Before the collection of a specimen, the surface of the wound is bathed with sterile normal saline to remove the superficial flora. Using a wound culture swab, the collection is made at the advancing margin of the wound. The swab is placed into a transport medium and the tip is pressed against the sponge at the bottom.

10. Genital specimens: Various female genital specimens are cultured for aerobes and anaerobes. Some specimens (e.g., endocervical, vaginal, urethra, vulva, and lochia) are processed only for aerobes as opposed to other specimens (e.g., uterus, fallopian tube, cervical aspirate, ovary, and Bartholin's gland) that are cultured for anaerobes.
Male genital specimens, namely urethral, prostatic fluid, and seminal fluid are processed only for aerobes.

11. Anaerobic cultures: Unlike aerobic cultures, anaerobic cultures need an anaerobic transport medium for maintaining their viability. Sources of specimens for anaerobic cultures are:

- deep wounds
- sterile fluids, e.g., synovial, pleural, and amniotic fluids
- abscess material, e.g., brain, lungs, and liver
- necrotic tissue, e.g., suspected cases of gas gangrene
- material from infected bites

Cultivation of bacteria

It is necessary to understand the environmental factors influencing bacterial growth before considering the growth media. These factors are:

(a) Nutrients
    1. Hydrogen donors and acceptors
    2. Carbon source
    3. Nitrogen source
    4. Minerals
    5. Growth factors
(b) pH
(c) Temperature
(d) Time
(e) Moisture
(f) Aeration
(g) Ionic strength and osmotic pressure
(h) Light

There are various types of culture media formulated to grow bacteria from a variety of pathological specimens. Some media are used in the liquid state, e.g., peptone sugar media can be used to know the ability of bacteria to ferment sugars to produce acid and/or gas. Thus, bacteria can be characterized and classified. On the other hand, the use of solid media is the only choice if one has to study the colony characteristics and to isolate the pathogen as a pure culture. Agar-agar powder is added as a solidifying agent to the liquid media. Media are designated according to the purpose of their use. They are briefly discussed below:

1. *Transport media:* Transport media preserve the viability of delicate organisms without promoting the growth of unwanted organisms during the transportation of clinical specimens from a collection center to the laboratory. Therefore, these media are designed (usually semi-solid) to include mainly buffers and salts, e.g., the inclusion of reducing agents to prevent oxidation. Some transport media and their intended uses are listed in Table 37.1.

Table 37.1: Some transport media and their intended uses

Transport medium	Purpose
Stuart	*Enterobacteriaceae*
Amies	*Enterobacteriaceae*
Cary-Blair	*Enterobacteriaceae*
Buffered glycerol saline	*Shigella* spp.
Pike's medium	*Streptococcus* spp. (throat specimens)
Activated charcoal transport medium	*Neisseria gonorrhoeae*
Alkaline peptone water	*Vibrio cholerae*
Venkatraman-Ramakrishnan (V-R)	*Vibrio cholerae*
Virus transport media (VTM)	Viruses

Apart from the use of an appropriate transport medium, it is equally important to immediately transport a clinical specimen in a leak-proof container at 4°-8°C (not CSF) with a completed requisition slip to a laboratory. If the culturing of CSF cannot be carried out immediately, it is preserved by placing the fluid in 3-7% CO_2 at 37°C or room temperature for no longer than 30 minutes.

2. Basal media: Basal media contain only basic nutrients, e.g., glucose, meat extract, NaCl, and water. Nutrient agar and trypticase soy agar (TSA) are classic and common examples of basal media that support the growth of a wide variety of bacteria, e.g., *Escherichia coli* and *Staphylococcus aureus.*

3. Enriched media: Enriched media contain additional nutrients (5% sheep blood) to facilitate the growth and multiplication of fastidious group of microorganisms. In other words, a fastidious group of bacteria fails to grow on basal media unless supplemented with special additives. Blood agar and chocolate agar are widely used as enriched culture media in clinical microbiology. For example, *Haemophilus influenzae* can be cultivated on chocolate agar but not on nutrient agar. (hemin-X factor and Isovitalex-V factor).

4. Selective media: Sometimes, it is required to use media that can favor the growth of only desired bacteria without supporting the growth of other organisms. This can be accomplished by the addition of an inhibitor to the medium. Inhibitors used for this purpose include antibiotics, stains, sodium taurocholate, phenylethyl alcohol (PEA), and so on in appropriate concentrations.

This can be well exemplified by several selective media used in the recovery of fecal pathogenic bacterial species. The sole purpose of any selective culture medium is to inhibit the overgrowing coliforms from stool samples in a selective manner. This is how enteric pathogen(s) finds better nutritional conditions to grow and multiply, thus helping in the process of their recovery. These selective culture media are tentatively grouped into three categories based on their degrees of selectivity:

1. Slightly selective, e.g., MacConkey II and eosin methylene blue (EMB), modified
2. Moderately selective, e.g., *Salmonella-Shigella* (S-S), xylose lysine deoxycholate (XLD), and Hektoen-enteric (HE)
3. Highly selective, e.g., Brilliant Green

Thus, the choice of a selective medium as a primary isolation selective medium depends on many factors, e.g., suspected enteric pathogen(s) and accompanying enteric normal flora in the given fecal specimen.

5. Differential media: Some media are specially designed just to help in the differentiation of bacteria. Usually, indicators are added to these media. For example, MacConkey's agar is a differential medium containing neutral red as an indicator. Key ingredients and their roles are as under:

1. Bile salts (sodium taurocholate): inhibits Gram-positive bacteria
2. Crystal violet: inhibits Gram-positive bacteria

3. Lactose: a fermentable sugar, allowing differentiation between lactose fermenters and lactose non-fermenters
4. Neutral red: turns acidic colonies (e.g., lactose fermenters) red/pink

Colonies of lactose fermenters (e.g., *Escherichia coli*) appear pink-red because of the precipitation of neutral red on these acidic colonies. But, the colonies of non-lactose fermenters (e.g., *Salmonella* spp. and *Shigella* spp.) remain colorless.

Blood agar is also a differential medium as it enables to differentiate between hemolytic and non-hemolytic bacteria.

6. Chromogenic media: It is a new approach that is increasingly becoming popular these days in the detection and identification of clinical isolates. Media are called chromogenic because they contain multiple chromogen-tagged substrates. Depending upon the target organism's enzyme system, a specific chromogenic substrate is used, turning the colony colored by a detached chromogen.

Chromogenic substrates, namely ONPG, X-Gal, or X-Glu are used in the formulation of such media. For example, colors of 6-chloro-3-indoxyl- and 5-iodo-3-indoxyl- are salmon and purple, respectively. Some chromogenic media and their uses are listed in Table 37.2.

Table 37.2: Some chromogenic media and their uses

Chromogenic medium	Use
ChromID MRSA	Methicillin-resistant *S. aureus*
Strepto B ID	*Streptococcus agalactiae*
CHROMagar 0157	*E. coli 0157:H7*
ChromID C. difficile	*Clostridium difficile*
CHROMagar Y. enterocolitica	*Yersinia enterocolitica*

Advantages
- Shorter turnaround time as compared to conventional media
- Ease of visual detection by direct observation of a distinct color change of the colony
- Additional tests (e.g., coagulase and fibrinolysin tests) can be performed simultaneously within the medium

7. Stool enrichment broths and media
It draws special attention to stool samples because there is a need to eliminate the normal flora of the intestinal tract. Before the inoculation on an appropriate selective culture medium, an appropriate selective enrichment broth is to be inoculated with the fecal specimen in question.

Gram-negative (GN) broth (sodium citrate and sodium deoxycholate as inhibitors) serves as the best stool enrichment broth for *Shigella* spp. Similarly, selenite F broth (selenite as an inhibitory agent) has proven to be an excellent stool enrichment broth for *Salmonella* spp. Both of these broths support the intestinal pathogens and suppress the coliforms at the same time. After about

18 hours of incubation, stool cultures are sub-cultured on appropriate selective media as shown in Table 37.3.

Table 37.3: Key ingredients of selective culture media for the isolation and identification of stool cultures

Medium	Sugar(s)	pH indicator(s)	Inhibitor(s)	Comment(s)
Brilliant Green agar	-Lactose -Sucrose	-Phenol red	-Brilliant green	-*Salmonella*: slightly pink-white opaque with red zone
Salmonella-Shigella (S-S) agar*	-Lactose	-Neutral red	-Brilliant green -Bile salts -Na-citrate	-*Salmonella*: transparent with black centers (H_2S production) -*Shigella*: transparent
Xylose lysine deoxycholate (XLD) agar	-Lactose -Sucrose -Xylose	-Phenol red	-Sodium deoxycholate	-*Salmonella*: red with black center (H_2S production) -*Shigella*: red or clear
MacConkey agar**	-Lactose	-Neutral red	-Crystal violet -Bile salts	-lactose fermenter: pink/red
Eosin methylene blue (EMB) agar, modified	-Lactose -Sucrose	-Eosin Y -Methylene blue	-Eosin Y -Methylene blue	Differentiation: Lactose fermenters from lactose non-fermenters
Hektoen-enteric (HE) agar	-Lactose -Sucrose -Salicin	-Acid fuchsin -Bromothymol blue	-Bile salts -Acid fuchsin	-*Salmonella*: blue-green with black center (H_2S production) -*Shigella*: green without black center
Campy agar	-Dextrose		-Cephalothin -Amphotericin B -Polymyxin B -Vancomycin -Trimethoprim	-*Campylobacter jejuni* and other spp. -*C. jejuni*: microaerophile that grows best at 42°C
Cefsulodin irgasan novobiocin (CIN) agar	-Mannitol	-Neutral red	-Cefsulodin -Irgasan -Novobiocin -Crystal violet -Na-deoxycholate	-*Yersinia enterocolitica*: colonies with deep-red centers with a "bull's-eye" appearance
Colistin nalidixic acid (CNA) agar			-Colistin -Nalidixic acid	-*Staphylococcus aureus*: white to golden-yellow colonies

* *Shig. sonnei* does not grow well on *Salmonella-Shigella (S-S)* agar. It can be used to recover *Yersinia enterocolitica*.
** MacConkey agar with sorbitol is used to differentiate *E. coli* 0157:H7 (colorless colonies).

Table 37.3 (cont.): Key ingredients of selective culture media for the isolation and identification of stool cultures

Medium	Sugar(s)	pH indicator(s)	Inhibitor(s)	Comment(s)
Thiosulfate citrate bile sucrose (TCBS) agar	-Sucrose	-Bromothymol blue -Thymol blue	-Ox gall -Sodium thiosulfate -Sodium citrate	*-Vibrio cholerae:* large yellow colonies
Cycloserine cefoxitin fructose agar (CCFA)	-Fructose	-Neutral red	-Cycloserine -Cefoxitin	*-Clostridium difficile:* large, circular, and yellow colonies
Deoxycholate citrate agar	-Lactose	-Neutral red	-Sodium deoxycholate -Sodium citrate	Differentiation: Lactose fermenters from lactose non-fermenters

Primary plating media include Hektoen-enteric agar (or XLD), MacConkey agar with sorbitol, Campy agar, and selenite F broth. In the case of *Yersinia* spp. and *Vibrio* spp. suspicion, selective media included are CIN agar and TCBS agar, respectively.

Enteric pathogens that are recovered during routine stool or rectal swab culture processing are:

- *Campylobacter* spp.
- *Salmonella* spp.
- *Escherichia coli* 0157:H7
- *Shigella* spp.
- *Clostridium difficile* (hospitalized patients on broad-spectrum antibiotics)
- less frequently isolated enteric pathogens include *Yersinia enterocolitica, Vibrio* spp., and *Aeromonas* spp.

8. Mycobacterial media: Some media for the primary isolation of mycobacteria contain inhibitory agents to suppress contaminants. These inhibitory agents include malachite green, lincomycin, cycloheximide, and nalidixic acid. Media used to grow mycobacteria are listed in Table 37.4.

Table 37.4: Media used to grow mycobacteria

Category	Specific culture media
Agar-based	- Middlebrook 7H10 - Middlebrook 7H11
Egg-based	- Lowenstein-Jensen - Wallenstein
Liquid	- Middlebrook 7H9 broth - Commercial broths, e.g., Bactec media

Except for sterile fluids (e.g., cerebrospinal fluid) and tissues, specimens need pretreatment before their transfer to growth media. This pretreatment step called the digestion-decontamination step helps kill any normal flora that may exist in the specimen. N-acetyl-L-cysteine (NALC)-NaOH procedure is a preferred concentration-digestion-decontamination method over zephiran-trisodium phosphate and 4% NaOH methods. Precautionary measures taken during the processing of clinical specimens include the use of a biosafety hood equipped with UV light and the use of screw-capped centrifuge tubes within screw-capped leak-proof centrifuge cups.

Thus, the possibility of aerosol formation can be avoided. After inoculation, culture media are incubated at 35°C in the dark with 5-10% CO_2 in the environment. However, media need to be incubated at 25°-30°C for *M. marinum* and *M. ulcerans*, if suspected in a given specimen. Since most mycobacteria have extended generation time (e.g., 15-22 hours for *M. tuberculosis*), culture media are incubated for 60 days, examining plates every week for the appearance of visible colonies.

Processing of specimens
Once the specimens are submitted to a microbiology laboratory, they should be processed without any delay. Processing of specimens is prioritized as under:

Urgent: In cases of life-threatening illnesses that require immediate attention, a preliminary report of laboratory results within 30-60 minutes is very crucial. Specimens treated as STAT:

- blood culture
- cerebrospinal fluid
- transtracheal aspirate
- bone marrow
- Pericardial fluid
- amniotic fluid

Routine: No immediate risk of life-threatening sequelae but require confirmatory laboratory diagnosis or observation of the efficacy of a chemotherapeutic agent. Specimens for routine processing include:

- throat
- pleural fluid
- peritoneal fluid
- burns
- eye
- genital, female (only aerobes)

Elective: Specimens that are processed expertly for confirmation rather than diagnostic purposes. Such specimens are:

- nose
- oral
- ear
- nasopharynx

- sinus
- stool/rectal swab
- genital, male

There are two methods for plating pathological specimens:

a. streak plate
b. pour plate

Usually, the streak plate method is used in clinical laboratories. The wire loop is used to streak the pathological specimens on an appropriate medium under aseptic conditions. A clinical microbiologist should take safety precautions while handling such specimens for microbiological study. Furthermore, specimens need to be autoclaved before their disposal. Usually, pathological specimens are streaked on special culture media as shown in Table 37.5.

Table 37.5: Use of different types of culture media (depending on the nature of pathological specimens)

Source	Blood agar	Chocolate agar	MacConkey agar	Modified Thayer Martin	CNA	CDC/PEA	CDC/KV	Thioglycolate broth	Lim broth	Gram stain	Hektoen-enteric	Campy agar	MacConkey with sorbitol	Comment (s)
Nose, Ear	x	x	x											
Eye	x	x	x	x										
Cord, Skin	x		x											
CSF	x	x	x					x		x				spin before plating
Body fluids	x	x	x			x	x	x		x				spin before plating
GC culture		x		x										
Genital, Placenta, Lochia, Bartholin cyst, CVE	x	x	x	x					x					
Throat	x													
Sputum, Trachea	x	x	x							x				
Bronchial washings	x	x	x											
Abscess	x	x	x		x			x						
Wound	x	x	x		x			x		x				
Urine	x		x											streak zigzag
Tissue	x	x	x		x				x	x				grind in sterile broth
Stool, Rectal					x						x	x	x	Inoculation of selenite F broth
Gallbladder, Bile	x		x		x						x		x	Inoculation of selenite F broth
Anaerobes						x	x							

283

Cultivation of anaerobes

Obligate or strict anaerobes are those bacteria that can grow only in the absence of oxygen. In other words, oxygen exerts its toxic effect on strictly anaerobic microbes. However, some anaerobic bacteria do tolerate a little exposure to oxygen called aerotolerant anaerobes. Unlike aerobic methods, special techniques are used to grow anaerobes in the laboratory. Anaerobic techniques for growing anaerobes in the oxygen-free environment are briefly outlined below:

1. *Anaerobic jar*: GasPak has been a very popular method in a clinical microbiology laboratory because it is easy to operate, quick, and inexpensive. Since the method takes its name GasPak, it uses a commercially made disposable chemicals-filled envelope. Upon the addition of water, chemicals produce gases namely, hydrogen and carbon dioxide. Hydrogen gas, in turn, reacts with atmospheric oxygen to form water. Palladium serves as a cold catalyst in this reaction. This is how oxygen disappears from the jar, creating anaerobiosis. To verify the anaerobic condition in the jar, wet methylene blue (an indicator) strip is placed in the jar. Methylene blue remains blue in the oxidized state whereas it turns colorless (leuko compound) in its reduced state.

Inoculated plates are stacked in the jar containing GasPak with added water and wet methylene blue strips. Thereafter, the lid is tightly screwed followed by the incubation of the jar. It is noteworthy that the jar should be opened after 48 hours because anaerobes are susceptible to atmospheric oxygen in their logarithmic growth phase.

2. *Anaerobic chamber* (glove box): Anaerobic chamber is a little sophisticated apparatus that is used to produce anaerobiosis. The key components of the anaerobic chamber are shown in Fig. 37.1.

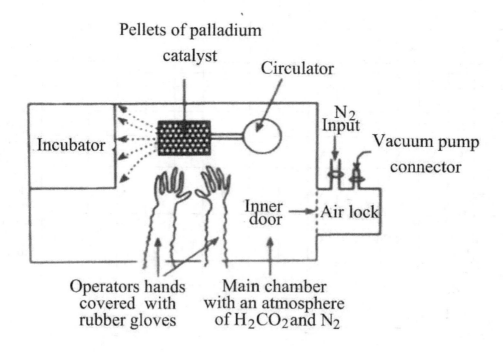

Fig. 37.1: The key components of the anaerobic chamber.

There are pressurized gas cylinders of N_2 and H_2 connected to the chamber to supply inside this flexible plastic glove box. There are sensors for oxygen as well as hydrogen to indicate their amounts within the chamber. Glove ports and rubber gloves are used by the bacteriologist to perform the manipulations. There is provision for the air circulation (circulator) through the palladium pellets to eliminate residual atmospheric oxygen if any.

An air-lock, equipped with inner and outer doors, plays a crucial role in an anaerobic chamber. Uninoculated culture media are placed inside an air-lock through the inner door. Thereafter, an air-lock is evacuated with the help of a vacuum pump followed by the refilling with N_2 through the outer door. This is how an air-lock and culture media therein become oxygen-free. These oxygen-free culture media are now moved from the air-lock to the chamber and inoculated. Inoculated plates are moved to the incubator fitted inside the chamber. The presence of a CO_2-rich atmosphere is essential in supporting the growth of anaerobes.

3. *Anaerobic bags or pouches*: Anaerobic bags are based on an oxygen removal system that contains calcium carbonate and a catalyst. Once the inoculated plates are placed inside these commercially made bags, bags are then sealed and the oxygen removal system is activated. This helps generate CO_2 within the bag. Thus, a CO_2-rich atmosphere (i.e., anaerobiosis) exists within the bag.

These bags are convenient to use in case of a small volume of anaerobic specimens. At the end of the incubation, colony characteristics can be studied without taking the plates out of the bag. Also, such bags can successfully be used in the transportation of samples containing anaerobes.

4. *Pre-reduced media*: Several anaerobic media have been formulated to support the growth of anaerobes. Anaerobic liquid media need to be boiled (in boiling water for 10 minutes) to expel any dissolved oxygen. Then, a non-toxic reducing agent (e.g., 0.1% sodium thioglycolate and 0.1% cysteine hydrochloride) is added to these media, thus lowering the oxidation-reduction (redox) potential or E_h. Also, the media are treated with oxygen-free N_2 for the maintenance of the anaerobic condition. Finally, these media are dispensed into tubes and autoclaved. A redox dye (e.g., methylene blue and resazurin) may also be used to monitor the E_h of the medium. Moreover, anaerobic media are supplemented with hemin, vitamin K, and yeast extract. For example, enriched thioglycolate broth can be used to grow aerobes, microaerophiles, and anaerobes in the process of detecting bacteria in normally sterile samples. Other anaerobic media include cooked meat broth (CMB), *Brucella* blood agar, *Bacteroides* bile esculin (BBE) agar, and phenylethyl alcohol (PEA) agar. CDC Anaerobe 5% sheep blood agar with PEA is an enriched selective medium developed by the Centers for Disease Control and Prevention (CDC) and is the preferred culture medium for the selective isolation of obligately anaerobic bacteria from mixed cultures. It contains 5% sheep blood agar and phenylethyl alcohol (PEA) as an inhibitor of facultatively anaerobic Gram-negative bacteria.

Conclusion

Cultivation of some bacterial pathogens remains an important challenge, e.g., *Mycobacterium leprae* and *Treponema pallidum.*

Chapter 38

Urine Culture and Susceptibility

Introduction

Normally, urine is sterile in the bladder. However, the urinary tract may be infected by bacteria and sometimes fungi. These infections are called urinary tract infections (UTIs). Usually, UTIs are caused by an enteric group of bacteria in certain conditions (e.g., entry of *Escherichia coli* from the intestinal tract into the urinary tract). Therefore, UTIs are categorized as opportunistic infections. The most common etiologic agent of UTIs is *Escherichia coli*. The involvement of *E. coli* as the main causative agent of UTIs is self-explanatory because it is a normal inhabitant of the intestinal tract and can easily reach the urinary tract via the anus. If an infection is limited to the kidneys, it is called pyelonephritis. In some instances, bacteria may invade the bladder (cystitis) or the urethra (urethritis).

The probability of contracting UTIs in females is much higher than in males because the urethra is closer to the anus in females. Interestingly, it is more prevalent in females (52%) as opposed to males (20%) of a similar age group (21-40 years). It is necessary to consider the predisposing factors of a patient while evaluating for the possibility of UTIs (e.g., diabetes and compromised immune system). These patients may be more easily infected by potential urinary pathogens in comparison to healthy individuals.

Urine specimens from pregnant women (the first trimester period) and patients scheduled for invasive urologic procedures are routinely tested for culture and susceptibility in the absence of symptoms.

The following symptoms are common in lower urinary tract infection:

- painful urination
- constant urge to urinate
- pain in the lower abdomen

Urine samples from UTI patients are usually cloudy and foul-smelling.

Sample collection and transportation

The first and most important step in performing a urine culture is the collection of an acceptable specimen. The specimen of choice for urine culture is referred to as a midstream clean catch urine. It is very important to avoid contamination of urine specimen. Therefore, instructions for obtaining these specimens must be strictly followed (e.g., cleansing of urinary opening).

There is no need for patient preparation for the test except to instruct the patient to drink 2-3 glasses of water 10 minutes before the collection of the urine specimen. The patient should wash his/her hands before and after the collection of urine specimens as both a safety measure and to minimize the chance of contaminating the specimen.

Depending on the circumstances, a specimen of urine may be collected in various ways as listed below:

1. *Midstream clean-catch specimen:* Void some urine into the toilet. Then stop urinating, and urinate the mid-portion into a clean and sterile cup and re-cap it immediately. Any remaining urine can be passed into a toilet. Anaerobic cultures should not be set up on routine clean-catch urine specimens.

2. *Catheterized specimen:* Inserting a soft narrow tube through the urethra into the bladder, i.e., catheter into the urethra. If it is required to collect urine from indwelling catheters, puncture the catheter line with a sterile needle and aspirate in a sterile syringe. Urine specimens collected from indwelling catheter bags should not be accepted for a culture test.

3. *Suprapubic aspirate:* Suprapubic aspiration is a procedure where a sterile needle and a sterile syringe are used to collect uncontaminated urine from the bladder. The procedure is rarely used for a routine urine culture test. This invasive procedure is performed if an anaerobic infection is suspected.

Urine specimens are transported to a microbiology laboratory as quickly as possible (<30 minutes). If delayed delivery beyond 2 hours of the collection is anticipated, urine specimens should be stored at 2°-8°C or on ice. The pre-analytical phase of the collection and transportation of urine specimens to a laboratory has a profound impact on test results.

Processing of urine cultures involve:

A. Culturing
B. Susceptibility

A. Culturing:

Upon receipt of urine specimens for culture and susceptibility test, a clinical microbiologist starts to work-up on acceptable urine specimens without any delay. In some cases, specimens are rejected if they do not meet the criteria set by the institution, e.g., unrefrigerated urine culture specimens stored for >2 hours.

1. Streaking: Different facilities have their strategies for processing urine specimens for a culture test. Each facility has its standard operating procedures (SOPs) in place to follow. Ideally, urine culture specimen is applied on 5% sheep blood agar (SBA) and MacConkey agar media as a part of preliminary processing protocol:

(i) Label plates on the bottom part with the patient's information, e.g., last name, date of birth, and the medical record number
(ii) Mix specimen well and remove the cap of the specimen container

(iii) Using a sterile disposable precisely calibrated loop (0.001mL[29]), charge the loop portion only with urine specimen

(iv) Make one line of inoculum across the plate touching opposite ends of a blood agar plate

(v) Perform streaking perpendicular to the line of inoculum to make nice tight streaks all across the inoculum line

(vi) Perform streaking on MacConkey agar plate by repeating the similar procedure used in a blood agar plate

(vii) Replace the cap of the specimen container

2. Incubation: Both the plates are incubated at 37°C for 24 hours in an inverted position.

3. Plate reading: Plates are read by experienced personnel and results are recorded, e.g., colony-forming units (CFUs)/mL and colony types (e.g., single or mixed) present on a blood agar plate. MacConkey agar, a selective and differential medium, allows only Gram-negative bacteria to grow. Also, differentiation between lactose-fermenting (e.g., *E. coli*) and lactose non-fermenting (e.g., *Proteus vulgaris*) bacteria can be made on this medium. Colony characteristics of commonly encountered urinary pathogens on MacConkey agar are listed in Table 38.1.

Table 38.1: Colony characteristics of commonly encountered urinary pathogens on MacConkey agar

Bacterial species	Lactose fermentation	Comment
E. coli	Pink/ red	Non-mucoid
Kleb. pneumoniae	Pink/ red	Mucoid
Acinetobacter baumannii	Colorless	Non-mucoid and opaque
Ps. aeruginosa	Colorless	Fluorescent growth
Pr. vulgaris	Colorless	No swarming
Staphylococcus spp.	Pale pink	Opaque

Besides blood agar and MacConkey agar media, some laboratories add colistin nalidixic acid (CNA) agar that favors the growth of only Gram-positive cocci, including yeasts. It is also a differential medium as it helps to differentiate between hemolytic and non-hemolytic bacteria.

The cystine-lactose-electrolyte-deficient (CLED) medium, accompanied by MacConkey agar, may also be used for urine cultures. The CLED medium supports the growth of both Gram-negative and Gram-positive bacteria while preventing the swarming growth of *Proteus* spp. The CLED medium also allows the differentiation between lactose fermenters and lactose non-fermenters. Various ingredients play their roles as stated below:

---

[29] With 0.001 mL loop, each colony (i.e., CFU) on SBA corresponds to several viable bacteria per mL of urine specimen. Fully automated systems are also available, e.g., spiral plating.

1. Cystine: a sulfur-containing amino acid, stimulates the growth of cystine-dependent dwarf colonies.
2. Lactose: a disaccharide, is fermented by lactose fermenting bacteria to form lactic acid.
3. Bromothymol blue: an indicator dye, displays its color in acidic/alkaline conditions. It turns bacterial colonies yellow in acidic conditions (i.e., lactose utilization by some bacteria) and deep blue in alkaline conditions (by decarboxylating cystine).

4. *Gram stain*: is performed as a part of the presumptive identification protocol.

5. *Biochemical tests*: Some instant biochemical tests using commercial kits are performed on isolated colonies to support the preliminary report that helps in the prompt management of the patient, e.g., oxidase test.

6. *Follow-up testing:* Following the preliminary work-up report, definitive identification testing may be carried out on automated analyzers (e.g., VITEK 2, Microscan, and MALDI-TOF MS), if warranted.

Interpretation

Based on CFUs/mL (semi-quantitative analysis) and types of bacterial species seen on culture plates, the following conclusions can be drawn:

1. No growth at the end of the incubation period (24 hours) constitutes a negative test result.
2. If the count is ≤10,000 CFUs/mL, it is an indication of either normal flora or possible contamination.
3. If the count exceeds 100,000 CFUs/mL, it denotes bacterial infection (bacteriuria) where definitive ID and susceptibility tests follow. However, quantitation is not useful in the laboratory diagnosis of *Candida*-associated UTIs (candiduria).
4. If the bacterial count lies between 10,000-100,000 CFUs/mL, the test result is considered to be borderline and it is recommended to repeat the test. Such borderline (indeterminate) counts are encountered in cases of chronic and relapsing infections.

While making a preliminary report (i.e. presumptive identification) for the ordering physician, one should consider the following parameters for complete evaluation:

- site of urine collection
- clinical diagnosis
- presence or absence of pus cells (i.e., pyuria)
- indication of any medication taken recently by the patient

Occasionally, UTIs occur without classic symptoms (e.g., painful frequent urination). Yet, a urine culture test shows the presence of bacteria. Such a UTI is called asymptomatic bacteriuria. Urinary etiologic agents isolated from urine specimens are listed in Table 38.2.

Table 38.2: Most commonly encountered urinary etiologic agents

Etiologic agent	Percent (%)
Escherichia coli	42.8
Klebsiella pneumoniae	16.8
Acinetobacter baumannii	12.9
Candida albicans	11
Citrobacter freundii	6.4
Staphylococcus aureus	3.2
Pseudomonas aeruginosa	1.9
Proteus vulgaris	0.6

Thus, it is evident that *Escherichia coli* is the principal causative agent of urinary tract infections, especially in women. Hospitalized patients with a long-term indwelling urinary catheter may be infected by resistant Gram-negative bacteria, namely *Pseudomonas* spp., *Providencia* spp., *Serratia* spp., and *Acinetobacter* spp. *Acinetobacter* spp. readily colonizes the urinary tract, especially in the presence of an indwelling catheter. This bacterial species continued to infect veterans and soldiers who served in Iraq and Afghanistan during the Iraq war.

B. Susceptibility:

   a. Manual method
   b. Automated method

a. Manual method

Antimicrobial susceptibility (sensitivity) testing can be performed by a manual method using a special medium called the Mueller-Hinton agar. It is equally important to that of bacterial identification. Modified Kirby-Bauer (KB) disk diffusion test is routinely used for non-fastidious aerobes and facultative anaerobes to determine the efficacy of antimicrobial compounds. Thus, the test helps select the best drug that can be used in treating a patient. In the Kirby-Bauer disk diffusion test, filter paper disks, impregnated with a defined strength of a specific antimicrobial agent suspension, are placed on a Mueller-Hinton agar already swabbed with a clinical culture in question. This is how confluent growth is produced. At the end of 16-18 hours of incubation, zones of inhibition are measured in mm using a ruler/caliper. Then, the diameter (in mm) of an inhibitory zone is correlated to the efficacy of an antimicrobial agent. The greater the zone of inhibition, the higher the potency of an antimicrobial agent. Based on the interpretive guideline chart from the manufacturer, antimicrobial agents are classified as sensitive, intermediate, or resistant.

The Clinical Laboratory Standards Institute (CLSI) is responsible for making improvements in the original procedure of Kirby-Bauer through a global consensus process, thus ensuring the uniformity of method and reproducibility of the test results.

The modified Kirby-Bauer disk diffusion technique has been recommended by the National Committee on Clinical Laboratory Services (NCCLS-USA) subcommittee on antimicrobial susceptibility testing. The most thoroughly scrutinized technique, with developed interpretive standards, is supported by laboratory and clinical data.

Procedure: (see Fig. 38.1)

1. Inoculate the Mueller-Hinton agar plate (i.e., 100 mm or 150 mm) with an appropriate inoculum density of a given clinical isolate in its log phase. Streaking is performed in three directions, turning the Petri dish by 60° between each streaking.
2. Using a pair of sterile forceps, place the paper disks one after the other and tap gently to ensure complete contact of a disk to the surface of the agar medium. Alternatively, a semi-automatic disk dispenser may also be used.
3. Incubate at 35°-37°C for 16-18 hours (in some cases 24 hours) in a CO_2-free atmosphere in an inverted position.
4. Measure the zones of inhibition by a ruler using the transmitted light. For sulfonamides and co-trimoxazole, 80% is read because there is a delay in diffusion. There is a correlation between the size of the inhibitory zone and the effectiveness of an antimicrobial agent.
5. Using the manufacturer's interpretive guidelines, report the susceptibility of a clinical isolate against various drugs as sensitive, intermediate, or resistant.

Factors that affect antimicrobial susceptibility are:

1. The density of an inoculum (0.5 McFarland standard)
2. Depth of medium (optimum 4 mm)
3. The pH of the medium (optimum pH 7.2-7.4)
4. The concentration of Ca^{++} and Mg^{++} (higher or lower concentration influences the size of the inhibition zone for *Pseudomonas aeruginosa* when tested against aminoglycoside and tetracycline)
5. The concentration of thymidine or thymine (Excessive concentration may reverse the inhibitory effects of sulfonamides and trimethoprim)
6. Diffusibility of a drug in question (molecular configuration-dependent)
7. Growth conditions (e.g., optimum incubation temperature of 35°C)

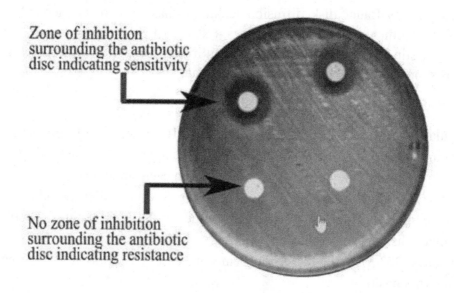

Zone of inhibition surrounding the antibiotic disc indicating sensitivity

No zone of inhibition surrounding the antibiotic disc indicating resistance

Fig. 38.1: Antimicrobial susceptibility testing.

Sources of error:

1. Inoculum too light
2. Antimicrobial agent too potent
3. Agar layer too thin
4. Reference strain mutated
5. Incorrect recording of assay results

Quality control:
Each laboratory must perform quality assurance testing preferably every week. Also, it is performed when a new lot of Mueller-Hinton medium and a new batch of antimicrobial disks arrive. The test includes the reference strains, namely *Escherichia coli* ATCC 25922, *Staphylococcus aureus* ATCC 25923, and *Pseudomonas aeruginosa* ATCC 27853 in parallel to the clinical isolate.

The modified Kirby-Bauer method proved to be a valuable technique to perform antimicrobial susceptibility testing on a fastidious group of microorganisms from specimens other than urine as well, provided a supplemented Mueller-Hinton agar medium is used. Bacteria, namely alpha-streptococci and *Streptococcus pneumoniae,* require complex nutrients for their growth without which they fail to grow. The Mueller-Hinton medium supplemented with 5% blood agar is recommended for *Streptococcus pneumoniae.* The modified GC agar base is a suitable medium for *Neisseria gonorrhoeae* (5% CO_2) to serve the purpose. For *Haemophilus influenzae,* a medium called Haemophilus test medium (HTM) is satisfactorily used for susceptibility testing. The HTM contains hemin(X factor), NAD (V factor), and yeast extract as complex nutritional additives in a Mueller-Hinton agar.

The modified Kirby-Bauer disk diffusion technique is not recommended for *Helicobacter pylori, Brucella* spp., and *Legionella* spp. However, the method may be used to screen for resistance. The minimal inhibitory concentration (MIC) method may be used for these bacteria.

b. Automated method

Automated instruments, e.g., VITEK 2 system (bioMerieux) also serve the purpose of antimicrobial susceptibility testing. The VITEK 2 system has this module to perform susceptibility testing of clinically significant isolates, namely Gram-positive cocci, Gram-negative bacilli, and yeasts against commonly used drugs. Here, micro-dilution cards are incubated overnight and read photometrically to measure the growth. The MIC means the highest dilution in µg/mL of a given antimicrobial agent without a visible growth of an organism in question. In this way, the MIC required to combat a microbe in question is determined.

The PCR-based automated machines for bacterial identification are also capable of detecting resistance-associated genes in a limited number of bacteria. Unfortunately, MALDI-TOF mass spectrometry lacks antimicrobial susceptibility testing (AST) features to date.

Antimicrobial susceptibility testing needs to be performed on each isolated urinary pathogenic strain. The susceptibility (%) pattern of most frequently isolated bacteria against routinely used antimicrobial agents is shown in Table 38.3.

Table 38.3: The susceptibility (%) pattern of most frequently isolated urinary pathogenic strains

Antibacterial agent	*Escherichia coli* (%)	*Klebsiella* spp. (%)	*Acinetobacter* spp. (%)
Ampicillin	0.9	13	11
Amikacin	71	37	47
Cotrimoxazole	31	23	28
Ciprofloxacin	11	31	40
Ceftriaxone	32	22	27
Gentamicin	27	15	29
Imipenem	37	39	13
Nitrofurantoin	82	20	18
Nalidixic acid	3	18	16
Norfloxacin	7	31	16

Drug resistance:
Urinary pathogens have developed resistance to routinely used antibiotics, namely ampicillin, norfloxacin, and nalidixic acid. The health care provider should wait until the susceptibility test is completed. In other words, only those patients with symptomatic UTIs should be treated with antibiotics, thus avoiding unnecessary exposure to antibiotics. Nowadays, an emerging multiple-drug resistant strain of *Acinetobacter baumannii* is a major threat in combating this hospital-acquired infection.

Conclusion

While interpreting the test results, the health care provider tries to gather information about the patient's history and use of any antimicrobial agent in the past. This information is crucial for the physician in the successful treatment of a patient. A "trial and error" method, while treating a patient, may favor the development of "drug-resistance". Clinically, the determination of drug-susceptibility is far more important than the identification of a clinical isolate.

Chapter 39

Biochemical Tests

Introduction

Biochemical tests are inexpensive and simple to perform in a microbiology laboratory. The biochemical test results are valuable in the characterization and identification of bacteria. The culture media are carefully designed to include certain ingredients, e.g., sugars as substrates for carbohydrate utilization studies. Such chemically defined media are inoculated with a pure culture of an unknown bacterial species followed by incubation for 18-24 hours at 37°C. At the end of the incubation period, reagents (e.g., indicator dyes) are added to some of these growth media to detect the metabolic end-products. Thus, biochemical reactions reflect the enzymatic makeup of a microbe in question. Some important biochemical tests and their applications are outlined in this chapter.

1. Indole production test: This biochemical test helps to detect tryptophanase in a bacterial species in question. The tryptone broth (1%) is inoculated with a pure unknown bacterial culture and incubated for 18-24 hours at 37°C. At the end of the incubation period, a few drops of Kovac's reagent (*para*-Dimethylaminobenzaldehyde in alcohol) is added down the inner wall of the test tube.

Alternatively, sulfide-indole-motility (SIM) medium can be used.

Principle: Cleavage of tryptophan through the activity of tryptophanase to form the key end-product, indole:

$$\text{Tryptophan} + H_2O \xrightarrow{\text{tryptophanase}} \text{Indole} + \text{Pyruvate} + NH_4^+$$

Interpretation: Development of a bright fuchsia red color at the interface of the reagent and the broth within seconds after adding Kovac's reagent indicates a positive test. On the other hand, no change in color after the addition of the reagent implies a negative test.

Expected results
Positive: *Escherichia coli* and *Proteus vulgaris*
Negative: *Enterobacter aerogenes*, *Proteus mirabilis*, *Klebsiella* spp., and *Salmonella* spp.

2. Methyl red (MR) test: This test makes use of a buffered glucose-peptone broth known as MR-VP broth since this broth is aliquoted after the incubation to perform the methyl red (MR) test and the Voges-Proskauer test as well. At the end of a mixed acid fermentation pathway, the production of stable organic acids, namely lactic acid, succinic acid, acetic acid, and formic acid is good enough to overcome the effect of a phosphate buffer. As a result of this, the pH of the broth drops to 4.4 or less.

Principle: Some members of the family *Enterobacteriaceae* follow a mixed acid fermentation pathway, producing stable acidic end-products, i.e., organic acids from the substrate, glucose:

Glucose ⟶ ⟶ ⟶ Pyruvate ⟶ Mixed organic acids
(pH 4.4 or below)

Interpretation: Development of a bright red color after the addition of methyl red (a pH indicator) constitutes a positive test. On the other hand, a yellow-orange color (pH 6.2) is indicative of a negative test.

Expected results
Positive: *Escherichia coli* and *Proteus mirabilis*
Negative: *Enterobacter aerogenes*

3. Voges-Proskauer (VP) test: The Voges-Proskauer test is completed using an aliquot of MR-VP broth after incubation. Some members of the enteric group of bacteria use an alternative route for glucose degradation called a butylene glycol (butanediol) fermentation, a type of glucose fermentation pathway. The test helps in the detection of an intermediary compound called acetyl methyl carbinol (acetoin). The reagents used before reading the test include Barritt's A (alpha-naphthol) and Barritt's B (40% KOH). Therefore, this qualitative test is valuable in differentiating some members of *Enterobacteriaceae*.

Principle: Conversion of acetyl methyl carbinol to diacetyl occurs in the presence of 40% KOH and atmospheric O_2:

(i) Glucose ⟶ ⟶ ⟶ Acetyl methyl carbinol (acetoin)

$$\text{(ii) Acetyl methyl carbinol} \xrightarrow[\text{atmospheric } O_2]{\text{40\% KOH}} \text{Diacetyl} + H_2O$$

So formed diacetyl reacts with guanidine components of peptone in the presence of alpha-naphthol (a catalyst and a color intensifier) to form a rose color:

$$\text{(iii) Diacetyl + Guanidine components of peptone} \xrightarrow{\text{alpha-naphthol}} \text{Pink (burgundy) color}$$

Interpretation: After shaking the broth and waiting for 15 minutes, the appearance of a pink color suggests a positive test. In the case of a negative test, there is no color change in the medium.

Expected results
Positive: *Enterobacter aerogenes* and *Klebsiella pneumoniae*
Negative: *Escherichia coli*

4. Citrate utilization test: This test helps to learn the presence or absence of citrate-permease needed to transport the exogenous citrate across the bacterial cell-wall. Technically, Simmon's citrate medium contains sodium citrate as the sole source of carbon and energy. Additionally, the medium is supplemented with inorganic ammonium dihydrogen phosphate as the sole source of nitrogen and a pH indicator, bromothymol blue. Thus, an uninoculated medium attains a pH of 6.9, displaying a green color.

Principle: A shift in pH from 6.9 to 7.6 by the virtue of citrate utilization and subsequent formation of sodium carbonate and bicarbonate (alkaline products) occurs:

(i) $Citrate \longrightarrow Pyruvate + CO_2$

(ii) $Sodium\ citrate + CO_2 + H_2O \longrightarrow Na_2CO_3$

Also, there is the formation of another alkali, ammonium hydroxide. Bromothymol blue at pH of 7.6 or above displays its Prussian blue (royal blue) color, indicating a positive test. In some cases, inoculated media need to be incubated at 37°C for 7 days (normal incubation period is 24-48 hours).

Interpretation: Development of a royal blue color after incubation constitutes a positive test. The green color similar to that of an uninoculated medium suggests a negative test.

Expected results
Positive: *Klebsiella pneumoniae, Enterobacter aerogenes, Citrobacter freundii, Salmonella* spp. other than *S. typhi* and *S. paratyphi A, Serratia marcescens, Proteus mirabilis* (the minority of strains give negative results*), and *Providencia* spp.
Negative: *Escherichia coli, Shigella* spp.*, Salmonella typhi, Salmonella paratyphi A, Morganella morganii,* and *Yersinia enterocolitica*

Note:
1. Tests with equivocal results need to be repeated.
2. Some bacteria show poor growth without changing the color of the medium. This test is to be considered a positive test.

Alternatively, Koser's citrate broth can be used to serve the same purpose. The broth needs to be inoculated with a test organism using a poor inoculum. The development of the turbidity implies the successful utilization of citrate (a positive test). In the case of a negative test, the broth remains clear.

All the four aforementioned tests form a test battery known as **IMViC** (**I** = indole production; **M** = methyl red; **V** = Voges Proskauer; **C** = citrate utilization; i is added for better euphony). They are of great significance in the differentiation between the two closely related Gram-negative bacterial species, namely *Escherichia coli* and *Enterobacter aerogenes* as shown in Table 39.1.

Table 39.1: Differentiation between *Escherichia coli* and *Enterobacter aerogenes*

Bacterial species	Indole	Methyl red	Voges-Proskauer	Citrate
Escherichia coli	+	+	-	-
Enterobacter aerogenes	-	-	+	+

5. Urease test: This test indirectly helps detect the presence or absence of urease in a given unknown bacterial culture. This can be accomplished by inoculating urea broth (pH 6.8) with an unknown bacterial culture and then incubating it at 37°C for 18-24 hours. Urea broth contains urea (as a substrate), very small amounts of other nutrients (e.g., yeast extract as a source of B vitamins), two pH buffers, and phenol red as a pH indicator.

Principle: Conversion of urea to ammonia and carbon dioxide is catalyzed by urease secreted by some members of the enterics. Though many enterics are capable of hydrolyzing urea, only a few can break it down rapidly. Thus, only rapid-urease producers can generate enough ammonia to overcome the effect of pH buffers, turning the pH indicator to bright pink (pH 8.4).

$$(NH_2)_2\,CO \ + \ H_2O \ \xrightarrow{\text{urease}} \ 2NH_3 \quad + \quad CO_2$$

Urea   Water   Ammonia   Carbon dioxide

Interpretation: Phenol red exhibits its bright pink color in alkaline environment (NH_3) developed by only rapid-urease producers, representing a positive test. Otherwise, the medium appears orange in color (pH 6.8), meaning thereby a negative test.

Expected results: The test proves its credibility in differentiating between the members of the genera, namely *Proteus, Morganella,* and *Providencia* from other enterics.
Positive: *Proteus vulgaris, Proteus mirabilis, Ureaplasma urealyticum,* and *Helicobacter pylori*
Negative: *Escherichia coli, Enterobacter aerogenes,* and *Serratia marcescens*

6. Phenylalanine deaminase test: This enzymatic test indicates the presence or absence of phenylalanine deaminase in the members of *Enterobacteriaceae*. This enzyme is present in members of the *Proteeae* tribe, e.g., *Proteus, Providencia,* and *Morganella*. The procedure includes the inoculation of phenylalanine agar (phenylalanine as a substrate) slant and then incubation at 37°C for 18-24 hours. Some bacteria may take 4-7 days to exhibit a positive reaction. At the end of the incubation period, 4-5 drops of 10% $FeCl_3$ reagent is added to detect the by-product, phenylpyruvic acid.

Principle: Phenylalanine undergoes oxidative deamination with the formation of a by-product, phenylpyruvic acid. In other words, there is a removal of an amino (-NH$_2$) group from phenylalanine (amino acid) to form phenylpyruvic acid:

$$\text{(i) Phenylalanine} \xrightarrow{\text{phenylalanine deaminase}} \text{Phenylpyruvic acid}$$

Then, 10% of FeCl$_3$ reagent is added to detect phenylpyruvic acid:

$$\text{(ii) Phenylpyruvic acid} + \text{FeCl}_3 \longrightarrow \text{Green color}$$

Interpretation: Development of a green or dark brown color upon the addition of 10% FeCl$_3$ reagent constitutes a positive test. No color change of the medium signals a negative test.

Expected results: Differentiation between the members of *Proteeae* tribe (*Proteus, Providencia,* and *Morganella*) and other members of *Enterobacteriaceae*

Positive: *Proteus vulgaris*
Negative: *Escherichia coli, Enterobacter aerogenes,* and *Serratia marcescens*

7. Nitrate reduction (nitratase) test: This biochemical test serves the purpose of detecting nitratase (nitrate reductase) in bacteria. The test results need a careful interpretation in comparison to other biochemical tests because there are two possible end-products:

(i.) nitrite (NO$_2$)
(ii.) nitrogenous products other than nitrite, e.g., molecular nitrogen (N$_2$), and ammonium (NH$_4^+$)

An uninoculated medium is included as a part of quality control. The slants are inoculated and incubated at 37°C for 48 hours. Then, reagents are added, namely sulfanilic acid (nitrate I), alpha-naphthylamine (nitrate II), and zinc dust. The reader needs to understand the two different mechanisms for the formation of nitrite while interpreting the test result:

The step (ii) is simply performed to justify the fate of nitrate other than nitrite formation. The nitrate (NO$_3$) is either unused in the first place or converted to nitrogenous compounds, e.g., molecular nitrogen (N$_2$) or ammonium (NH$_4^+$).

Principle: Some bacteria are capable of converting nitrate (NO$_3$) to either nitrite (NO$_2$) or some other nitrogenous compounds:

$$\text{(i) NO}_3 \xrightarrow[\text{(bacteria)}]{\text{nitratase}} \text{NO}_2 \text{ (true bioconversion by a bacterial enzyme)}$$
Nitrate   Nitrite

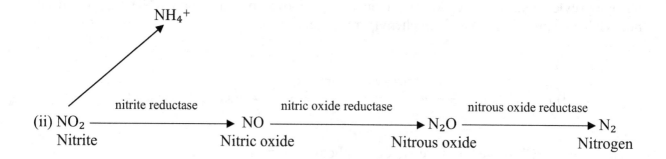

(ii) NO_2 —[nitrite reductase]→ NO —[nitric oxide reductase]→ N_2O —[nitrous oxide reductase]→ N_2

Nitrite   Nitric oxide   Nitrous oxide   Nitrogen

Nitrite is a stable end-product in some bacteria. This truly formed nitrite is detected by adding two reagents in the correct order:

  (i) sulfanilic acid
  (ii) alpha-naphthylamine, causing a red color (positive test)

or

NO_2 (nitrite) ——————→ N_2 (nitrogen gas) or NH_4^+ (ammonium)

This is a stable end-product in some bacteria and is the second possibility for the reaction to be a truly positive test.

Interpretation: It is very important that laboratory personnel should record and report the final results with caution. The development of a red color upon the addition of sulfanilic acid and alpha-naphthylamine in their correct order establishes the truly formed nitrite, i.e., a positive test. Alternatively, the test can truly be positive if the color of the medium remains unchanged after the addition of a third reagent, zinc powder in the second medium. This confers that nitrate is converted to nitrogenous products (N_2 or NH_4^+) other than nitrite.

On the other hand, the development of a red color after the addition of a pinch of zinc powder as a third reagent in the third tube justifies that unused nitrate is converted to nitrite through a chemical reaction (i.e., zinc), constituting a negative test.

Expected results
Positive: *Escherichia coli, Proteus vulgaris,* and *Pseudomonas aeruginosa*
Negative: *Streptococcus pneumoniae*

8. Carbohydrate fermentation test: This is a simple qualitative biochemical reaction included in the test package meant for the characterization and classification of the members of *Entero-bacteriaceae*. Phenol red broth equipped with an inverted Durham vial contains only one specific sugar (substrate) at a time, e.g., glucose, lactose, or sucrose. After inoculating with a given unknown pure bacterial culture under aseptic conditions, phenol red broth needs to be incubated at 37°C for 18-24 hours. Upon the completion of the incubation period, the broth is checked for any change in color and presence or absence of gas bubbles trapped in the Durham vial. Bacteria capable of fermenting sugar form only acidic end-products (e.g. lactic acid and acetic acid) which are symbolized as 'A'. Additionally, some bacteria generating gas (e.g. carbon dioxide and hydrogen) along with the organic acids are designated as 'A' and 'G'. Thus, sugar fermentation reactions help to provide some clues regarding the metabolic activities of bacteria.

Principle: Phenol red (a pH indicator) exhibits its red color at a neutral pH (uninoculated broth) as it can be noticed in case of a negative test (failure to produce acids from sugar by some bacteria). It turns yellow in an acidic environment as evidenced during successful carbohydrate fermentation, constituting a positive test. Trapping of gas bubbles in the inverted Durham vial signals the by-product of the carbohydrate fermentation. In general, sugar fermentation results are shown below:

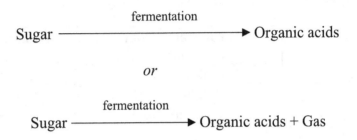

Interpretation: The development of yellow color in the broth medium is indicative of a positive test because phenol red displays a yellow color in the presence of acidic end-products. The generation of gaseous products is concluded from gas bubbles in the Durham vial. No change in color (i.e., red) signals a negative test.

Over incubation may result in the formation of NH_3 (alkaline) from amino acids (peptone) following the carbohydrate depletion in the phenol red broth. This causes the change in phenol red indicator color from yellow (truly positive) to red (falsely negative). This reaction is referred to as reversion.

Expected results: Based on carbohydrate fermentation tests, members of *Enterobacteriaceae* are assigned to a specific category, e.g., lactose-fermenters versus lactose non-fermenters. Glucose fermentation by some enterics is outlined in Table 39.2.

Table 39.2: Glucose fermentation by some enterics

Gram-negative small rods	Acid ('A')	Gas ('G')
Escherichia coli	+	+
Enterobacter aerogenes	+	+
Klebsiella pneumoniae	+	+

9. Oxidative/fermentative (O/F) metabolism: This test (Hugh and Leifson, 1953) aids in the determination of the pathway used by an organism of interest during carbohydrate utilization. It requires a semisolid (2% agar) medium that contains both glucose (1%) and bromothymol blue as a pH indicator (pH 7.1). An organism is inoculated in two tubes by stabbing followed by overlaying one tube with sterile mineral oil. The tube layered with mineral oil creates anaerobiosis, an environment suitable for strict anaerobes and facultative anaerobes to grow.

Principle: Microorganisms that utilize glucose fermentation pathway produce acid in both media as opposed to the failure of oxidative microorganisms to produce acid in an oil-covered tube.

Interpretation:
Following incubation at 37°C for 48 hours, both tubes are examined for acid formation as shown in Table 39.3.

Table 39.3: Fermentative and oxidative pathways

Pathway	Aerobic conditions (without mineral oil)	Anaerobic conditions (with mineral oil)
Fermentative	yellow (acid)	yellow (acid)
Oxidative	yellow (acid)	green (alkaline)
Nonsaccharolytic	green (alkaline)	green (alkaline)

Expected results
Fermentative: *Escherichia coli, Staphylococcus* spp.
Oxidative: *Pseudomonas aeruginosa, Micrococcus* spp.
Nonsaccharolytic:: *Alcaligenes faecalis, Moraxella* spp.

10. Gelatin hydrolysis test: This test aids in understanding the ability of an organism to break down gelatin (animal protein). Thus, gelatin hydrolysis test is employed to differentiate bacteria as gelatinase positive versus gelatinase negative. The nutrient gelatin (12% gelatin) is used for the test.

Principle: Gelatinase hydrolyzes gelatin (collagen) to stable end products called amino acids, thus causing the gelatin to liquefy. During this bioconversion, intermediary polypeptides are formed in the first place:

$$\text{(i) Gelatin} + H_2O \xrightarrow{\text{gelatinase}} \text{Polypeptides}$$

$$\text{(ii) Polypeptides} + H_2O \xrightarrow{\text{gelatinase}} \text{Amino acids}$$

Interpretation: At the end of the incubation period of 48 hours at 37°C, test tubes need to be placed in an ice bath or a refrigerator for 30 minutes before reading them. If tubes remain in a liquid state (i.e., liquefaction) after refrigeration, the test result is reported as gelatinase positive. Oppositely, if the nutrient gelatin medium solidifies after the refrigeration, it is suggestive of gelatinase negative. The gelatin medium needs further incubation for one week to include some organisms with poor gelatinase activity. Results are simply read based on the physical state of the gelatin medium after refrigeration (4°C).

Expected results
Positive: *Bacillus anthracis, Staphylococcus aureus, Clostridium tetani, Proteus vulgaris,* and *Serratia marcescens*
Negative: *Escherichia coli, Enterobacter aerogenes,* and *Staphylococcus epidermidis*

Note: Gelatin was used as a solidifying agent in routine microbiological media in the early days. Later, gelatin was replaced by agar agar powder as a solidifying agent because of the following two reasons:

1. Gelatin is in a liquid state at 28°C and above. This property makes it unfit to use as a solidifying agent because a majority of microbial cultures need to be incubated at 37°C (optimum temperature for growth).
2. Some microbial agents produce gelatinase, turning the solid medium to a liquid state during the incubation period. This undesirable change from solid to liquid state does not allow the medium to form colonies.

11. Starch hydrolysis (α-amylase test): This test is useful in detecting the bacterial extracellular enzyme called α-amylase. This enzyme-mediated breakdown of starch produces di- and monosaccharides surrounding the bacterial growth. The technique includes the inoculation of a starch plate by making a small streak line of the bacterial culture. Then, the plate is incubated at an appropriate temperature for 24-48 hours.

Principle: α-amylase brings about the bioconversion of starch (amylum) to maltose and glucose:

$$\text{(i) Starch (polysaccharide)} + H_2O \xrightarrow{\text{α-amylase}} \text{Maltose (disaccharide)}$$

$$\text{(ii) Maltose} + H_2O \xrightarrow{\text{maltase}} \text{2 Glucose (monosaccharide)}$$

Interpretation: The development of a yellow color upon flooding the starch plate with Lugol's or Gram's iodine interprets the disappearance of the starch surrounding the bacterial growth. This type of reaction is called a positive test. On the other hand, the development of a blue-black color is an indication of the negative test, leaving the starch in its intact form. For a better reading, it is advisable to view the plate on an illuminated box.

Expected results
Positive: *Bacillus subtilis*
Negative: *Escherichia coli*

12. DNA hydrolysis (DNAse) test: This is a valuable test in evaluating the DNAse-catalyzed hydrolysis of deoxyribonucleic acid (DNA) by some bacteria. This is accomplished by culturing the bacterial species on a medium supplemented with bacterial DNA (substrate). Thereafter, the DNA medium is incubated at an appropriate temperature for 24-48 hours followed by the addition of enough 0.1 *N* hydrochloric acid (HCl) to cover the surface of the medium. Thus, the DNAse agar medium serves as a differential medium.

Principle: Cleavage of DNA by an exoenzyme (DNAse), leading to the formation of free nucleotides:

$$DNA + H_2O \xrightarrow{\text{DNAse}} \text{Free nucleotides}$$

Interpretation: The appearance of a clear zone (zone of hydrolysis) surrounding the bacterial colonies constitutes a positive test. In other words, DNA is digested/hydrolyzed by the bacterial species in question. Oppositely, the cloudy area (precipitated DNA by HCl) around the bacterial growth signals a negative test.

Expected results
Positive: *Staphylococcus aureus,* and *Serratia marcescens*
Negative: *Staphylococcus epidermidis*

13. Decarboxylase test: This test is very valuable in the detection of an enzyme called decarboxylase. Decarboxylase plays a crucial role in the metabolism of many amino acids. As the name implies, it catalyzes the detachment of the carboxylic acid (-COOH) from an amino acid, ending up in the formation of an alkaline end product, amine. Each tube of Moeller's broth base is supplemented with 1% of one amino acid in question, 0.1% of glucose, pyridoxal, and two pH indicators (bromocresol purple and cresol red). The pH of the medium is adjusted to 6.2. Unlike the deaminase test, anaerobic conditions are essential in the test. This is why media are overlaid (depth of at least 1 cm) with sterile mineral oil. Also, the use of screw-capped tubes is recommended for air exclusion.

Principle: Decarboxylase, in the presence of pyridoxal (coenzyme), mediates the removal of a carboxylic acid (-COOH) from an amino acid. It should be remembered here that each decarboxylase secreted by a microbe is amino acid-specific. This can be clarified from the following biochemical reactions, involving a specific decarboxylase for each amino acid:

$$\text{1. Lysine} \xrightarrow[\text{decarboxylase}]{\text{lysine}} \text{Cadaverine} + CO_2$$

$$\text{2. Ornithine} \xrightarrow[\text{decarboxylase}]{\text{ornithine}} \text{Putrescine} + CO_2$$

304

3. Arginine undergoes hydrolysis in the presence of arginine dihydrolase, thus forming ornithine and urea:

(i) Arginine + H_2O $\xrightarrow[\text{dihydrolase}]{\text{arginine}}$ Ornithine + Urea

(ii) Ornithine $\xrightarrow[\text{decarboxylase}]{\text{ornithine}}$ Putrescine + CO_2

Interpretation: The interpretation of the test results is a little bit tricky. It would be wise to deal with fermenters and non-fermenters separately at the time of reporting the results.

1. Initially, glucose fermenters produce acid and turn the color of the pH indicator to yellow. Afterwards, if decarboxylase is present, the development of a purple color occurs due to the accumulation of an alkali (positive). Medium lacking the specified amino acid exhibits a yellow color.

2. Glucose non-fermenters fail to form acids and maintain the original purple color of the medium. In the case of a positive reaction, the medium turns deep purple as compared to an uninoculated tube (control).

Expected results Expected test results for each of an individual specific amino acid decarboxylase by some members of *Enterobacteriaceae* are outlined in Table 39.4.

Table 39.4: Expected results of decarboxylation of some key amino acids by Gram-negative bacteria

Decarboxylase	Positive	Negative
Lysine decarboxylase	*Klebsiella pneumoniae*	*Shigella flexneri*
Ornithine decarboxylase	*Enterobacter aerogenes*	*Proteus vulgaris*
Arginine decarboxylase	*Enterobacter cloacae*	*Klebsiella pneumoniae*

14. Catalase test: This test is very easy and quick to perform. However, laboratory personnel needs to take some precautions to eliminate false results. Unlike strict anaerobes, aerobic bacteria use oxygen as a final electron acceptor in an electron transport chain (ETC) to generate energy. During this energy-yielding activity, a harmful compound known as hydrogen peroxide is formed. Fortunately, these bacteria secrete catalase to degrade hydrogen peroxide to harmless products.

There are three different methods to perform this test:

1. Emulsifying a few bacterial cells with 2-3 drops of 3% hydrogen peroxide on a clean microscope slide.
2. Addition of a few drops of 3% hydrogen peroxide directly to colonies on an agar plate.
3. Addition of a few drops of 3% hydrogen peroxide directly to an actively growing broth culture.

Principle: Breakdown of hydrogen peroxide to water and molecular oxygen is catalyzed by catalase:

$$2H_2O_2 \xrightarrow{\text{catalase}} 2H_2O + O_2$$

Hydrogen peroxide   Water   Oxygen

Interpretation: Upon mixing of some cells of a test organism with 2-3 drops of hydrogen peroxide, immediate and rapid bubbling (foaming) constitutes a positive test. If bubbles are not formed, the test is interpreted as negative.

Precautions: Though the test is easy to perform and interpret, the technician needs to exercise certain precautions to avoid false positive/negative results:

1. Avoid the test colonies from blood agar plates since red blood cells do contain catalase
2. Avoid iron- or nichrome-made wire loops
3. Use sterile wooden applicator sticks for picking bacterial cells up from a colonial growth
4. Use overnight incubated cultures
5. Use a freshly prepared 3% hydrogen peroxide reagent
6. Store 3% H_2O_2 in a dark and cold place to protect from its decomposition
7. Use safety glasses at all times to protect against the corrosive effect of hydrogen peroxide

Expected results
Positive: *Staphylococcus aureus, Micrococcus luteus, Bacillus subtilis, Escherichia coli*, and *Pseudomonas aeruginosa*
Negative: *Streptococcus pyogenes, Enterococcus faecalis,* and *Clostridium* spp.

The superoxol (30% H_2O_2) test is performed as a rapid presumptive test for *Neisseria gonorrhoeae* (quick and strong bubbling = positive) recovered from modified Thayer-Martin (MTM) Chocolate agar. Some other species of *Neisseria (*e.g., *N. sicca)* do demonstrate a weak or delayed bubbling and is interpreted as a negative reaction.

15. Oxidase test: Like a catalase test, the oxidase test is a simple and rapid test that detects the presence or absence of cytochrome *c* oxidase (the last enzyme of some bacterial plasma membrane-associated electron transport chains). It catalyzes the transfer of electrons from a reduced ferrocytochrome c to oxygen:

$$\text{Compound}_{(red.)} + O_2 \xrightarrow{\text{cytochrome c oxidase}} \text{Compound}_{(oxi.)} + 2H_2O$$

Aerobic respiration involves three steps, namely glycolysis, citric acid cycle, and electron transport chain (ETC). Both NADH (from glycolysis and citric acid cycle) and $FADH_2$ (from citric acid cycle) are oxidized by donating electrons to molecular oxygen (a terminal electron acceptor) via ETC. While electrons pass from reduced molecules (i.e, NADH and $FADH_2$) to oxygen through a series of redox reaction complexes, they deliver energy to form ATP molecules, a process called oxidative phosphorylation. Thus, three and two molecules of ATP are generated for every NADH and $FADH_2$ oxidized, respectively.

Principle: N,N,N',N',-tetramethyl-p-phenylenediamine dihydrochloride, artificial indicator, acts as an electron donor (colorless) and cytochrome c oxidase (electron acceptor), causes the oxidation of an indicator dye. This oxidized form of dye exhibits a dark purple color within 15 seconds, denoting a positive test. In a negative test, the indicator remains in reduced form (colorless).

Interpretation: Development of a purple or violet color indicates a positive test as opposed to a negative test where the indicator remains an unchanged leuco compound (colorless).

Precautions: It is necessary to take the following precautions to eliminate the erroneous results:

1. Avoid the use of metallic wire loops for making the transfer of bacterial cells. Use either pointed glass rods or wooden applicator sticks instead
2. Use overnight incubated unknown cultures
3. Use freshly prepared indicator reagent
4. Read the test within 15 seconds (a weak slow reaction continues, turning the indicator to blue color (false positive))
5. Autoclave the tested filter paper disc as it is a biohazardous material

Expected results
Positive: *Pseudomonas aeruginosa, Neisseria gonorrhoeae, Vibrio cholerae, Aeromonas* spp., and many more.
Negative: All members of *Enterobacteriaceae, e.g., Escherichia coli*

16. Coagulase (tube) test: Actually, there are two forms of coagulase found in a pathogenic *Staphylococcus aureus*: free versus bound ("clumping factor"). A bound form of coagulase can be detected by a rapid slide technique as a screening test. Free coagulase can be detected by a confirmatory tube technique, including a positive control and negative control. Citrated rabbit plasma (1mL of 1:10 diluted) is inoculated with a suspension (0.2mL) of a bacterial isolate in question. Similarly, both positive control (0.2mL of *Staphylococcus aureus*) and negative control (0.2mL of nutrient broth) tubes are also inoculated. Then, all the test tubes are incubated at 37°C and examined at half-hourly intervals until a period of four hours for clotting. A positive test shows a plasma clot as opposed to the absence of coagulation in a negative test. The presence of coagulase in *Staphylococcus aureus* is associated with the virulence of the organism since coagulases activate prothrombin, thereby converting fibrinogen to fibrin and a fibrin meshwork around the bacterial cells offers protection against the host defense system.

Principle: Coagulase-mediated transformation of fibrinogen (soluble) to fibrin (clot) occurs:

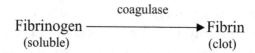

$$\text{Fibrinogen} \xrightarrow{\text{coagulase}} \text{Fibrin}$$
$$\text{(soluble)} \qquad\qquad\qquad \text{(clot)}$$

Interpretation: The formation of a clot is checked by gentle tilting of the inoculated and incubated (37°C) test tubes in front of a black background. A test tube demonstrating a clot within four hours constitutes a positive test. On the other hand, the failure of a coagulation reaction implies a negative test.

Expected results: Coagulase test is of great value in separating coagulase-positive *Staphylococcus aureus* from other coagulase-negative staphylococci, e.g., *Staphylococcus epidermidis*.

17. Bile Esculin test: This is a widely used presumptive test that differentiates group D streptococci and enterococci from non-group D viridans group streptococci. The medium includes esculin and peptone as nutrients whereas 2% oxgall ((equivalent to 40% bile) is added to inhibit Gram-positives other than enterococci and group D streptococci. Ferric citrate is added as a color indicator.

Principle: The hydrolysis of esculin (glycoside) leads to the formation of esculetin which, in turn, reacts with ferric citrate to form a phenolic iron complex (black precipitate):

(i) Esculin $\xrightarrow{\text{acid}}$ β-D-Glucose + Esculetin

(ii) Esculetin $+ Fe^{3+}$ (Ferric citrate) $\longrightarrow$ Phenolic iron complex
$$\qquad\qquad\qquad\qquad\qquad\qquad\qquad\qquad\qquad \text{(dark brown to black)}$$

Interpretation: If more than half of the agar slant turns dark brown to black in less than 48 hours of incubation, it indicates a positive test. If less than half of the agar slant turns dark brown to black after 48 hours of incubation, it indicates a negative test.

Expected results
Positive: *Enterococcus faecalis*
Negative: *Streptococcus pyogenes*

Triple sugar iron (TSI) agar

Occasionally, Triple sugar iron (TSI) agar is used to support the results of identification. This medium contains the following constituents:

1. Peptone
2. Meat extract
3. Yeast extract
4. Sodium chloride
5. Three sugars, namely lactose, sucrose, and glucose (10:10:1)

6. Ferric ammonium citrate
7. Sodium thiosulfate
8. Phenol red (indicator)
9. Agar powder
10. pH adjusted to 7.4 ± 0.2

Key for interpretation

Key	Observation	Interpretation
No change (-)	Pink slant and butt	No fermentation of sugars and no formation of H_2S
Alkaline (Alk.)	Deep red	No fermentation of sugars; alkaline products formed
A	Yellow slant	Fermentation of sucrose and/or lactose with the formation of acid
A	Yellow butt	Fermentation of glucose
G	Upward displacement of the whole medium or cracking of the medium	Formation of gas by heterofermentative bacteria
H_2S	Blackening of the medium	Formation of H_2S

Characteristic reactions of some species of *Enterobacteriaceae* on triple sugar iron (TSI) agar are shown in Table 39.5.

Table 39.5: Characteristic reactions of some species of *Enterobacteriaceae* on TSI

Genus/Species	Butt	Slant	H₂S production
Escherichia coli	AG	A	-
Enterobacter aerogenes	AG	A	-
Enterbacter cloacae	AG	A	-
Citrobacter freundii	AG	A	+
Klebsiella pneumoniae	A/AG	-/Alk	-
Alcaligenes faecalis	-	-/Alk	-
Proteus vulgaris	AG*	A	+
Proteus mirabilis	AG*	Alk/A	-
Morganella morganii	AG*	-/Alk	-
Providencia spp.	A/Alk	-/Alk	-
Salmonella typhi	A	-/Alk	+
Salmonella typhimurium	AG	-/Alk	+
Salmonella enteritidis	A/G	-/Alk	+
Shigella spp.	A	-/Alk	-
Pseudomonas aeruginosa	-	-/Alk	-

*Some strains can be A without gas formation.

Rapid tests

Advanced technology has greatly contributed to the development of commercial kits, as revealed in Fig. 39.1 (a), (b). These cost-effective kits are very convenient to use in the definitive identification of clinical isolates. These kits contain dehydrated substrates in miniature compartments (cupules), allowing multiple biochemical tests to be performed at a time. Some tests need the addition of the reagent(s) before reading. However, tube tests are still used in the student laboratories at teaching institutions.

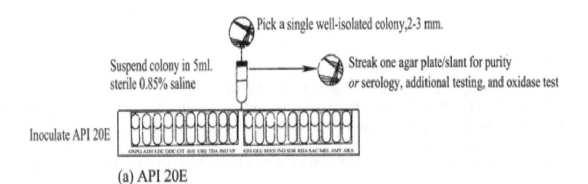

Pick a single well-isolated colony, 2-3 mm.

Suspend colony in 5ml.
sterile 0.85% saline

Streak one agar plate/slant for purity
or serology, additional testing, and oxidase test

Inoculate API 20E

(a) API 20E

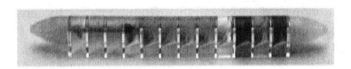

(b) Enterotube II

(a) API 20E
(b) Enterotube II

Fig. 39.1: Commercial miniaturized, rapid, and
ready-to-use identification systems.

Chapter 40

Gram-Positive Bacteria and Mycobacteria

Introduction

It is beyond the scope of this book to include a detailed account of Gram-positive bacteria. Clinically significant Gram-positive bacterial species are briefly described in this chapter. Therefore, only the key features of Gram-positive bacteria are summarized below.

The schematic structure of the cell wall of Gram-positive bacteria is depicted in Fig. 41.1(a).

1. Possess thick peptidoglycan (murein) layer that measures 20-80 nm
2. Contain teichoic acids and lipids in the peptidoglycan layer
3. Contain a cytoplasmic phospholipid membrane
4. Have a much smaller volume of periplasm than Gram-negative bacteria
5. Retain crystal violet-iodine complex during Gram's staining
6. Have only two basal body rings in some flagellated species

Prokaryotic taxonomy and *Bergey's Manuals*

Bergey's Manual of Determinative Bacteriology was first published in 1923 based on phenotype (non-evolutionary approach). The Manual was so-named to honor the first chairman, Dr. David H. Bergey, of its editorial board. Bergey's Manual of Determinative Bacteriology (9th Edition, 1994) is an authoritative reference for prokaryotic classification and taxonomy. However, *Bergey's Manual of Systematic Bacteriology* (2nd Edition, 5 Volumes, 2001-2012) is based on the 16S rRNA gene sequence data (Garrity and Holt, 2001; Ludwig *et al.*, 2009, 2011). Thus, it is an evolutionary approach, thereby providing a phylogenetic backbone of the prokaryotes (bacteria and archaea domains). About 15,000 names of prokaryotic taxa had been published till December 2012 and this number is increasing at a constant rate of about 750 names per year since 2006. There are still problems in establishing well-defined taxonomic classes and orders for many bacteria.

The collaborative efforts of the Bergey's Manual Trust and nearly one thousand microbiologists from all over the world has resulted in the publication of these Manuals. The Manuals serve microbiology researchers, students, clinicians, and other professionals to provide reliable detailed descriptions of each of the prokaryotic groups compiled by experts. *Bergey's Manual of Systematic Bacteriology* (2nd edition, 5 Volumes) is available online since April 2015.

Spectrum of biochemical tests used

The author prefers to use the term "rod" and not bacillus throughout the discussion for the rod-shaped bacteria. The term "bacillus" will only be limited to the genus *Bacillus* to avoid confusion. The following list of routine biochemical tests is valuable while characterizing Gram-positive bacteria:

1. Catalase
2. Growth characteristics on blood agar plate (BAP)
3. Growth characteristics on mannitol salt agar (MSA)

4. Bacitracin sensitivity
5. Optochin sensitivity
6. Growth in 6.5% NaCl
7. CAMP test
8. Bile esculin agar
9. Nitrate reduction
10. Starch (amylum) hydrolysis
11. Motility agar
12. Coagulase (bound and free)

A. Cocci (see Fig. 40.1)

Cocci (singular coccus) are round- or ovoid-shaped bacteria. Depending on patterns of their cell-division, they exhibit different types of cellular arrangements as shown in Table 40.1.

Table 40.1: Classical cellular arrangements of cocci

Arrangement	Microscopic appearance	Example
diplococci	in pairs	*Streptococcus pneumoniae*
streptococci	in chains	*Streptococcus pyogenes*
staphylococci	irregular clusters	*Staphylococcus aureus*
sarcinae	cubical pockets of eight	*Sarcina aurantiaca*
tetrads	clusters of four	*Micrococcus luteus*

This characteristic of typical arrangement is useful in the process of identification. Also, most cocci are non-motile and non-spore-formers. Gram-positive cocci are classified into two major families:

1. *Micrococcaceae* (catalase-positive)
2. *Streptococcaceae* (catalase-negative)

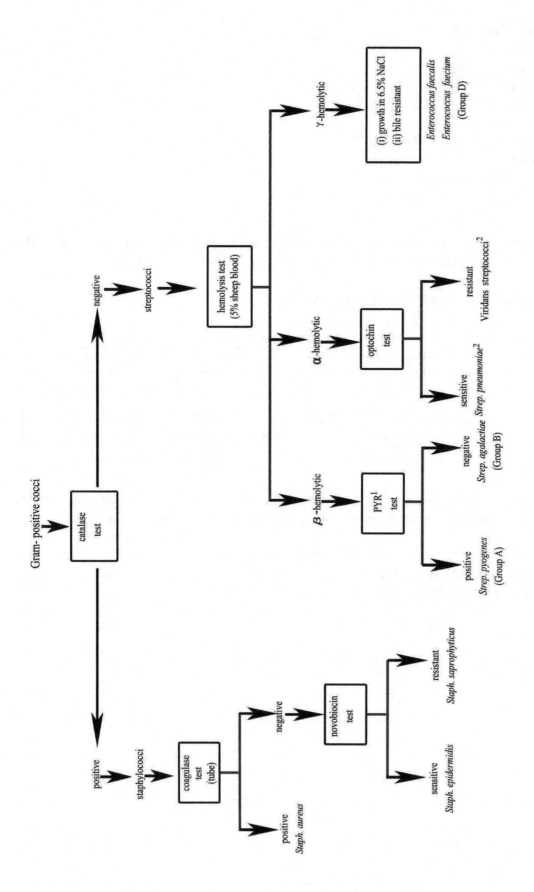

Fig.40.1: Differentiation of Gram-positive cocci up to species level on the basis of biochemical tests.

[1] PYR = pyrrolidonyl aminopeptidase; a test preferred over bacitracin
[2] Do not belong to any Lancefield groups

Staphylococcus aureus
- Golden yellow pigment
- Beta-hemolytic (only at 4°C)
- Coagulase = positive
- Resistant to penicillin (beta-lactamase production)
- Ferments glucose, sucrose, lactose, maltose, and mannitol
- Catalase = Positive
- Oxidase = Positive
- DNAse = Positive
- Urease = Positive
- Toxins produced by *S. aureus:* hemolysin, leukotoxin, exfoliative toxin, enterotoxin, and toxic-shock syndrome toxin-1 (TSST-1)
- Cause of boils, furuncles, carbuncles, bacteremia, toxic shock syndrome, scalded skin syndrome, and food poisoning
- Methicillin-resistant *Staphylococcus aureus* (MRSA) infections are difficult to treat

Staphylococcus epidermidis
- Non-hemolytic and produces white pigment
- Mostly capsulated
- Glucose = Positive
- Mannitol = Negative
- Oxidase = Negative
- Coagulase = Negative
- Catalase = Positive
- Urease = Positive
- Sensitive to novobiocin
- Forms a biofilm
- Causes infections relating to prosthetic devices

Staphylococcus saprophyticus
- Non-hemolytic
- Coagulase = Negative
- Mannitol = Negative
- Catalase = Positive
- Urease = Positive
- Resistant to novobiocin
- Causes uncomplicated cystitis in young sexually active females

Streptococci are classified based on hemolysis on 5% sheep blood agar as under:
1. Beta-hemolytic = Complete hemolysis
2. Alpha-hemolytic = Partial hemolysis
3. Gamma-hemolytic = No hemolysis

(i) Beta-hemolytic (complete hemolysis)

Lancefield grouping of streptococci: An American microbiologist, Rebecca Lancefield, classified streptococci based on their group-specific antigenic differences into 20 serological groups and named as group A-V (except I and J). Streptococcal cell wall contains C-carbohydrate that is species-specific. Rapid latex agglutination can help identify the C- carbohydrate antigen. These group-specific antigens differentiate the streptococci into different groups, namely A, B, C, F, and G. Some tests used in further differentiation of these streptococci are outlined in Table 40.2.

Table 40.2: Characterization and differentiation among group D streptococci, enterococci, and viridans streptococci

	Group D streptococci	Enterococci*	Viridans streptococci
Bile esculin	+	+	0
PYR	0	+	0
6.5% NaCl	0	+	0

Enterococcus species generally are resistant to cephalosporins and withstand heating at 60°C for 30 minutes.

Streptococcus pyogenes (Group A)
- Beta-hemolytic (larger zones)
- Catalase = Negative
- >85% susceptible to 0.04 units bacitracin
- L-pyrrolidonyl-beta-naphthylamide (PYR) = positive
- Associated with pharyngitis, scarlet fever, erysipelas, acute glomerulonephritis, necrotizing fasciitis (also called flesh-eating disease), and toxic shock syndrome
- ASO test to identify streptolysin O

Streptococcus agalactiae (Group B)
- Beta-hemolytic (small zones)
- Hydrolysis of sodium hippurate = Positive
- Associated with puerperal sepsis and neonatal sepsis and meningitis
- Catalase = Negative
- Bacitracin-resistant
- CAMP factor = Positive
- PYR = Negative

(ii) Alpha-hemolytic (partial hemolysis - "greening" of the medium)

Streptococcus pneumoniae (does not belong to any Lancefield groups)
- Mucoid colonies by encapsulated strains
- Lancet-shaped diplococci
- Bile solubility = Positive
- Catalase = Negative
- Susceptible to optochin
- Inulin = Positive

- Leading cause of lobar pneumonia, otitis media in children and meningitis in all age groups
- Quellung reaction: serotyping of capsular types (90 serotypes known)

Viridans streptococci (do not belong to any Lancefield groups)
- A group of streptococci without serological specificity
- Are commensals of mouth and upper respiratory tract
- Bile solubility = Negative
- Resistant to optochin
- Inulin = Negative
- Implicated in subacute bacterial endocarditis
- Penicillin-resistant

Streptococcus mitis
- Facultative anaerobe
- Present in throat, nasopharynx, and mouth
- Mesophile
- Alpha-hemolytic
- Catalase = Negative
- Causes bacteremia and infective endocarditis
- 16S rRNA sequencing used for species identification

Streptococcus mutans
- Present in human oral cavity
- Forms a sticky polysaccharide using sucrose (facilitates in plaque formation)
- Ferments glucose, fructose, and lactose producing lactic acid as an end-product
- Causes dental caries

(iii) Gamma-hemolytic (no hemolysis)

Enterococcus faecalis (Group D)
- Facultatively anaerobic, non-motile, and lacks a capsule
- Can grow at 10°C as well as 45°C, at a pH of 9.6, and culture media containing 40% bile or 6.5% NaCl
- Catalase = Negative
- Sugars (most) = Acid; no gas
- PYR = Positive
- Penicillin-resistant
- Acquired through contaminated food or water, air-droplets, and inanimate objects
- causes bacteremia, endocarditis, UTIs, and nosocomial infections

Enterococcus faecium
- Causes neonatal meningitis and endocarditis
- Causes device-associated infections (e.g., ventilators) by vancomycin-resistant enterococcal (VRE) strains
- Ferments glucose, maltose, ribose, mannitol, and D-mannose
- 22 sequenced *Enterococcus faecium* genomes

Streptococcus bovis
- Produces lactic acid from fermentable sugars, e.g., starch (called lactic acid bacterium)
- Non-hemolytic
- Cannot grow on culture media containing 6.5% NaCl
- Bile-esculin = Positive
- A member of the Lancefield group D streptococci (non-enterococci)
- Causes endocarditis, urinary tract infections, bacteremia, and colorectal cancer

B. Rods (see Fig. 40.2)

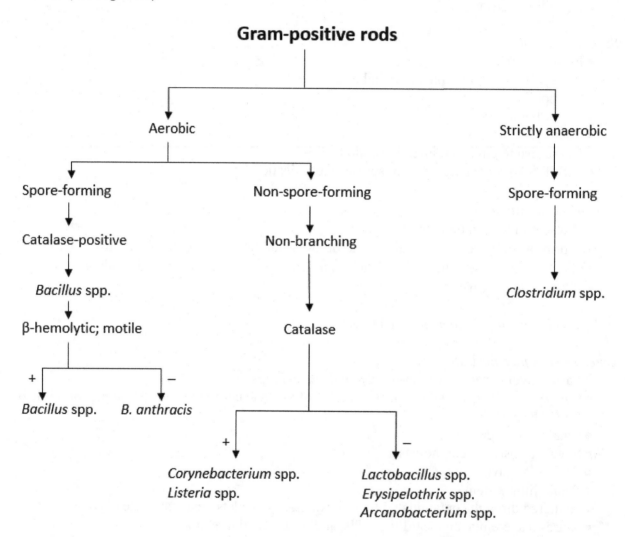

Fig. 40.2: An overview of medically important Gram-positive rods other than branching filamentous rods.

Actinomycetes are widely distributed in nature, e.g., soil and water. They are slow growing unicellular organisms that contain peptidoglycan layer in their cell wall. However, they show fungus-like growth pattern in tissues or in culture. Unlike the industrially important *Streptomyces* spp., some members of *Actinomyces* and *Nocardia* are associated with human infections.

(i) Aerobic spore-formers

*Bacillus subtilis (*hay-bacillus or grass-bacillus)
- Found in soil and gastrointestinal tract of ruminants and humans
- Used in quality control programs of microbiological testing
- Industrial applications, e.g., α-amylase production
- Catalase = Positive

Bacillus anthracis
- Non-hemolytic large colonies with irregular margin ("Medusa head" colonies)
- Tenacious consistency
- Large Gram-positive rods with squarish ends
- Central or subterminal endospores
- Encapsulated and non-motile
- Gamma phage lysis assay (a common diagnostic method)
- McFadyean's reaction = Positive
- Penicillin-resistant
- Produces potent exotoxin
- Causes:
  - (i) Pulmonary (inhalation) anthrax (contracted from handling contaminated wool called "wool sorter" disease)
  - (ii) Cutaneous anthrax (contracted by spores entering through the abraded skin (i.e., zoonotic)
  - (iii) Gastrointestinal anthrax (contracted by ingestion of carcasses of animals dying of anthrax containing spores)
- Most common agent of bioterrorism

Bacillus cereus
- Facultatively anaerobic and motile
- Beta-hemolytic and "waxy" appearance
- Isolation and identification on mannitol-egg yolk-polymyxin (MYP) medium
- Acid production from glucose
- Sugars, namely mannitol, xylose, and arabinose not fermented
- Voges Proskauer = Positive
- Citrate = Positive
- Lecithinase = Positive
- Causes food poisoning:
  - (i.) Diarrheal toxin (secreted only after entering into the intestine, causing a prolonged incubation period of 8-16 hours)
  - (ii.) Emetic toxin (heat-stable preformed toxin that acts immediately with a short incubation period of 1-6 hours)

(ii) Anaerobic spore-formers

Clostridium spp.
- Strictly anaerobic to aerotolerant

319

- Extremely powerful exotoxin producers
- Usually, stain Gram-positive may stain Gram-negative or Gram-variable
- Endospores may be central, subterminal, or terminal

Clostridium tetani
- Obligate anaerobe, motile bacillus (drumstick-like appearance)
- Swarming growth in culture
- Spores ubiquitous globally
- Genome consists of a circular chromosome with 2,799,250 base pairs with a G-C content of 28.6%
- TetX gene (encodes tetanus neurotoxin) detected by PCR technique
- Produces two types of toxins: tetanospasmin and tetanolysin
- H_2S = Positive
- DNase = Positive
- Amylase, lipase, nitrate reductase, and lecithinase = Negative
- Causative agent of tetanus (lockjaw): an acute disease that is manifested by skeletal muscle spasm and autonomic nervous system disturbance

Clostridium botulinum
- Obligate anaerobe and motile bacillus
- Causes three types of botulism: (i) infant (ii) food-borne (iii) wound
- Botulinum neurotoxins (BoNTs) are the most poisonous substances known to mankind
- *Clostridium botulinum* isolation (CBI), a selective medium, may be used

Clostridium perfringens (formerly known as *Cl. welchii*)
- Non-motile and spore-former
- Exceptionally generation time (6.3 minutes)
- Lecithinase = Positive (opalescence on an egg yolk medium called Nagler's reaction)
- Shows double zone hemolysis
- Lipase = Negative
- Catalase = Negative
- Spot indole test = Positive
- Reverse CAMP test = Positive
- Produces lecithinase on egg-yolk agar
- Causes gas gangrene
- Leading cause of food poisoning in the United States and Canada

Clostridium difficile
- Motile
- Catalase = Negative
- Superoxide dismutase = Negative
- Produces multiple toxins (e.g., enterotoxin A and cytotoxin B)
- Grows on cycloserine-cefoxitin-fructose agar, producing yellow ground-glass colonies.
- Causes antibiotic-associated diarrhea and pseudomembranous colitis

(iii) Non-spore-formers

Corynebacterium spp.
- Facultative anaerobes and non-motile
- Pleomorphic and club-shaped (V and Y configurations)
- Catalase = Positive
- Urease = Positive
- Grows slowly on most media, e.g., trypticase soy agar (TSA), blood agar, and Loeffler's medium
- Non-spore formers and non-capsulated
- Presence of metachromatic (volutin) granules (composed of polymetaphosphates)

Corynebacterium diphtheriae (Klebs-Loeffler bacillus)
- Non-motile, non-capsulated, non-sporulating with high G:C content
- Black colonies with dark brown halos on modified Tinsdale agar
- Four biotypes: gravis, intermedius, mitis, and belfanti
- Metachromatic granules formation on Loeffler's medium
- MALDI-TOF-MS technique for species identification
- Modified Elek test for the detection of toxigenicity
- Causative agent of diphtheria associated with necrosis of throat (pseudomembranous) and systemic toxemia

Corynebacterium jeikeium
- Ferments glucose
- Resistant to antimicrobial agents, especially macrolide antibiotics
- Susceptible to vancomycin and tetracycline
- Causes nosocomial infections in immunocompromised patients with catheters, prosthetic devices, and bone marrow patients

Lactobacillus spp.
- Highly pleomorphic rods that form chains in thioglycollate broth
- Catalase = Negative
- Alpha-hemolytic and pin-point colonies on blood agar, resembling *streptococcus viridans*
- Predominant flora of the vagina during reproductive years

Listeria monocytogenes
- Facultative anaerobe
- Lacks capsule
- Shows tumbling motility if grown at 20°-25°C in nutrient broth but non-motile at 37°C
- Beta-hemolytic on 5% sheep blood agar
- Glucose = Positive
- Catalase = Positive
- Oxidase = Negative
- Transmitted by contaminated food
- Invades neonates, pregnant women, and immunocompromised individuals (e.g., AIDS)
- Causes bacteremia, meningitis, and septic abortion

- Laboratory diagnosis needs culturing of blood, CSF, or wounds

Erysipelothrix rhusiopathiae
- Found in wild and domestic animals
- Causes occupational disease (erysipeloid), e.g., farmers and slaughterhouse workers
- Facultatively anaerobic
- Pleomorphic
- Non-motile
- Grayish and alpha-hemolytic colonies on blood agar after 2-3 days of incubation
- Catalase = Negative
- Coagulase = Positive (most strains)
- H2S = Positive

C. Branching filamentous rods (see Fig. 40.3)

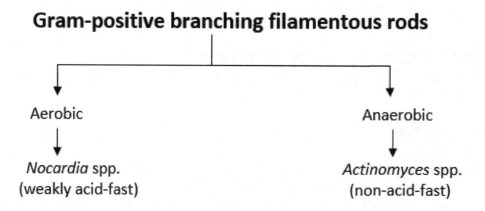

Fig. 40.3: A flowchart of Gram-positive branching filamentous cells of medical interest.

(i) Aerobic and partial acid-fast

Nocardia spp.
- Obligate aerobes
- Beaded branching filamentous rods
- Catalase = Positive
- 85 species known
- High G-C content
- 16S rRNA gene sequencing, a "gold standard" technique, for routine identification
- Accurate identification to species level by multilocus sequence analysis (MLSA) technique as a reference method (expensive and laborious)
- Optimized VITEK® MS database associated with a suitable sample preparation protocol enables a rapid, accurate, and robust identification of clinically relevant *Nocardia* species

Nocardia asteroides
- Causes a severe pulmonary infection in immunocompromised patients, e.g., HIV and organ transplant cases
- Found in the environment, e.g., soil and vegetation (exogenous source)
- Filaments may be demonstrated from sputum by a modified Kinyoun acid-fast technique
- Grows on 5% blood agar and chocolate agar (2-7 days), forming rough colonies of varied colors, e.g., white, orange, and red

Nocardia brasiliensis
- Causes a chronic skin infection (e.g., mycetoma)
- Laboratory diagnosis involves an examination of exudate, pus, and deep biopsy tissue

Nocardia farcinica
- Least common species of clinical importance
- Opacification of Middlebrook 7H10 agar, growth at 45^0C, and resistance to cefotaxime, tobramycin, and erythromycin provide a consistent differentiation between isolates *Nocardia asteroides* complex strains
- Has one circular chromosome (6, 021,225 bp) and two circular plasmids (i.e., pNF1=184,027 bp; pNF2=87,093 bp)

(ii) Anaerobic and non-acid-fast

Actinomyces israelii
- Non-acid-fast and anaerobic branching filamentous bacterium
- Found as a scanty normal commensal in the vagina, colon, and mouth
- Transmission is endogenous (opportunistic infections)
- Indole = Negative
- Catalase = Negative
- Ferments arabinose, maltose, sucrose, xylose, trehalose, and lactose
- Urease = Positive
- Nitrate = Positive
- Produces "sulfur granules" surrounded by neutrophils
- "Molar-tooth" colony on agar
- 16S rRNA sequencing useful in indirect detection (a reference method for identification)
- MALDI-TOF-MS technique accurately identifies at genus level to date
- Most common causative agent of actinomycosis

Propionibacterium acnes
- An aerotolerant, anaerobe, pleomorphic rod
- Forms a part of the microbiota of the skin, oral cavity, gastrointestinal and genitourinary tracts
- An opportunistic pathogen, causing implant-associated infections (e.g., breast fibrosis and periprosthetic knee joint infections)
- Grows on blood (glistening, circular, and opaque), chocolate, brucella, and brain heart infusion agar under anaerobic-to-microaerophilic conditions
- Catalase = Positive

- Indole = Variable
- Detected in tissue cultures (10 days) and sonication cultures (7 days)
- Good efficacy of rifampin against *P. acnes* biofilms

Mycobacteria

Mycobacteria are acid fast, non-motile, non-sporing, noncapsulated, weakly Gram-positive, straight or slightly curved rod-shaped bacteria, which are obligate aerobes (or microaerophilic). They sometimes show branching filamentous forms, resembling fungal mycelium and hence the name mycobacteria. These weakly Gram-positive bacilli have high mycolic acids (lipid) content in their cell walls. Owing to this type of cell wall composition, mycobacteria are resistant to many physical and chemical agents. Mycobacteria can be classified into:

a. *Mycobacterium tuberculosis* complex (MTC): causative agent of tuberculosis in humans
b. *M. leprae* : causative agent of leprosy
c. Nontuberculous mycobacteria (also called atypical mycobacteria or environmental mycobacteria): a diverse group of mycobacteria isolated from soil, animals, and water and occasionally cause opportunistic infections in humans
d. Saprophytic mycobacteria: present in soil, water, and other environmental sources

Unlike strict pathogens namely, *M. tuberculosis*, *M. leprae*, and *M. bovis*, potentially pathogenic mycobacteria are called "environmental mycobacteria", "atypical mycobacteria", or "nontuberculous mycobacteria" (NTM). More than 190 species of nontuberculous mycobacteria have been identified so far. Nontuberculous mycobacteria are routinely identified based on some biochemical tests, e.g., niacin, nitrate, catalase, Tween-80 hydrolysis, and more. However, reference laboratories perform sequencing (i.e., molecular) to identify mycobacteria. According to Neuschlova et al. (2017) from Slovakia, MALDI-TOF-MS can reliably be used in the routine identification of mycobacteria. A botanist named Ernest Runyon (1959) classified these non-tuberculous mycobacteria into four major groups based on their pigmentation and the rate of growth as shown in Table 40.3.

Table 40.3: Major groups (Runyon) of nontuberculous mycobacteria (NTM)

Group	Characteristics	Examples
Photochromogens	– buff-colored if grown in the dark, changes to yellow pigment after exposure to light – colonies appear after 7 days of incubation	*M. kansasii* *M. marinum* *M. simiae*
Scotochromogens	– yellow pigment if grown in dark or light – growth appears after 7 days of incubation	*M. gordonae* *M. scrofulaceum*
Non-photochromogens	– no pigment production in dark or light – colonies appear after 7 days of incubation	*M. avium-intracellulare* *M. ulcerans* *M. xenopi* *M. haemophilum* *M. terrae* *M. szulgai* *M. genavense*
Rapid growers	– colonies appear within 7 days of incubation	*M. smegmatis* *M. fortuitum* *M. chelonae* *M. abscessus* *M. peregrinum*

Mycobacterium tuberculosis
- Niacin = Positive
- Nitrate = Positive
- At 37°C catalase = Positive; at 68°C catalase = Negative
- Pyrazinamidase test = Positive
- Thiophene carboxylic acid hydrazide (TCH) = Resistant
- Prolonged generation time (i.e., 15-22 hours)
- Acquired by inhalation of airborne droplet nuclei from infected persons
- First-morning sputum is the specimen of choice
- On Lowenstein-Jensen medium, colonies appear small, rough, dry, buff-colored, and
- Eugonic after 4-6 weeks
- Direct detection from clinical specimens by a polymerase chain reaction
- Can spread to kidneys, spleen, bone marrow, central nervous system (CNS), and gastrointestinal (GI) tract called miliary tuberculosis
- PPD skin test (>10 mm positive; < 5 negative)

Mycobacterium leprae (Hansen's bacillus)
- Obligately intracellular
- Gram-Positive
- Acid-fast (less acid fast as compared to tubercle bacilli)

- Aerobic, non-motile, and non-spore-forming bacilli
- Fails to grow *in vitro* (i.e., artificial media); but can be grown in the footpads of mice and the armadillos
- Transmitted through inhalation and direct or indirect contact with infectious skin lesions
- Invades mucous membranes of the nose and peripheral sensory nerves
- Prolonged generation time (i.e., 12-13 days)
- Incubation period is measured in years
- Two forms of leprosy: tuberculoid (Th1 response) and lepromatous (Th2 response)
- Laboratory diagnosis: AFB smears of skin scrapings (positive only in lepromatous cases), histopathological (punch biopsy) examination, serological test (phenolic glycolipid I), and molecular test (PCR)

Mycobacterium bovis
- Microaerophilic
- Niacin = Negative
- Nitrate = Negative
- Pyrazinamidase test = Negative
- Susceptible to 5 μg/mL of thiophene-2-carboxylic acid hydrazide (T2H)
- Causes TB in cattle, rarely found in humans

Mycobacterium avium–intracellulare
- Infects gastrointestinal tract in patients with AIDS
- Stool specimens for smear and culture
- Niacin = Negative
- Nitrate = Negative
- Pyrazinamidase test = Positive
- Reduction of potassium tellurite to metallic tellurium (black precipitate) in 3-4 days

Mycobacterium kansasii
- Photochromogen
- Niacin = Negative
- Nitrate = Positive
- Pyrazinamidase test = Negative
- Hydrolysis of Tween 80 = Positive (development of pink color in approximately 5 days)
- Causes pulmonary infection

Mycobacterium marinum
- Photochromogen
- Optimum growth temperature between 25°-32°C
- Nitrate = Negative
- Pyrazinamidase test = Positive
- Hydrolysis of Tween 80 = Positive
- Contracted through abraded skin upon exposure to contaminated water
- Causes "swimming pool granuloma"
- Colonizes on the extremities (the lowest favorable skin temperature) and produces granulomatous skin lesions

Mycobacterium gordonae
- Scotochromogenic tap water bacillus
- Nitrate = Negative
- Urease = Negative
- Tween 80 hydrolysis = Positive
- Not pathogenic for humans
- Can be found as a specimen contaminant

Mycobacterium fortuitum
- Rapid grower (less than 7 days)
- Nitrate = Positive
- Reduces potassium tellurite to metallic tellurium (black precipitate)
- Iron uptake = Positive
- Arylsulfatase = Positive
- Grows on crystal violet-deficient MacConkey's agar
- Causes pulmonary infection

Mycobacterium chelonae
- Rapid grower (less than 7 days)
- Nitrate = Negative
- Iron uptake = Negative
- Causes pulmonary infection

Mycobacterium scrofulaceum
- Scotochromogen (yellow pigment in dark/light)
- Nitrate = Negative
- Urease = Positive
- Hydrolysis of Tween 80 = Negative
- Causes cervical adenitis, mainly in children

Chapter 41

Gram-Negative Bacteria, Spirochetes, and Rickettsiae

Introduction

Unlike the cell wall of Gram-positive bacteria, the Gram-negative bacteria have a more complex structure as depicted in Fig. 41.1 (b).

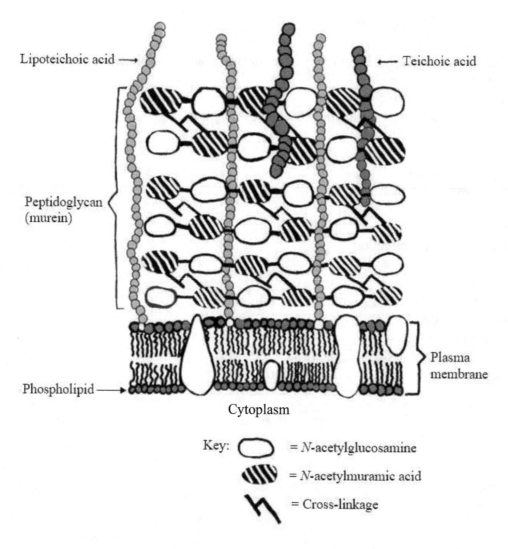

Lipoteichoic acid →

← Teichoic acid

Peptidoglycan (murein) {

Phospholipid →

Plasma membrane

Cytoplasm

Key: ⬭ = *N*-acetylglucosamine

〰 = *N*-acetylmuramic acid

ꀷ = Cross-linkage

(a) Cell wall of Gram-positive bacteria

Fig. 41.1: Chemical composition of bacterial cell wall.

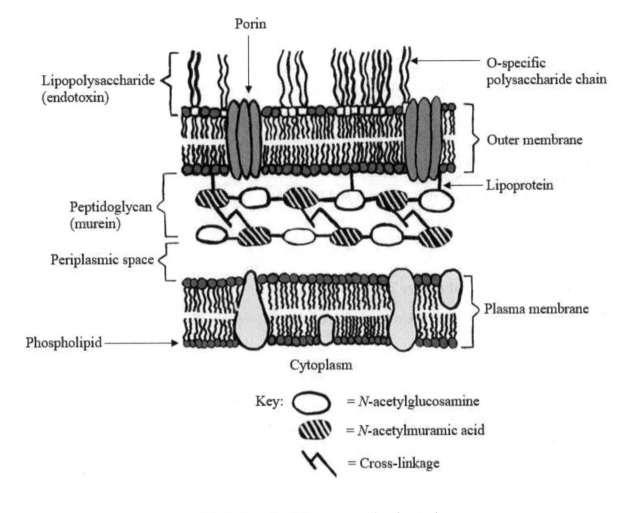

Porin

Lipopolysaccharide
(endotoxin)

O-specific
polysaccharide chain

Outer membrane

Lipoprotein

Peptidoglycan
(murein)

Periplasmic space

Plasma membrane

Phospholipid

Cytoplasm

Key: ⬭ = N-acetylglucosamine

= N-acetylmuramic acid

= Cross-linkage

(b) Cell wall of Gram-negative bacteria

Fig. 41.1: Chemical composition of bacterial cell wall.

Key features of Gram-negative bacteria are listed below:

1. Have a thin layer of peptidoglycan (2-3 nm) between the two membranes, namely plasma (cytoplasmic or cell) membrane and outer membrane
2. Have a larger periplasmic space compared to that of Gram-positive bacteria
3. Get decolorized following 95% alcohol treatment
4. Stain by a counterstain (safranin)
5. Have four basal body rings in some flagellated Gram-negative species

The following list of routine biochemical tests are valuable while characterizing Gram-negative bacteria:

1. Oxidase
2. Growth characteristics on MacConkey agar
3. Indole production
4. Methyl red (MR)
5. Voges-Proskauer (VP)
6. Utilization of citrate
7. Production of H_2S
8. Utilization of sugars (e.g., glucose and lactose)
9. Urease
10. Nitrate reduction
11. Motility agar

Prokaryotic taxonomy and *Bergey's Manuals* (see chapter 40)

A flowchart of medically relevant Gram-negative bacteria (see Fig. 41.2).

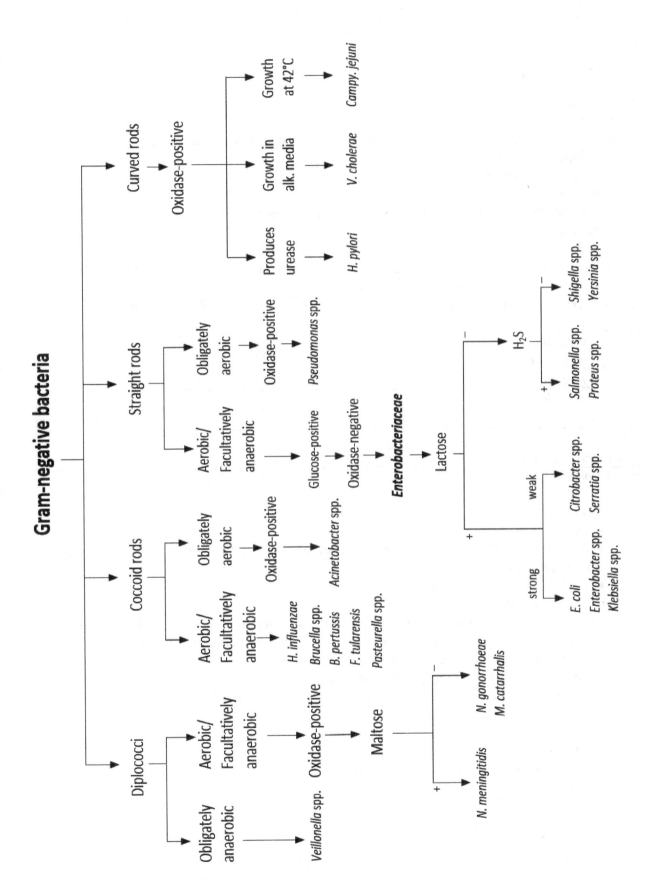

Fig.41.2: Flowchart of medically relevant Gram-negative bacteria.

A. Cocci

a. Aerobic/facultatively anaerobic

Neisseria spp.
- Aerobic
- Gram-negative diplococci with adjacent sides flattened (coffee-bean shaped)
- Oxidase = Positive
- Catalase = Positive (most)
- Non-motile
- Form the only acid from oxidation of sugars (non-fermentative)
- Pathogens are capnophilic (CO_2 lovers)

The utilization of some sugars by *Neisseria* spp. and *Moraxella catarrhalis* is shown in Table 41.1.

Table 41.1: Utilization of some sugars by *Neisseria* spp. and *Moraxella catarrhalis*

Gram-negative diplococci	Glucose	Maltose	Lactose
Neisseria gonorrhoeae	+	-	-
N. meningitidis	+	+	-
*N. lactamica**	+	+	+ (slow)
N. sicca	+	+	-
Moraxella catarrhalis	-	-	-

*Growth on MTM agar; β-D-galactosidase = positive.

Neisseria gonorrhoeae
- Kidney-shaped diplococci
- Media used include modified Thayer-Martin (MTM), Martin-Lewis (ML) agar, and New York City agar
- Oxidase, catalase = Positive
- Superoxol (30% H_2O_2) = Positive
- Causes gonorrhea (a sexually transmitted disease that commonly manifests as cervicitis, urethritis, and conjunctivitis), salpingitis in women, ophthalmia neonatorum (uncommon as all neonates are treated with $AgNO_3$ or antibiotic)
- Causes bacteremia leading to septic arthritis
- Increasingly resistant to penicillin (beta-lactamase = Positive)
- Nucleic acid probes available for detection

Neisseria meningitidis
- Diplococci with adjacent sides flattened like half moon-shaped
- Produces a thick capsule
- Normal flora of nasopharynx
- Mode of transmission: Inhalation of droplets
- Oxidase and catalase = Positive
- Causes epidemic meningitis in young adults (early childhood, i.e., 3 months to 5 years with a second episode occurring in adolescents, i.e., 15-25 years of age)

- Fastidious and very delicate cocci that do not grow in basal media. But, they can be cultured on chocolate agar or modified Thayer-Martin medium
- Quellung reaction used for serotyping
- Rapid identification by PCR technique

Moraxella catarrhalis
- Gram-negative, fastidious, non-motile diplococci
- Morphologically resemble *Neisseria* spp.
- Grows poorly on MTM medium
- Catalase, oxidase, DNase = Positive
- Glucose, fructose, lactose, maltose, sucrose = Negative
- Tributyrin hydrolysis = Positive
- Causes otitis media and sinusitis in infants and children, infections of the lower respiratory system, central nervous system, and joints in humans

Chlamydiae
- Obligate intracellular parasites
- Cell wall resembles to that of Gram-negative bacteria, although they lack a peptidoglycan layer
- Cannot be grown in artificial culture media

Chlamydia trachomatis
- Causes a variety of infections, e.g., trachoma, lymphogranuloma venereum, and non-gonococcal urethritis and neonatal infections
- Nucleic acid amplification tests and nucleic acid hybridization tests useful for detection
- Divided in to two biovars:
  1. Trachoma-inclusion conjunctivitis (TRIC)
  2. Lymphogranuloma venereum (LGV)

Chlamydia pneumoniae
- Exclusively human pathogen
- Associated with atherosclerosis
- Causes walking pneumonia, asthma, and chronic obstructive pulmonary disease (COPD)

Chlamydia psittaci
- Pathogen of parrots and other psittacine birds
- Causes psittacosis

b. Obligately anaerobic

Veillonella spp.
- Non-motile, non-sporulating bacteria
- Of the four species found in humans: *Veillonella parvula, V. dispar, V. atypica,* and *V. alcalescens,* only *V.parvula* and *V. alcalescens* have been recovered from clinical specimens
- *V. parvula* causes dental caries, sinusitis, osteomyelitis, endocarditis, and meningitis

- Ability to utilize lactate
- Unable to ferment carbohydrates or amino acids
- Reduce nitrate to nitrite
- Produce red fluorescence under UV light in specific growth media

B. Aerobic rods

Enterobacteriaceae
- Gram-negative non-spore-forming rods
- Facultative anaerobes
- Glucose = Positive
- Oxidase = Negative
- Nitrate = Positive
- Catalase = Positive (except one species of *Shigella*)

a. Lactose fermenters

Escherichia coli
- Motile (peritrichous flagella) small rods
- Normal flora of the gastrointestinal (GI) tract
- Indole = Positive
- Methyl red = Positive
- Voges-Proskauer = Negative
- Citrate = Negative
- Green metallic sheen on EMB plate (i.e., lactose fermenter)
- TSI = A/A; gas
- Causes urinary tract infections (UTIs), diarrhea, and neonatal meningitis

  o Urinary tract infections caused by Uropathogenic *E. coli* (UPEC)
  o Diarrhea
     i. Infantile diarrhea caused by Enteropathogenic *E. coli* (EPEC)
     ii. Traveler's diarrhea caused by Enterotoxigenic *E. coli* (ETEC)
     iii. Bacillary dysentery caused by Enteroinvasive *E. coli* (EIEC)
     iv. Hemorrhagic colitis and hemolytic uremic syndrome caused by Enterohemorrhagic *E. coli* (EHEC *E coli* 0157: H7 which is sorbitol = negative)
     v. Persistent and acute diarrhea caused by Enteroaggressive *E. coli* (EAEC)

Enterobacter spp.
- Form mucoid colonies
- Motile
- Lactose = Positive
- Indole = Negative
- Methyl red = Negative
- Voges-Proskauer = Positive
- Citrate = Positive
- Oxidase = Negative
- Catalase = Positive

- DNase = Negative
- Ornithine decarboxylase = Positive
- H_2S = Negative
- TSI = Acid/Acid;gas
- Associated with opportunistic and nosocomial infections
- Two species, namely *E. aerogenes* and *E. cloacae* are most common

Klebsiella pneumoniae[30]
- Facultative anaerobe and non-motile rods
- Ability to form thick capsule (virulence factor)
- Lactose = Positive
- Urease = Positive
- Indole = Negative
- Methyl red = Negative
- Voges-Proskauer = Positive
- Citrate = Positive
- TSI = A/A; gas
- Causative agent of lobar pneumonia and many nosocomial infections, e.g., urinary tract infections and chronic obstructive pulmonary disease
- Most of hospital strains are multi-drug resistant

Citrobacter freundii
- Facultatively anaerobic
- Occurs in feces of humans and lower animals
- Motile
- *o*-Nitrophenyl-*β*-D-galactosidase (ONPG) = Positive
- Indole = Negative
- Methyl red = Positive
- Voges-Proskauer = Negative
- Citrate = Positive
- TSI = K/A; gas (H_2S)
- Opportunistic pathogen

---

[30] *K. pneumoniae* is closely related to *K. oxytoca* and differentiated by its ability to grow on melezitose but not 3-hydroxybutyrate and negative indole test.

Serratia marcescens
- Facultative anaerobe
- Opportunistic pathogen
- Produces non diffusible red-pigment called prodigiosin on nutrient agar at RT
- Motile by peritrichous flagella
- Glucose = Positive (acid; ±gas)
- Voges-Proskauer = Positive
- Citrate = Positive
- DNAse = Positive (most)
- Gelatin = Positive
- Nitrate = Positive
- Causes urinary tract infections and septicemia in immunosuppressed persons

b. Lactose non-fermenters

(i) oxidase-positive

Vibrio spp.
- Facultative anaerobes
- Glucose = positive
- Curved or straight Gram-negative rods
- Motile by one or more polar flagella
- Commonly found in marine environments

Vibrio cholerae
- Comma-shaped Gram-negative rods
- Non-halophile
- Cholera red reaction = Positive
- Produces yellow colonies on thiosulfate citrate bile salts sucrose (TCBS) medium
- Sucrose = Positive
- Venkatraman Ramakrishnan (VR) medium may be used to transport feces from suspected cholera patients
- Motility demonstrable by a dark-field microscopy
- Produces an enterotoxin that causes the release of fluids and electrolytes into the intestinal lumen (watery diarrhea)
- Causative agent of Asiatic cholera ("rice-water stools") which is a food- or water-borne disease
- Confirmation of O1 or O139 antigen[31] in rice-water stool by a serological test

---

[31] *V. cholerae* O1 and O139 serotypes cause epidemic cholera.

Vibrio parahaemolyticus
- Major causative agent of food poisoning (gastroenteritis) related to contaminated fish or raw shellfish
- Capsulated
- Halophile (grows in 8% NaCl)
- Produces green colonies on TCBS
- Sucrose = Negative
- Kanagawa phenomenon: It causes β hemolysis on Wagatsuma agar (high salt blood agar)

Vibrio vulnificus
- Lactose = positive {the only lactose fermenting (L^+) *Vibrio* spp.}
- Halophile
- Mostly produces deep green colonies on TCBS
- May cause septicemia, especially in people with liver disorder

Campylobacter jejuni
- Microaerophilic and motile
- Curved, slender, Gram-negative rods ("seagulls")
- Found in the GI tract of dogs, cats, and poultry
- Grows at 42°C but not 35°C with increased CO_2 on campy-blood agar
- Microaerophilic condition for growth (5% O_2, 10% CO_2, and 85% N_2)
- Exhibits darting corkscrew motility
- Oxidase = Positive
- Catalase = Positive
- Nitrate reductase = Positive
- Sugars = Negative
- Susceptible to nalidixic acid
- Produces heat-labile enterotoxin (stimulates cAMP)
- Most common cause of bacterial diarrhea in the US (invasive gastroenteritis)

Helicobacter pylori
- Microaerophilic and motile
- Recovered from gastric biopsy
- Grows on chocolate agar and Campy agar (28°C)
- Catalase = Positive
- Oxidase = Positive
- Rapid urease = Positive
- Colonization in acidic environment (i.e., stomach) is favored due to abundant urease that catalyzes urea hydrolysis to produce ammonia. So formed ammonia buffers the gastric acid
- Causative agent of peptic ulcer, gastric carcinoma, and gastritis in humans

Pseudomonas spp.
- Aerobe
- Oxidative
- Oxidase = Positive
- Possess genes coding for resistance to several antimicrobial agents

Pseudomonas aeruginosa
- Strict aerobe that grows at 42°C
- Grape-like odor
- Produces large, translucent, and flat colonies with feathered edges on blood agar (β-hemolytic)
- Produces pyocyanin (a water-soluble pigment) and fluorescein
- Cetrimide agar: a selective medium
- All fermenting sugars = Negative
- Infects burns and wounds
- Oxidase = Positive
- Causative agent of cystic fibrosis
- Most common cause of nosocomial infections

Alcaligenes faecalis
- Strict aerobe and motile
- Oxidase = Positive
- Catalase = Positive
- Fails to grow in 6.5% NaCl; non-hemolytic and grows luxuriantly on MacConkey agar
- Linked with nosocomial infections

Burkholderia (Pseudomonas) cepacia
- Nosocomial pathogen
- Slender Gram-negative rods
- Grows best at 30°C.
- Produces yellow or green pigment
- Causative agent of pneumonia in cystic fibrosis patients

Aeromonas hydrophila
- Present in the sea and freshwater
- Straight Gram-negative rods
- Usually beta-hemolytic
- Oxidase = Positive
- Causes wound infections and gastroenteritis

Legionella pneumophila
- Flagellated, non-capsulated, and non-spore-forming pleomorphic rods
- Stains positive with Dieterle silver stain and easily visualized
- Obligate aerobes grow facultatively inside the macrophages (i.e., facultative intracellular parasite)
- Aerial transmission (no human-to-human transmission known)
- Found in water sources, e.g., cooling towers
- Causes Legionnaires' disease and Pontiac fever
- Sugars not fermented
- Oxidase, catalase, and β-lactamase = Positive

- Requires cysteine and iron for growth, e.g., Mueller-Hinton agar with hemoglobin and IsoVitaleX and buffered charcoal-yeast extract (BCYE) agar media (takes 3-5 days) are used
- Immunofluorescence technique for the detection
- Nucleic acid probes available

(ii) oxidase negative

Shigella dysenteriae sonnei
- Out of four species *(Shigella dysenteriae flexneri, S. dysenteriae boydii, S. dysenteriae sonnei and S. dysenteriae dysenteriae),* S. dysenteriae sonnei is most common in the US
- Motility = Negative
- TSI = K/A; no gas; no H_2S
- Lysine decarboxylase = Negative
- IMViC reactions = ±, -, -, -
- Transmitted by the fecal-oral route
- Causes diarrhea (bacillary dysentery) with blood and mucus (dysentery)

Salmonella spp.
- More than 2000 serotypes based on 0 and H antigens (Kauffman-white scheme)
- Motility = Positive (peritrichous flagella)
- TSI = K/A; gas (H_2S)
- Oxidase = Negative
- Catalase = Positive
- Nitrate = Positive
- IMViC reactions = - ; + ; - ; +
- Peculiar growth on Salmonella–Shigella, Hektoen enteric, and xylose lysine tergitol-4 (XLT4) agar media
- Causes gastroenteritis, septicemia, food poisoning (poultry and eggs), and osteomyelitis
- Clinical classification: It divides *Salmonella* into two groups as under:
  o *Typhoidal Salmonella:* It includes serotypes namely, S. *typhi* and S. *paratyphi.* They cause enteric fever (typhoid/paratyphoid fever).
  o *Non-typhoidal Salmonella:* They are associated with food-borne gastroenteritis and septicemia.

Salmonella typhi
- Can be cultured from stool, blood, and urine during an enteric fever
- Colonizes the gallbladder, leading to a carrier state
- TSI = K/A; no gas; little H_2S
- Causative agent of typhoid fever and rose-spot rashes
- Infective dose of Salmonella is 103 – 106 bacilli to initiate the infection
- Laboratory diagnosis: Widal test (serum antibody detection)

Proteus spp.
- Swarm on most agar surfaces
- TSI = K/A; gas (H_2S)
- Urease = Positive

- Phenylalanine deaminase = Positive
- Oxidase = Negative
- Catalase = Positive
- Methyl red = Positive
- Facultatively anaerobic and motile
- Associated with gastrointestinal infections, UTIs, sepsis in burn cases, and struvite stones in kidneys[32]

Proteus vulgaris
- Swarming growth in culture
- Indole = Positive
- Catalase = Positive
- Urease = Positive
- H_2S = Positive
- NO_3 reduction = Positive
- Causes urinary tract infections (10-15% of hospital-acquired UTIs) .

Proteus mirabilis
- Facultative anaerobe
- Frequently isolated from humans
- Indole = Negative
- Urease = Positive
- Swarming motility

Acinetobacter baumannii
- Coccoid rods
- Strict aerobe
- Biofilm formation
- Swarming motility
- Oxidase = Negative
- Catalase = Positive
- Linked with nosocomial infections (e.g., UTI)

Acinetobacter calcoaceticus
- Aerobe
- Oxidase = Negative

o two subspecies:
  (i) Acinetobacter calcoaceticus var. *anitratus*
  - Saccharolytic

  (ii) Acinetobacter calcoaceticus var. *Iwoffi*
  - Asaccharolytic

---

[32] *Proteus* species produce urease which splits urea to form ammonia, making the urine alkaline. Then, alkaline urine predisposes to the deposition of phosphate and leads to the formation of kidney stones (also called renal calculi, urolithiasis, or nephrolithiasis).

Yersinia spp.
- Exhibits bipolar staining
- Lactose = Negative
- Indole = Negative
- TSI = A/A; no gas
- Catalase = Positive
- Urease = Negative
- Nitrate = Positive
- Voges-Proskauer = Negative
- Citrate = Negative

Yersinia pseudotuberculosis
- Causes Yersiniosis
- Some strains express a super antigen mitogen which has caused scarlet-like fever
- Rhamnose, salicin, and melibiose = Positive

Yersinia enterocolitica
- Causes Yersiniosis, a food and water-borne infection
- Causes enterocolitis in children; mimics acute appendicitis
- Cefsulodin-irgasan-novobiocin (CIN) medium for isolation purposes (pink to red at 25°C.)
- Sucrose, cellobiose, and sorbitol = Positive

Yersinia pestis
- Facultative intracellular parasite
- Transmitted by bite of infected rat fleas
- Causes plague (black death): (i) bubonic (ii) pneumonic (bloody sputum) (iii) septicemic
- Blood, sputum, and spinal fluid can be used as specimens for identification
- Special transport medium to protect handlers

Morganella morganii
- Facultatively anaerobic and non-motile
- Oxidase = Negative
- Catalase = Positive
- Urea = Positive
- H_2S = Negative
- IMViC reactions= +, +, –, –
- Associated with UTIs, respiratory infections, and wounds

Other Gram-negative rods

Haemophilus spp.
- Coccoid rods
- Pleomorphic
- Non-motile
- Growth stimulated by CO_2

- Need growth factors (X and/or V)
- Grow on chocolate agar
- Normal flora of upper respiratory tract

Different species of *Haemophilus* are characterized in Table 41.2.

Table 41.2: Identification of different species of *Haemophilus*

Haemophilus spp.	Requirement for X factor (hemin)*	Requirement for V factor (NAD)**	Hemolysis on rabbit or horse blood agar	Porphyrin (ALA)***
H. influenzae	+	+	0	0
H. parainfluenzae	0	+	0	+
H. haemolyticus	+	+	+	0
H. parahaemolyticus	0	+	+	+
H. aphrophilus	V/0	0	0	+
H. ducreyi	+	0	0	0

*Hemin = found in hemoglobin.
**NAD = nicotinamide adenine dinucleotide (coenzyme).
***ALA = delta-aminolevulinic acid (substrate for the synthesis of hemin).

H. influenzae (Pfeiffer's bacillus)
- Short pleomorphic rods
- Requires X and V factors
- Grows on a chocolate agar plate (CAP) with a "mousy" odor
- Demonstrates "satellitism" on a blood agar plate containing *Staphylococcus aureus*
- Causes infantile meningitis in kids (6-24 months old)

H. ducreyi
- Fastidious coccoid rods
- Exhibits "school of fish" appearance on Gram-stain
- Can be cultured on chocolate agar
- Requires X factor but not V factor for growth
- Oxidase = Positive
- Causes a sexually transmitted disease called chancroid or soft chancre (painful sores on genitalia

Bordetella pertussis
- Strict aerobe and motile coccoid rods
- Causes an acute respiratory infection called pertussis (whooping cough or 100 days fever), particularly in children
- Colonizes the ciliated cells of the mucous membrane of the respiratory tract
- Produces various virulence factors, including adhesins, capsule, and toxins
- Four overlapping stages of the disease are: incubation (7-10 days), catarrhal stage, paroxysmal coughing stage (lymphocytosis), and convalescent stage
- Transmitted by airborne droplets

- Needs special culture media, e.g., Regan-Lowe (charcoal blood agar) and Bordet-Gengou media
- Convex, glistening, and pearl-like (mercury drops) colonies on Bordet-Gengou medium
- No growth on MacConkey agar
- Catalase = Positive
- Oxidase = Positive
- Urease = Negative
- Nitrate reductase = Negative
- Citrate utilization = Negative
- Diagnosis includes bacterial cultures of respiratory secretions (nasopharyngeal swab) and a fluorescent antibody test (FAT)
- PCR more sensitive than culture method

Brucella spp.
- Four species pathogenic for humans are: *Br. abortus* (cattle), *Br. melitensis* (goats and sheep), *Br. suis* (swine), and *Br. canis* (dogs)
- Causes undulant fever (brucellosis) and Malta fever, leading to abortion, sterility, and decreased milk formation
- Brucellosis is primarily a zoonotic disease affecting various domestic animals, e.g., sheep, goat, or cattle
- Strictly aerobic and non-motile
- Isolated from blood and biopsies of RE tissue
- Requires tryptose in enriched culture media (Brucella agar containing erythritol), increased CO_2, and prolonged incubation time (2-3 weeks)
- Oxidase = Positive
- Catalase = Positive
- Urease = Positive
- H_2S = Positive
- The accomplishment of distinction at species level based on responses to dye-impregnated disks and biochemical reactions
- Serological tests are used for laboratory diagnosis

Mycoplasmas
- The smallest microbes capable of free living in the environment and self-replicating on artificial culture media
- Belong to the Mollicutes class (mollis = soft; cutis = skin)
- Absence of a cell wall which is replaced by a triple-layered cell membrane containing sterol
- Difficult to culture; pleuropneumonialike organisms (PPLO) selective agar medium can be used (weeks to months before tiny "fried-egg" colonies appear)
- Pleomorphic
- Fully resistant to antibiotics acting on cell wall, e.g., β lactams
- Non-sporing and non-flagellated
- Usually non-motile (some species exhibit gliding motility)
- Pleuropneumonia-like organisms (PPLO)

- Family *Mycoplasmataceae* comprises two genera, namely *Mycoplasma* and *Ureaplasma*

Mycoplasma pneumoniae (Eaton's agent)
- Requires cholesterol and nucleotides for growth
- Cold agglutination with O blood group cells antigen
- Causative agent of walking pneumonia

Mycoplasma hominis
- Analysis of the *M. hominis* PG21 genome sequence indicates that this bacterial species has the second smallest genome among self-replicating free organisms
- Incubation period is unknown
- Causes acute pyelonephritis, post-partum and post-abortum fever
- May increase the risk for tubal occlusion and infertility
- Found in blood cultures, respiratory specimens, and cerebrospinal fluid (CSF) of newborns through vertical transmission at birth
- Detection by real time PCR technique from genital swabs and urine samples
- Safe sex practices (e.g., use of condom) help to prevent the infection

Mycoplasma genitalium (also called Mgen)
- The smallest prokaryote (approximately 200-300 nm) among self-replicating free organisms
- Flask-shaped appearance
- Motile (gliding motility)
- Transmitted by genital-to genital contact
- Causes non gonococcal urethritis in men and mucopurulent cervicitis in women (STI)
- Detected by nucleic amplification assay test (NAAT) from urine, endometrial biopsies, and urethral, vaginal, and cervical swab

Ureaplasma urealyticum
- Requires cholesterol and nucleotides for growth
- Also called T-forms
- Urea hydrolysis = Positive (for energy production)
- Colonizes sexually active males without urethritis
- Causes urogenital tract disease

Ureaplasma parvum
- Commensal in female genital tract
- Hydrolyzes urea for energy production
- Not considered as a classic sexually transmitted infection (STI) due to its low degree of pathogenicity
- Detected by Real-Time PCR technique from urine samples or genital swabs

Streptobacillus moniliformis
- Cells occur singly or in long, wavy chains called a string of beads
- Requires enriched media for best growth e.g., blood agar
- Colonies may spontaneously transform to L forms with a "fried egg" appearance

- The "puffball" appearance in broth culture
- Glucose = Positive (only acid)
- Oxidase = Negative
- Catalase = Negative
- Nitrate reductase = Negative
- Causes rat-bite fever
- Transmitted by rat bite or ingestion of contaminated milk by rat feces

Francisella tularensis
- Facultative intracellular parasite and an aerobe
- Transmitted through unbroken skin or the conjunctiva from infected animals or animal products, ingestion of improperly cooked meat, and from the bites of infected wood ticks and deer flies
- Laboratory workers acquire through aerosol inhalation
- Agent of bioterrorism (classified as category A)
- Biochemical tests are of little importance in the identification
- Highly fastidious that requires special media e.g., cystine-blood-glucose agar (small, smooth, and grayish colonies in 2-3 days)
- Immunofluorescent method or agglutination reaction helpful in the diagnosis
- Causes tularemia (rabbit fever) with ulcer formation and enlargement of lymph nodes

Pasteurella multocida
- Facultatively anaerobic and non-motile
- Luxurious growth on serum bovine albumin (SBA)
- Oxidase = Positive
- Catalase = Positive
- Nitrate reductase = Positive
- Methyl red = Negative
- Voges-Proskauer = Negative
- Sugars (most) = Positive (acid; no gas)
- Usually, humans acquire infections from the bite/scratch of a domestic dog/cat

Gardnella vaginalis
- Gram-negative or Gram-variable, Gram-positive type cell-wall and may appear Gram-positive
- Needs special media and a CO_2 incubator for culture
- Non-motile
- Catalase = negative
- Oxidase = negative
- Implicated in bacterial vaginosis
- Vaginal epithelial cells covered by small Gram-negative rods known as "Clue cells"

Bacteroides fragilis
- Obligately anaerobic, rod-shaped, and encapsulated (polysaccharide) bacterium present as normal flora of the human colon
- Helps to convert complex compounds into simpler ones in the colon

- Causes opportunistic infections following surgery/trauma, e.g., sustained bacteremia and peritonitis
- Resistant to many antibiotics, especially to beta-lactam ring antimicrobial agents
- Anaerobic transport medium required
- Can grow in the presence of 20% bile
- Sucrose = Positive
- Catalase = Positive
- Identified by polymerase chain reaction (PCR)

Spirochetes

The spirochetes are Gram-negative, thin, and long spring-shaped motile bacteria. The salient feature of spirochetes is the presence of endoflagella. The endoflagella are present in the periplasmic space between the outer membrane and the peptidoglycan layer. These unicellular and slow-growing spirochetes may be anaerobes, facultatively anaerobic, or aerobes. Since culturing these exceptionally fastidious bacteria is a difficult task, microscopic techniques such as dark-field microscopy, electron microscopy, or other similar techniques are used for identification purposes. Clinically significant spirochetes belong to one of these three genera: *Treponema*, *Borrelia*, and *Leptospira*. Important species of these genera are briefly outlined below:

Treponema pallidum
- Causative agent of a sexually-transmitted disease syphilis
- Divided into four types: primary, secondary, latent, and tertiary
- The corkscrew appearance of bacterial cell
- Cannot be cultured
- VDRL and RPR can be used as screening tests
- Diagnosed by dark-field microscopy, immunofluorescence microscopy, or antibody detection, e.g., fluorescent treponemal antibody absorption test (FTA-ABS) and microhemagglutination test for *T. pallidum* (MHAP-TP)
- More diseases caused by species other than *T. pallidum* include: yaws, bejel, and pinta

Borrelia burgdorferi
- Causes a tick-borne disease known as Lyme disease (the most prevalent in the US)
- Rodents and deer are main reservoirs of Lyme disease
- Different stages of the disease depending upon the incubation time: early localized stage, spreading stage, and late-stage
- Microaerophiles
- Needs blood agar media to culture

Borrelia recurrentis
- Causes relapsing fever
- Human-to-human transmission by body lice
- Large and microaerophilic spirochetes that can be cultured on a variety of media containing long-chain fatty acids
- Can be visible under a light microscope amongst blood cells in blood smears

Leptospira interrogans
- Natural reservoirs include domestic animals and rodents
- Consists of fine tightly wound spirals with hook-like ends
- Causes leptospirosis (zoonotic disease) in two phases: Phase 1 and Phase 2
- Severe form of leptospirosis is called Weil's disease
- There are three important epidemiological determinants for Leptospirosis, namely exposure to rodents, rainfall, and rice field.
- Blood is a specimen of choice during the first week, urine is the best specimen after a week
- Aerobes that can be grown in certain enriched media (pH 6.8 -7.8); β-hemolytic

Bartonella spp.
- Facultatively intracellular, Gram-negative, and aerobes
- Non-motile
- Grows on chocolate agar or trypticase soy, or brain-heart infusion agar plus 5% sheep blood and CO_2 rich environment
- Catalase = Negative
- Oxidase = Negative
- Urease = Negative
- Sugars = Non-reactive
- Risk factors include immunocompromised patients, e.g., HIV infection and organ transplant cases
- Detected by culturing on enriched media, staining tissue biopsies, and polymerase chain reaction (PCR)

Bartonella henselae
- Causes bacillary angiomatosis, cat scratch fever disease (usually a benign or self-limiting), and persistent bacteremia

Bartonella quintana
Incubation period varies from 5 to 20 days
- Causes trench fever (transmitted by body louse), bacillary angiomatosis, and endocarditis
- Include nonspecific signs and symptoms including fever, malaise, headache, and body pain

Bartonella bacilliformis
Causes Oroya fever or Carrion's disease

Rickettsiae

The rickettsiae are Gram-negative obligate intracellular parasites of endothelial cells. They naturally parasitize arthropods (notably, ticks, lice, fleas, and mites). They are transmitted to humans or the other vertebrates through the bites of arthropods. Like viruses, they cannot be cultivated on artificial culture media. These filterable bacteria have a generation time of 9-12 hours.

These organisms, formerly classified with viruses, are now reclassified as Gram-negative coccoid rods because of the following characteristics:

1. Binary fission as a mode of multiplication
2. Both DNA and RNA present
3. The presence of a thin electron-dense rigid cell-wall i.e. can be stained by Gram's method
4. Susceptibility to antibiotics
5. Presence of metabolic enzymes

The family *Rickettsiaceae* has four genera as depicted in Table 41.3.

Table 41.3: Four genera of the family *Rickettsiaceae* with corresponding diseases

Genus	Disease(s)
Rickettsia	Typhus and spotted fever
Orientia	Scrub
Coxiella	Q-fever (no arthropod vector involved for spread)
Ehrlichia	Ehrlichiosis and febrile illness

Among these genera, *rickettsia* is the most prominent genus from the clinical aspect. Surprisingly, the pattern of the clinical symptoms seen in different rickettsial infections is similar. These signs and symptoms are:

- fever
- malaise
- a particular type of rash
- severe headache

It is very important to be aware of the fact that Rickettsial infections take several days for a characteristic rash to appear. This is why Rickettsial infections in their early stages can be mistaken for viral infections, e.g., influenza. Since Rickettsiae share an alkali-stable polysaccharide antigen with some strains of *Proteus* spp., laboratory diagnosis has become easier.

The patient's serum is tested for the specific antibody followed by the determination of the rising titer after a week or so. A well-known reaction termed the Weil-Felix test is performed as a primary test as shown in Table 41.4.

Table 41.4: Weil-Felix* reaction as a diagnostic test for Rickettsial diseases

Disease	Organism	Pr. vulgaris OX-19	Pr. vulgaris OX -2	Pr. mirabilis OX-K
Rocky Mountain spotted fever**	R. rickettsii	+	+	-
Rickettsial pox	R. akari	-	-	-
Epidemic typhus	R. prowazekii	+	+/-	-
Murine typhus	R. typhi	+	+/-	-
Scrub typhus	Orientia tsutsugamushi	-	-	+
Trench fever	Bartonella quintana	-	-	-

* False-positive reactions in case of infections by *Proteus* spp. and *Salmonella typhi*.

** The most severe and most frequently reported in the United States.

Further differentiation can be made by other serological tests namely, complement fixation test, latex agglutination, and enzyme immunoassay.

Chapter 42

Microbiology and Automation

Introduction

Like chemistry, hematology, and immunohematology, clinical microbiology is also equipped with fully automated instruments, especially for the identification of microorganisms. These automated systems perform several operations without human intervention, thus minimizing the risk of exposure of laboratory workers to potential pathogens.

The author believes that this is a "transitioning" era because microbial identification is undergoing a rapid transformation from conventional methodologies to genomics-based (molecular-based) methodologies and most recently, proteomics-based technology. For example, the detection of *Chlamydia trachomatis* was performed using a tissue culture method in the past. This necessitated transportation of the specimen to a laboratory through a cold-chain and the subsequent processing in less than 24 hours. These painstaking steps were aimed at the viability of culture for the successful recovery of the potential pathogen. With the availability of molecular diagnostics (i.e., nucleic acid amplification tests), it has become possible to complete the identification of non-viable organisms. In developing automated machines, one should not ignore the role of bioinformatics, including software and appropriately-built database libraries needed to match a particular pattern of an isolated microbial strain.

The author discusses the identification techniques for microbes in two major categories listed below:

A. Conventional
B. Innovative

A. Conventional: The conventional *versus* methods have been used for decades to identify microorganisms. They are listed below:

1. *Morphological characteristics*: Stained smears reveal morphologies (shape, size, and arrangement) as discussed in chapter 36.
2. *Cultural characteristics*: Growth characteristics on a variety of culture media as dealt in chapter 37.
3. *Biochemical characteristics*: Indirectly, these tests measure enzymes or metabolic pathways of microbes as outlined in chapter 39.
4. *Serological characteristics:* These tests disclose antigenic profiles of microorganisms or antibody titers (e.g., convalescent stage of infection) as summarized in chapters 33 and 34.

B. Innovative: The reader will find only the elaboration of automated procedures for the identification of microbes, comparing their advantages and disadvantages. Importantly, genomics- and proteomics-based approaches are discussed extensively since these principles are fairly innovative with short turnaround time. However, a phenotypic approach to characterize the clinically isolated strains is still used today because no single technique is free from its shortcomings to date. Today, manual kits (e.g., API 20 E) that contain dry chemical reagents are still in use as a backup tool.

1. Automated biochemical tests

The characterization and the subsequent identification of clinical strains are based on staining characteristics, colony characteristics, and biochemical tests. Ready-to-use biochemical cards of different groups of bacteria are commercially available. According to a suspected strain isolated from a clinical specimen, the choice of a card may be made, e.g., Gram-negative and -positive.

The major steps include sample preparation, inoculation, incubation, and reading the end-point reactions. It is important that one prepares a suspension of optimum density in 3.0 mL normal saline using isolated colonies (e.g., grown on sheep blood agar) and is equivalent to the appropriate McFarland standard. For example, VITEK 2 requires an inoculum that is visually equivalent to a McFarland standard of 0.5-0.63 for Gram-negative and Gram-positive bacteria. Finally, a reaction pattern is matched with a database library, generating a report. The generated report also indicates an additional test(s) to be performed, if warranted.

Microbial enzymes bring about bioconversion of substrates to end-products. Such end-products are then detected using indicator dyes and/or chemical reagents. This is how we learn useful metabolic characteristics to classify them. Manually performed biochemical reactions and their mechanisms are briefly outlined in chapter 39.

Preliminary culturing of specimens on appropriate media (e.g., 5% sheep blood agar) and incubation of inoculated cards inside an automated machine are time-consuming steps. Also, there has to be a set level of confidence for each system. For example, all VITEK 2 identification systems must have a confidence level of 90% or higher.

Automated instruments, e.g., VITEK 2 system (bioMérieux), also serve the purpose of antimicrobial susceptibility testing. The VITEK 2 system has this module to perform susceptibility testing of clinically significant isolates, namely Gram-positive cocci, Gram-negative bacilli, and yeasts against commonly used drugs. Micro-dilution cards are incubated overnight and read photometrically to measure the growth. The minimal inhibitory concentration (MIC) means the highest dilution in µg/mL of a given antimicrobial agent without a visible growth of an organism in question. Thus, MIC required to combat a microbe in question is determined.

Available phenotype-based instruments

1. VITEK 2 (bioMérieux Inc.)
2. BD Phoenix Automated Microbiology System (BD)
3. Microscan (Siemens Healthcare Diagnostics Inc.)
4. Other manufacturers

2. Genomics-based approach

Genotypic identification of an unknown clinical isolate is a breakthrough in the field of clinical microbiology. Specifically, the technique is referred to as a partial 16S ribosomal RNA gene sequencing because a segment of RNA of an etiological agent is subjected to amplification. The polymerase chain reaction (PCR) has reduced the turnaround time from days to hours. This especially benefits those patients needing immediate treatment. A clinician must start treatment as soon as possible. Therefore, this innovative tool has become so popular these days because it allows direct identification of various microorganisms (e.g., bacteria, fungi, parasites, and viruses) from a variety of specimens (e.g., serum, plasma, whole blood, cerebrospinal fluid, stool, and respiratory specimens).

Polymerase chain reaction (PCR)

Polymerase chain reaction is a powerful analytical tool in molecular biology. The technique was invented by Kary Mullis (1983) while working at Cetus Corporation (California, USA). This revolutionary tool has aided to meet the challenges of the conventional phenotypic identification systems, e.g., the difficulty of culturing *in vitro*. In this technique, there is an exponential amplification through the repetitive replication of the original DNA in the presence of DNA polymerase. PCR-based identification uses commercially designed gene probes (preferably primers) to identify the unknown bacterial DNA. Thus, complementarity and the subsequent binding between the base sequence of a gene probe and a target DNA of unknown bacterium indicate the positive identity. Therefore, knowledge of a base sequence of DNA from unknown bacteria is necessary for designing commercial gene probes. Thus, PCR is a specific, sensitive, and rapid method. Also, PCR is faster and more convenient than recombinant DNA-based cloning methods. The PCR involves the following three steps depicted in Fig. 42.1.

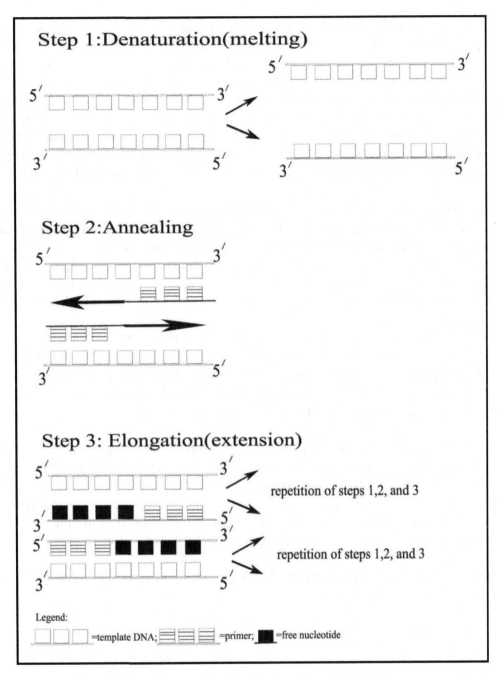

Fig 42.1: Polymerase chain reaction (PCR).

a. *Denaturation*: Denaturation, also called melting, brings about the separation of two strands of a template DNA. This is accomplished when the temperature of the reaction chamber is 90°-95°C for 30-60 seconds.

b. *Annealing:* Upon the addition of primers (usually two) made up of synthetic oligonucleotides at 40°-65°C for 30-60 seconds, each complementary template DNA strand binds to it at the 3'-hydroxyl terminus of the primer. The length of designed primers in most primer design protocols is 18-24 nucleotides, thus decreasing the possibility of non-specific binding. Longer primers increase the likelihood of the formation of secondary structures. In contrast, the shorter primers reduce the specificity of binding to a gene and make it difficult to select the annealing temperature.

c. *Elongation*: Following the binding of a primer to the template DNA, it extends in length while it reads the sequence of the template DNA strand. This cycle is effected at 75°-80°C in the presence of free nucleotides and a thermo-stable (heat-resistant) DNA polymerase. For example, Taq DNA polymerase catalyzes the elongation at 70°-75°C (optimum 72°C). The time required for elongation depends on the type of enzyme in use. For example, Taq DNA polymerase requires 40-50 seconds and 8 minutes for elongation per every 1 and 10 kilobase pairs (kbps), respectively.

Once the replication cycle is completed, the reaction mixture needs to be heated again to separate the DNA strands. Repeated temperature changes called thermal cycles of the reaction chamber at specified time intervals are programmed. Each newly synthesized strand, i.e., template DNA, in turn, binds a complementary synthetic primer followed by the elongation step. Usually, 20-30 consecutive cycles are required to run to reach the goal of amplification. The formula to calculate the number of template DNA copies formed at the end of a given number of cycles is 2^n.

The universal PCR has successfully been designed to detect and identify commonly encountered pathogenic bacteria (a total of 18 species) in cerebrospinal fluid. In this universal PCR, a fraction of the 16S rRNA gene is used in the process of amplification. It is used in conjunction with restricted endonuclease digestion. A satisfactory sensitivity of 92.3% (included 150 CSF samples) has been reported as compared to that of cultural methods.

Microarray-based bacterial identification system uses fluorescent dye-tagged DNA probes. Upon successful hybridization of pre-amplified bacterial DNA to arrayed species-specific synthetic probes, the dye fluoresces. The fluorophore, Cy3, is a bright orange-fluorescent dye that is commonly used in the labeling of nucleic acids. Species-specific synthetic oligonucleotide probes are available for designated locations of targeted genes, e.g., the gene probe for *Staphylococcus aureus* (K) emits a blue signal (K_1) upon binding with target DNA.

Apart from its use in bacterial identification, PCR technique is also used in forensic investigations and bio-terrorism threats.

Drug-resistance and genes

Limited to some bacteria, sequencing-based identification is coupled with the detection of genes associated with drug-resistance. Rapid panels are assembled based upon the likelihood of the clinically significant etiological agent in a given sample. For example, broad molecular panels to test positive blood cultures are available from the manufacturer.

Available genotypic-based instruments

1. The FilmArray Blood Culture Identification Panel (Biofire Diagnostics, LLC)
2. The Verigene Gram-positive Blood Culture Test and Gram-negative Blood Culture Test (Nanosphere, Inc.)
3. Cepheid (GeneXpert System)
4. GEN-PROBE TIGRIS DTS System (*Chlamydia trachomatis* and *Neisseria gonorrhoeae*)

3. Proteomics-based approach

Mass spectrometry is the most recent and diverse approach to microbial identification. It is a simple, rapid, reliable, and cost-effective proteomic technique compared to the conventional phenotypic methods.

The technique is called "matrix-assisted laser desorption/ ionization time-of-flight" (MALDI-TOF) mass spectrometry, depicting its underlying principle as shown in Fig.42.2 (a), (b).

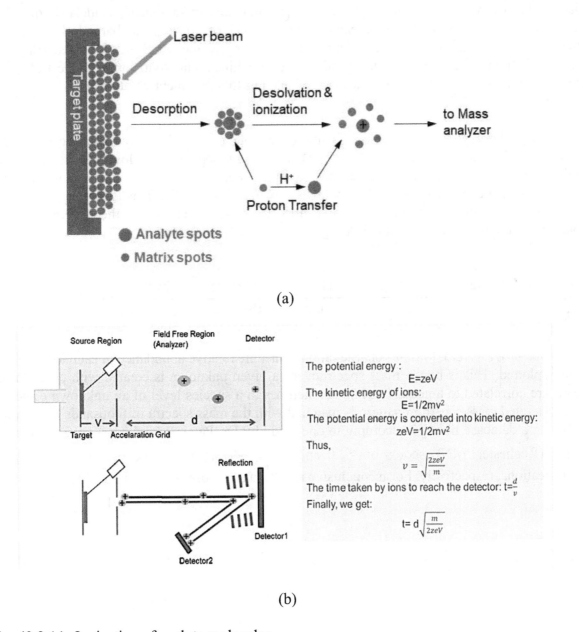

(a)

(b)

Fig. 42.2 (a): Ionization of analyte molecules.
   (b): Separation of charged ions based on mass-to-charge ratio.
   (Reproduced with permission from Creative Proteomics; Shirley, New York)

Working

(i) The ion source: Matrix-assisted laser desorption and ionization is a crucial step of the technique. The so-called soft ionization brings about the ionization of the biomolecules (e.g., ribosomal protein) with minimal degradation. When a laser light falls on the matrix, heat is generated and thus causes the ionization of proteins. This effect generates typically singly charged ions of two forms, namely high mass and low mass.

The matrix contains a saturated solution of alpha-cyano-4-hydroxycinnamic acid (CHCA) dissolved in a solvent consisting of 50% acetonitrile and 2.5% trifluoroacetic acid. A single colony of an unknown organism (1μL) is smeared to a single well of a disposable, barcode-labeled target slide overlaid with matrix (1-2 μL), and air dried. After drying, the target slide is placed in a plating chamber (a high vacuum environment) and then the machine is started to complete the assay. Both matrix and analyte undergo co-crystallization, leading to subsequent ablation and desorption of cellular proteins.

(ii) Mass analyzer: Before entry into a flight tube, a cloud of ions (i.e., proteins) is accelerated by the constant kinetic energy (KE = ½ mv²). Mass analyzer separates the low mass ions from the high mass ions whereby the low mass ions fly at a faster rate in a flight tube of known length toward the magnetic field of known strength as shown in Fig.42.2(b). This is how lighter ions are separated based on the mass/charge (m/z) ratio. Usually, the charge of the generated ions is constant. The ions' time of flight recording uses the following formula:

$$\frac{\text{Mass}}{\text{Charge}} = \frac{2\,(\text{elementary charge})(\text{acceleration voltage})}{\text{path length}^2} = \text{time}^2$$

(iii) Detector (receiver): Mass-to-charge ratio against the relative abundance of each low mass ion type is plotted. This is how a mass spectrum for a given unknown is created with peaks. These peaks are correlated to a genus level and sometimes to a species level of an unknown organism. The generated mass spectrum pattern is matched with the mass spectra of thousands of reference strains in a database library. According to one study by Dr. Patel, R. and her associates at Mayo Clinic (Rochester, MN), scores of ≥2.0 and 1.7-1.999 are indicative of species and genus identifications, respectively. For inconclusive results, a score of < 1.7 was indicative.

Hui-Fen WU et al. successfully identified *Streptococcus mutans* from dental samples using the MALDI-TOF-MS technique (Microflex). The sample was suspended in 200 µL water followed by vortexing combined with centrifugation led to the successful detection of the bacterial signals by MALDI-TOF-MS {Fig.42.3 (b). The sample spectrum was matched against a standard BCRC 10793 *Streptococcus mutans* (isolated from human dental caries}. The matching spectra were collected in linear mode with laser energy of 63.2 µJ as shown in Fig. 42.3 (a), (b).

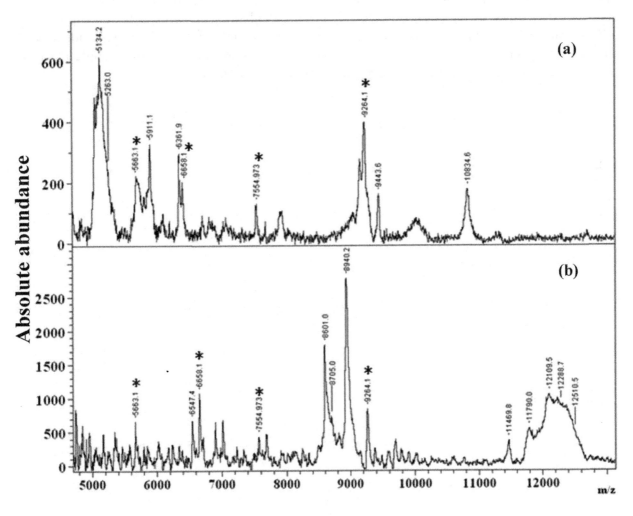

(a) before sample pretreatment
(b) after sample pretreatment

Fig. 42.3: A sample spectrum of *Streptococcus mutans* marked with an asterisk(*).
(Reproduced with permission from Hui-Fen WU).

Apparatus (see Fig. 42.4)

The revolutionary version of MALDI-TOF-MS-based technology, VITEK® MS (bioMérieux), is an advanced instrument for robust and accurate microbial identification. This machine has seamless integration of identification (ID) and antimicrobial susceptibility testing (AST) when using the VITEK®2. This is a little different from other similar machines in that a created spectrum is carefully digitized utilizing bioMérieux's proprietary Advanced Spectra Classifier algorithm. The system reads an individual spectrum as a series of peaks followed by sortation based on mass and intensity. Since every peak is included in the calculation, allowing a better approach of differentiation. Such translation to a digital format uses a Weighted Bin Matrix while identifying an unknown spectrum of an organism. In other words, there is no comparison of a sample spectrum with database reference spectra (i.e., reference spectra-free system).

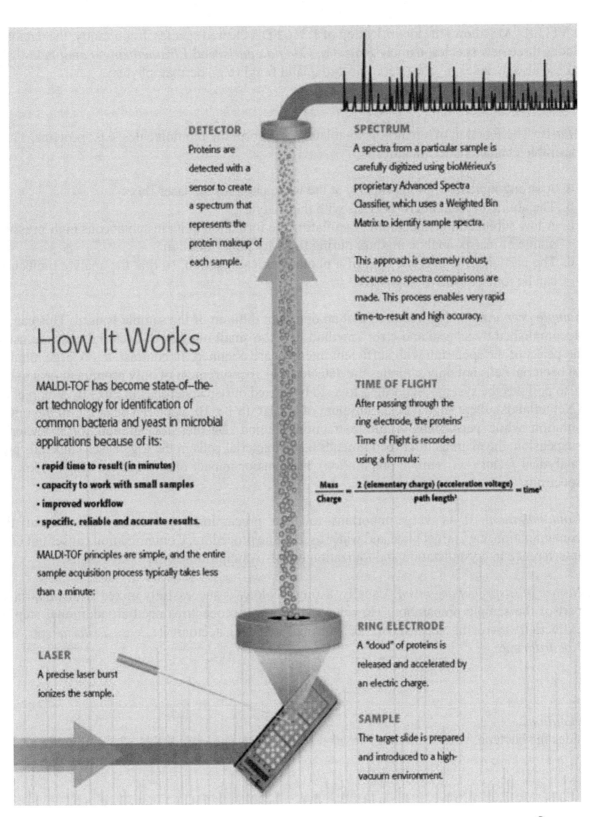

Fig. 42.4: A revolutionary version of MALDI-TOF-MS-based technology, VITEK®-MS
(Reproduced with permission from bioMérieux, Inc.)

The VITEK® MS allows the identification of 1,316 FDA cleared species. Importantly, the database includes three new species, namely *Brucella*, *Candida auris*, and *Elizabethkingia anopheles*. The database also includes mycobacteria, nocardia, and fungi (e.g., dermatophytes).

Factors that influence the mass spectrometry

1. *Matrix:* The function of a matrix is to ablate and desorp the biomolecules, e.g., proteins. The desirable characteristics include:

   a. A strong light absorption property at the wavelength of the laser flux
   b. The ability to form micro-crystals with the analyte
   c. A low sublimation temperature, facilitating the formation of an instantaneous high-pressure plume of matrix-analyte mixture during the laser pulse duration
   d. The participation in some kind of a photochemical reaction, so that the analyte molecules can be ionized with high yields

2. *Sample preparation:* It is required that an optimum dilution of the sample is used. This can be accomplished by a "trial and error" method. If a too small number of bacterial cells are used, no peaks of the spectrum with sufficient intensity are obtained. In contrast, a too large number of bacterial cells not only saturates the detector (i.e., measurement of only prominent peaks) but also pollutes the system. According to a study carried out on anaerobes in 2014 by Veloo et al. (Netherlands), there should be a minimum of 5×10^6 to 1×10^7 bacterial cells/mL in the initial solution while performing a full extraction method. Besides the strength of a bacterial suspension, the manufacturer recommends using bacterial cells in the log phase. Thus, this pre-analytical factor (i.e., sample preparation) has a major impact on the quality of the unknown spectrum.

3. *Contamination:* It is very important to take precautionary measures to prevent the contamination, e.g., target plate and water used in the procedure. Contamination causes not only interference in crystallization and ionization but also compromises the assay results.

4. *Nature of suspected organism*: Usually, a single colony is successfully mixed with a matrix as part of the sample preparation. However, some assay procedures need an additional step of extraction, involving the use of 70% formic acid and acetonitrile, e.g., *Listeria* spp. and *Nocardia* spp.

Applications
Besides the bacteria, yeasts and fungi are also identified as shown in Table 42.1 and Table 42.2.

Table 42.1: Reportable yeasts for the FDA-approved/cleared Vitek MS and MALDI Biotyper CA systems as of October 2018. Those entries marked with "V" are FDA-approved/cleared for the Vitek MS system only and those marked with "B" are FDA-approved/cleared for the MALDI Biotyper CA system only. Those with marked with neither a "V" nor a "B" are FDA-approved/cleared on both systems
(Reproduced with permission from Dr. Patel, R., Mayo Clinic, Rochester, MN., USA, and Ms. Man Luo)
(Managing editor, Journal of Fungi).

Candida albicans	Candida krusei	Candida tropicalis	Kodamaea/Pichia ohmeri ***
Candida boidinii[B]	Candida lambica	Candida utilis/Cyberlindnera jadinii *	Malassezia furfur
Candida dubliniensis	Candida lipolytica	Candida valida[B]	Malassezia pachydermatis
Candida duobushaemulonii[B]	Candida lusitaniae	Candida zeylanoides	Rhodotorula mucilaginosa
Candida famata	Candida metapsilosis[B]	Cryptococcus gattii[B]	Saccharomyces cerevisiae
Candida glabrata	Candida norvegensis	Cryptococcus neoformans[V]	Trichosporon asahii
Candida guilliermondii	Candida orthopsilosis[B]	Cryptococcus neoformans var grubii[B]	Trichosporon inkin
Candida haemulonii	Candida parapsilosis	Cryptococcus neoformans var neoformans[B]	Trichosporon mucoides[V]
Candida inconspicua	Candida pararugosa[B]	Geotrichum candidum[B]	
Candida intermedia	Candida pelliculosa	Geotrichum capitatum/Saprochaete capitate **	Trichosporon mucoides group [B]
Candida kefyr	Candida rugosa[V]	Kloeckera apiculata	

* *Cyberlindnera jadinii* (teleomorph) is approved/cleared on the MALDI Biotyper CA system, whereas *Candida utilis* (anamorph) is approved/cleared on the Vitek MS system

** *Geotrichum capitatum* is approved/cleared on the MALDI Biotyper CA system, whereas *Saprochaete capitate* is approved/cleared on the Vitek MS system

*** *Kodamaea ohmeri* is approved/cleared on the Vitek MS system whereas *Pichia ohmeri* is approved/cleared on the MALDI Biotyper CA system.

Table 42.2. Reportable filamentous and dimorphic fungi for the FDA-approved/cleared Vitek MS system as of October 2018

(Reproduced with permission from Dr. Patel, R., Mayo Clinic, Rochester, MN., USA, and Ms. Man Luo (Managing editor, Journal of Fungi).

Acremonium sclerotigenum	*Blastomyces dermatitidis*	*Histoplasma capsulatum*	*Rhizopus arrhizus* complex
Alternaria alternata	*Cladophialophora bantiana*	*Lecythophora hoffmannii*	*Rhizopus microsporus* complex
Aspergillus brasiliensis	*Coccidioides immitis/posadasii*	*Lichtheimia corymbifera*	*Sarocladium kiliense*
Aspergillus calidoustus	*Curvularia hawaiiensis*	*Microsporum audouinii*	*Scedosporium apiospermum*
Aspergillus flavus/oryzae	*Curvularia spicifera*	*Microsporum canis*	*Scedosporium prolificans*
Aspergillus fumigatus	*Epidermophyton floccosum*	*Microsporum gypseum*	*Sporothrix schenckii* complex
Aspergillus lentulus	*Exophiala dermatitidis*	*Mucor racemosus* complex	*Trichophyton interdigitale*
Aspergillus nidulans	*Exophiala xenobiotica*	*Paecilomyces variotii* complex	*Trichophyton rubrum*
Aspergillus niger complex	*Exserohilum rostratum*	*Penicillium chrysogenum*	*Trichophyton tonsurans*
Aspergillus sydowii	*Fusarium oxysporum* complex	*Pseudallescheria boydii*	*Trichophyton verrucosum*
Aspergillus terreus complex	*Fusarium proliferatum*	*Purpureocillium lilacinum*	*Trichophyton violaceum*
Aspergillus versicolor	*Fusarium solani* complex	*Rasamsonia argillacea* complex	

Mycobacteria can be routinely identified by MALDI-TOF-MS (Neuschlova et al.; 2017). The applicability of MALDI-TOF-MS for viral identification is challenging because viruses have low biomass.

Advantages and disadvantages
Mass spectrometric bacterial identification outperforms over the conventional methods. However, some shortcomings need to be addressed:

Advantages
1. Short turnaround time
2. High throughput
3. Cost-effective
4. Easy cross-training
5. Complete traceability
6. Identification of non-viable cultures
7. Inclusion of anaerobes, mycobacteria, yeasts, and fungi for identification
8. Green (environmentally-safer)

Disadvantages
1. It requires backup testing in case of discrepancies, e.g., failure to discriminate closely related species, namely *Klebsiella pneumoniae* and *Klebsiella variicola*. Furthermore, it misidentifies *Shigella* spp. as *Escherichia coli*. Therefore, this technique is not a standalone test
2. Initial capital equipment investment is very high
3. No antimicrobial susceptibility testing
4. Requires a repetitive analysis on some occasions
5. Occasionally, extraction is needed as a part of specimen preparation
6. Except for urine specimens, direct testing of clinical specimens cannot be performed

Available MALDI-TOF mass spectrometry-based instruments

1. Microflex LT (Bruker Daltonics)
2. VITEK® MS V.3.2.0 (bioMérieux)
3. Anagnos Tec GmbH
4. Andromas (limited to Europe)

Conclusion

For accurate identification of an unknown organism using MALDI-TOF-MS, an extensive database is needed. Researchers are still engaged in resolving these issues. For example, available databases on anaerobes need to be optimized for their routine identification.

An integrated approach of each of these three different methodologies, namely phenotypic, genomics, and proteomics, should be used in case of discrepancies encountered during microbial identification.

Chapter 43

Human Pathogenic Fungi

Introduction

Unlike the prokaryotic bacteria, eukaryotic fungi are much larger and contain the organelles typical of eukaryotic cells. Also, the cell walls of most fungi contain chitin $\{(C_8H_{13}O_5N)_n\}$ and glucans. The fungal cell membrane contains ergosterol that provides flexibility and stability to it. Based on recent genetic analysis, fungi are more closely related to animals than to plants. Thousands of species of fungi exist in nature, e.g., soil, decaying vegetation, and water. Most fungi are decomposers because hyphae secrete extracellular enzymes that degrade biopolymers such as cellulose and lignin. Fungi are chemoheterotrophic (non-photosynthetic), and aerobic or facultatively anaerobic organisms. They can grow in moist and acidic environments. They can be parasitic, saprophytic, or symbiotic. Fungi include microscopic molds and yeasts as major groups of medical importance. About a few hundred of them are known to be pathogenic to humans and are studied in medical mycology. However, some fungi are industrially important and used in the production of antibiotics, organic acids, brewer's and baker's yeasts, and the biological control of pests.

Structure of fungi

Fungi may be unicellular or multicellular structures. The unicellular yeasts are round or oval and reproduce asexually by a process termed 'budding'. On the contrary, multicellular fungi form long, branching filaments. Each filament is designated as a hypha (plural, hyphae). The hypha can be coenocytic (aseptate or nonseptate) or septate {see Fig. 43.1 (a), (b)}. These hyphae, in turn, intertwine forming a meshwork called a mycelium (plural, mycelia).

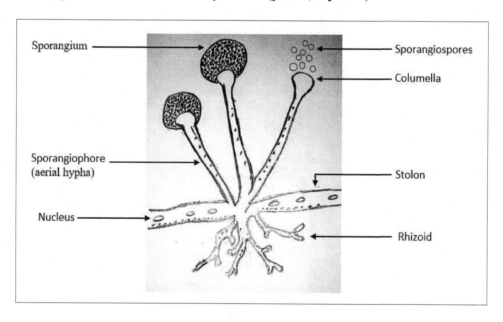

(a) Coenocytic hypha of *Rhizopus stolonifer.*

Fig. 43.1: Structure of fungi.

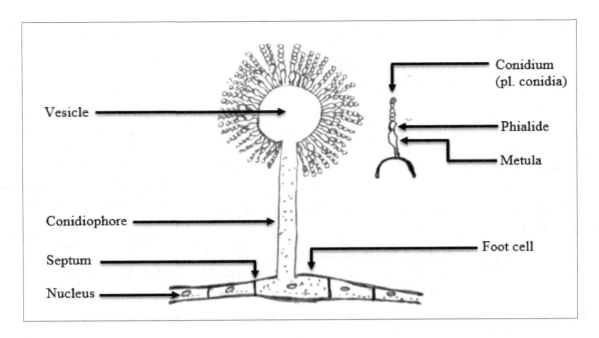

(b) Septate hypha of *Aspergillus niger*.

Fig. 43.1: Structure of fungi.

Dimorphism

Dimorphism means the ability of some fungi to grow in two different forms, namely unicellular and filamentous. Such fungi are referred to as dimorphic fungi. Usually, dimorphism is a temperature-dependent phenomenon seen in some pathogenic fungi. For instance, *Blastomyces dermatitidis* grows as a yeast (unicellular) at 37°C (body temperature) and as a mold (filamentous) at 25°C (room temperature).

Types of fungal spores

Fungi reproduce both asexually and sexually. Asexual reproduction in fungi is carried out by fragmentation, budding, or asexually (mitosis). All sexual reproduction methods in fungi include the following three stages:

1. Plasmogamy
2. Karyogamy
3. Meiosis

Different asexual and sexual fungal spores are enlisted in Table 43.1 and Table 43.2, respectively.

Table 43.1: Types of asexual fungal spores (see Fig. 43.2)

Type of asexual spores	Brief description	Typical representative(s)
Arthroconidia (arthrospores)	- Formed by fragmentation of a septate hypha	- *Coccidioides immitis* - *Geotrichum candidum* - *Trichosporon* spp.
Blastoconidia (blastospores)	- Buds out from a parent cell (found in some yeasts)	- *Cryptococcus* * *neoformans* - *Histoplasma capsulatum* - *Saccharomyces cerevisiae*
Chlamydoconidia (chlamydospores)	-Produced by enlargement, rounding off, and development of thick walls within a hyphal segment during unfavorable conditions	- *Candida albicans*
Conidia (conidiospores)**	- Produced in a chain at the end of an aerial hyphae	- *Aspergillus* spp.
Microconidia	- Smallest of two types of conidia produced by a single species of fungus	- *Trichophyton* spp.
Macroconidia	- Multi-compartment structures separated by internal cross-walls - Different morphological characteristics that help in species identification	- *Microsporum gypseum* - *T. rubrum* - *Epidermophyton floccosum*
Sporangiospores	- Formed within a sac (sporangium). Sporangium, in turn, is produced at the end of aerial hyphae called sporangiophore	- *Rhizopus* spp.

*Also called *Filobasidiella*.
**Also called phialoconidia.

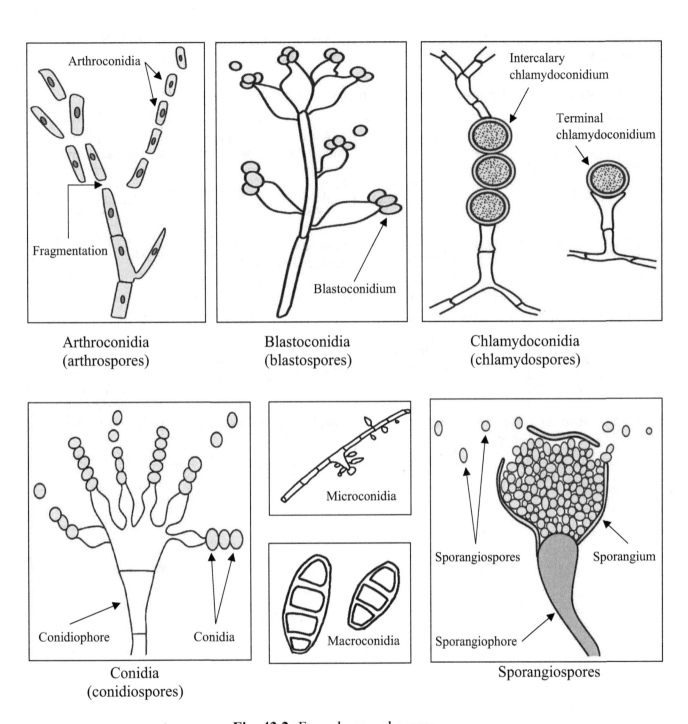

Fig. 43.2: Fungal asexual spores.

The classes of fungi are based mainly on the types of sexual spores produced. Different classes and their general properties are summarized in Table 43.2.

Table 43.2: Different classes of fungi and their sexual spores (see Fig. 43.3)

Taxonomic group	Common name	Hypha	Asexual structure(s)	Type of sexual spores	Typical representative(s)
Zygomycetes	Bread molds	Coenocytic (non-septate)	Spores, conidia	Zygospore	- *Mucor* spp. - *Rhizopus* spp.
Ascomycetes	Sac fungi	Septate	Conidia, blastoconidia	Ascospores	- *Trichophyton* spp. - *Neurospora* spp. - *Morchella* spp. - *Saccharomyces* spp.
Basidiomycetes	Club fungi	Septate	Conidia	Basidiospores	- *Cryptococcus* spp.
Oomycetes	Water molds	Coenocytic (non-septate)	Spores, conidia	Oospore	- *Allomyces* spp.
Deuteromycetes	The imperfect fungi	Septate	Conidia	Unknown	- *Penicillium* spp. - *Aspergillus* spp. - *Epidermophyton* spp. - *Candida* spp.

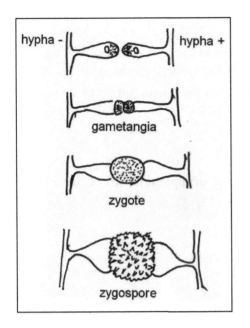

Zygospore

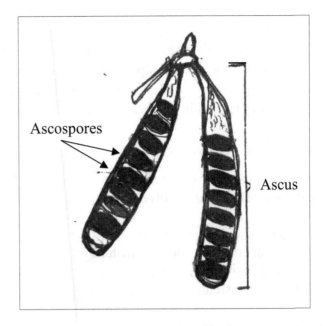

Ascospores

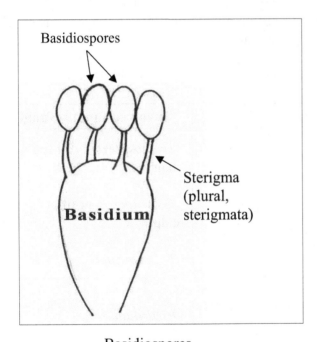

Basidiospores

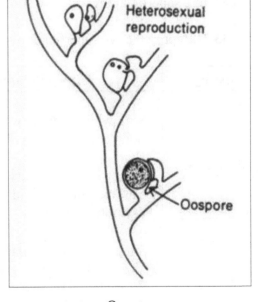

Oospore

Fig. 43.3: Fungal sexual spores.

Modes of transmission

(i) *Air-borne*: Because fungal spores are found in soil and environment, most fungal infections can easily be acquired through inhalation of spores, e.g., *Blastomyces dermatitidis, Coccidioides immitis,* and *Histoplasma capsulatum.*

(ii) *Direct contact:* The causative agents of superficial and cutaneous mycoses (dermatophytoses) are generally acquired through direct contact with infected individuals or other animals.

(iii) *Fomites:* Fomites (inanimate objects) can play a role in the transmission of fungal infections. For example, tinea can be spread via shared towels, clothing, or bedding.

(iv) *Sexual contact: Candida albicans* infection can be acquired from direct mucosal contact with lesions in others.

Spectrum of mycoses

The fungal infections are referred to as mycoses. Mycoses are grouped into four categories based on the tissue or organ involvement:

1. Superficial mycoses
2. Cutaneous mycoses (dermatophytoses)
3. Subcutaneous mycoses
4. Deep (systemic) mycoses

1. Superficial mycoses

Those infections that involve only the outermost layers of the skin or parts of hair shafts are categorized as superficial mycoses. These infections occur predominantly in tropical climates. The representative superficial mycoses are summarized in Table 43.3.

Table 43.3: Representative superficial mycoses and associated clinical manifestations

Disease	Clinical manifestations	Involved fungus (fungi)
White piedra	- Soft, white, creamy white, or light brown nodular concretions along the terminal hair shaft - Affects pubic, axillary, and facial hair - Chronic infection and typically asymptomatic	- *Trichosporon inkin* (pubic hair) - *T. ovoides* (hair of the scalp) - *T. cutaneumi*
Black piedra	- Small, stone-hard, black, and gritty nodules (1-2 mm) tightly adherent to the hair shafts - Restricted to scalp hair - Asymptomatic	- *Piedraia hortae*
Tinea nigra	- Affects the skin of the soles or palms - Persistent, brown or black patches - Patches are slightly scaly that do not sting or itch	- *Hortaea werneckii* (formerly *Phaeoannellomyces werneckii* and others)

2. Cutaneous mycoses (Dermatophytoses)

The cutaneous mycoses (dermatophytoses) are infections of keratin-containing tissues such as skin, nails, or hair caused by fungi. Such fungi infect and are limited to the keratinized tissues and are called dermatophytes. Sometimes, the terms ringworm and tinea are used to indicate dermatophytoses. The clinical manifestations of some representative dermatophytoses are summarized in Table 43.4.

Table 43.4: Clinical manifestations of some representative dermatophytoses

Disease	Clinical manifestations	Most frequently involved fungi
Tinea barbae (ringworm of the beard)	Circular patches on bearded part; some loss of hair	- *Trichophyton rubrum* - *T. mentagrophytes*
Tinea capitis (ringworm of the scalp)	Involvement of scalp hair; scaly lesions on hair	- *Microsporum canis* - *Trichophyton tonsurans*
Tinea corporis (ringworm of the body)	Ringlike lesions and central scaling, pruritic	- *Trichophyton rubrum* - *T. mentagrophytes* - *Microsporum canis*
Tinea pedis (ringworm of the feet)	Fluid-filled lesions, itching, scaling, peeling, and fissures	- *Epidermophyton floccosum* - *Trichophyton mentagrophytes* - *T. rubrum*
Tinea cruris (ringworm of the groin)	Ringlike patches and itching in skin folds of the pubic area, pruritic	- *Trichophyton rubrum* - *T. mentagrophytes* - *Epidermophyton floccosum*
Tinea unguium (ringworm of the nails)	Hardening and discoloration of the nails	- *Trichophyton rubrum* - *T. mentagrophytes* - *Epidermophyton floccosum*

3. Subcutaneous mycoses

Subcutaneous mycoses are caused when the causative fungal agents gain access beneath the skin through tissue injury. Two dimorphic fungi that can cause subcutaneous mycoses are summarized in Table 43.5.

Table 43.5: Two representative subcutaneous mycoses and their clinical manifestations

Disease	Clinical manifestations	Involved fungus (fungi)
Chromoblastomycosis*	- Initially a small pink papule that progresses to a verrucous plaque on the lower legs - Itching - Mucous membranes not affected -May evolve into a variety of skin lesions leading to a polymorphic appearance: *nodular, tumor-like, verrucous hypertrophic plaques, cicatricial, and scaly papules*	- *Fonsecaea pedrosoi* - *F. compacta* - *Phialophora verrucose* - *Cladophialophora carrionii* - *Rhinocladiella aquaspersa*
Sporotrichosis	- Numerous nodules (pink to purple) under the skin along with the lymph nodes - Often the hand or forearm affected - Nodules may develop abscesses and ulcers that drain clear fluid -Rarely extends to other parts of the body, e.g., bones, joints, lungs, and the central nervous system (CNS)	- *Sporotrichum (Sporothrix) schenckii*

* The KOH preparation may show typically copper-colored muriform bodies.

4. Deep (systemic) mycoses

Several fungal agents can infect some deeper tissues and organs, e.g., lungs, abdominal viscera, bones, joints, and brain. Portals of their entry can be the respiratory tract, gastrointestinal tract, and bloodstream. Most cases of primary deep mycoses are asymptomatic or clinically mild infections in normal individuals following exposure to endemic areas. Important representative fungal species associated with deep mycoses are summarized in Table 43.6.

Table 43.6: Some important representative fungal agents associated with deep mycoses

Disease	Clinical manifestations	Involved fungus (fungi)
Coccidioidomycosis (San Joaquin Valley Fever)	- *Self-limited form*: cough, chest pain, loss of appetite, headache, fatigue, and myalgia -*Disseminated form*: affects the meninges and visceral organs	- *Coccidioides immitis*
Blastomycosis	-*A mild form*: fever, weight loss, malaise, and a productive cough -*Disseminated form*: affects the skin, bones, joints, prostate gland, and testes	- *Blastomyces dermatitidis*
Histoplasmosis	-Infects the reticuloendothelial system -*Severe form*: may show chills, chest pain, and malaise -*Progressive pulmonary form*: similar to pulmonary TB (sputum production, weight loss, and night sweats) - *Disseminated form*: involves the skin, CNS, lungs, adrenal glands, and gastrointestinal tract	- *Histoplasma capsulatum*

Opportunistic mycoses

Opportunistic mycoses are caused by fungal agents that do not harm healthy individuals. Fungal infections occur frequently in individuals with weakened immune systems popularly known as opportunistic infections, e.g., individuals having HIV/AIDS, diabetes mellitus, cancer, or organ transplants. Opportunistic mycoses are usually systemic. Some fungal representatives of opportunistic infections are summarized in Table 43.7.

Table 43.7: Key fungal representatives associated with opportunistic infections

Disease	Clinical manifestations	Involved fungus (fungi)
Candidiasis	*Neonatal thrush:* white patches in and around the mouth, difficulties with feeding, possibly cracking of the skin at the corners of the mouth, and diaper rash *Vulvovaginitis:* itching in the vagina and the vulva, an itchy rash on the vulva and surrounding skin, white curd-like vaginal discharge, and burning while urinating	- *Candida albicans*
Cryptococcosis	*Lungs:* cough, shortness of breath, chest pain, and fever *Brain:* headache, fever, neck pain, nausea and vomiting, sensitivity to light, and confusion	- *Cryptococcus neoformans* - *C. gattii*
Pneumocystis pneumonia (PCP)	Dry cough, fever, shortness of breath, chest pain, and progressive respiratory failure	- *Pneumocystis jirovecii* (*P. carinii*)
Aspergillosis*	*Invasive aspergillosis:* fever, chest pain, cough, coughing up blood, shortness of breath	- *Aspergillus fumigatus*
Talaromycosis	- Small and painless bumps on the skin (usually on the face and neck) - Fever, malaise, weight loss, cough, dyspnea, diarrhea, and abdominal pain - Swollen lymph nodes	-*Talaromyces marneffei*
Mucormycosis	- A rare but serious infection - May involve sinuses, brain, lungs, skin, bloodstream, or gastrointestinal tract - Does not spread from person to person	-*Mucor* spp. -*Rhizopus* spp. -*Rhizomucor* spp. -*Cunninghamella bertholletiae* -*Apophysomyces* spp. -*Lichtheimia* spp.

* Other symptoms depend on the part of the body affected, e.g., bone pain, chills, headache, malaise, weight loss, wheezing, decreased urine output, and vision problems.

Some fungi of medical interest are diagrammatically shown in Fig. 43.4.

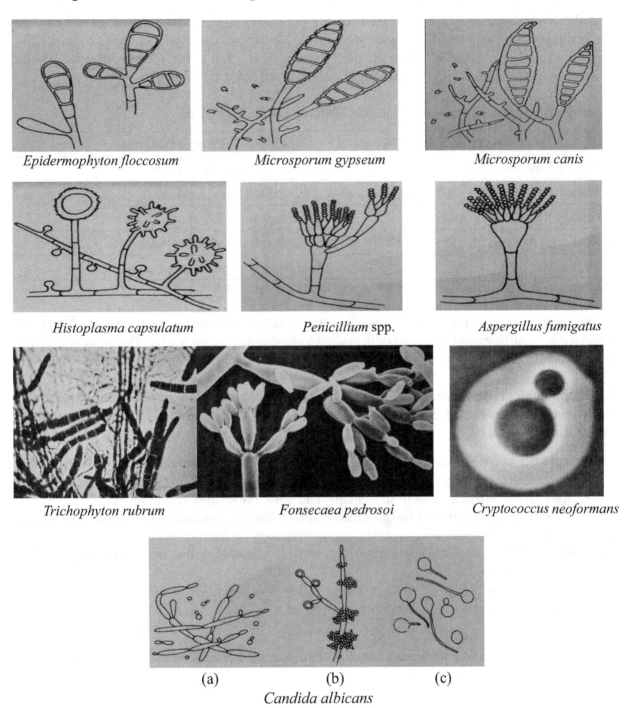

Epidermophyton floccosum

Microsporum gypseum

Microsporum canis

Histoplasma capsulatum

Penicillium spp.

Aspergillus fumigatus

Trichophyton rubrum

Fonsecaea pedrosoi

Cryptococcus neoformans

(a)   (b)   (c)

Candida albicans

(a) Blastoconidia and pseudohyphae in exudate
(b) Pseudohyphae and chlamydoconidia in culture at 20°C
(c) Germ tube when placed in sheep or human serum for 3 hours at 37°C (presumptive test)

Fig. 43.4: Microscopic views of some fungi of medical interest.

Laboratory diagnosis

Sample: Various samples are processed for the laboratory diagnosis of fungal infections. The specimens routinely received for fungal isolation and identification include scrapings of skin, nails, hairs plucked from the infected areas, pus, sputum, CSF, and other related materials. Some commonly used samples with typical fungal isolate(s) are listed in Table 43.8.

Table 43.8: Some commonly used samples with typical fungal isolates

Sample	Fungal isolate(s)
Bone marrow	*Histoplasma capsulatum**
Cerebrospinal fluid	*Cryptococcus neoformans*
Draining sinus tract of foot	*Pseudallescheria boydii*
Interdigital lesion of the foot	*Trichophyton mentagrophytes*
External ear	*Aspergillus niger, A. fumigatus*

* Demonstration of intracellular yeast cells in smears stained by Wright's stain.

Liquid samples, e.g., urine, bronchoalveolar lavage (BAL), or transtracheal aspirate (TTA), are subjected to centrifugation to obtain pellets used to inoculate culture media. Tissue samples need to be macerated by chopping with a sterile scalpel blade to release the fungal elements.

A. Morphological approach: This is a time-consuming approach that needs a well-experienced professional to characterize fungi. The key criteria which can be used for the identification of clinical isolates include:

1. Direct microscopic examination of a specimen (e.g., nail, skin, or hair) in a 10% KOH mount for fungal elements (e.g., chains of arthroconidia of *E. floccosum* in a nail specimen).
2. Colony characteristics, namely size, shape, and color on various fungal media.
3. Microscopic examination of fungal growth using a lactophenol cotton blue stain to search for mycelium, spores (sexual or asexual), and morphology of fruiting structures.
4. Dimorphic fungi, e.g., *Sporotrichum (Sporothrix) schenckii* grow as a small yeast form at 36°C and as a mold at 25°C.
5. Germ-tube formation at 37°C after 3-hour incubation in animal serum, e.g., positive for *C. albicans* (presumptive identification).

a. Wet preparation technique
Principle: Ten percent of potassium hydroxide dissolves the keratinized tissues, thus making visually clear the fungal structure.

Procedure

1. Add a few drops of 10% KOH on a clean and dry glass slide.
2. Place the pathological specimen in KOH and place the coverslip. (Pieces of nails are allowed to react with a few mL of 10% KOH in the test tube).
3. Warm the slide or tube, as the case may be, over the Bunsen flame for rapid clearing.
4. Remove excess of KOH with the help of a blotting paper.
5. Examine the slide under a low-power followed by a high-power objective lens.

6. Record the results.

Results
Spores or branching refractile mycelium or both which cross the epithelial outlines can be seen.

Limitations

1. The fungal cells are not stained.
2. Wet preparation is examined under low- and high-power objectives instead of the oil-immersion lens.
3. If it is allowed to dry, the formation of crystals makes the reading difficult.
4. KOH can damage the objectives of the microscope and the stage.

b. Lactophenol cotton blue stain
Lactophenol cotton blue (LPCB) stain is a widely used stain for the characterization and the subsequent presumptive identification of fungi.

Principle: Different ingredients present in the stain play their roles as shown below:

- *Lactic acid (clearing agent)*: preserves the fungal structures
- *Phenol (disinfectant)*: kills the living organisms
- *Cotton blue (stain)*: stains chitin and cellulose of the fungal cell wall

Procedure

1. Place a good-sized drop of lactophenol cotton blue on a clean microscopic glass slide.
2. Using a sterile inoculating needle, transfer a small piece of fungal growth (2-3 mm) from the margin of the isolated colony followed by a gentle teasing.
3. Place a coverslip without pressing/taping to avoid dislodging of conidia from conidiophores.
4. Examine the slide under a low-power followed by a high-power objective lens to characterize the mycelial structures as well as the fruiting structures.

Note: Stain cannot be used if there are any signs of contamination or deterioration.

c. India ink preparation
This staining technique can be performed to demonstrate capsules. The capsular material repels the carbon particles of the India ink. Therefore, yeast cells appear as cells surrounded by a clear halo-like capsule, e.g., detection of a polysaccharide capsule in *Cryptococcus neoformans* from cerebrospinal fluid (CSF).

In fluorescence microscopy, mold structures and yeasts exhibit bright apple-green fluorescence with typical morphology when stained by calcofluor white stain (fluorochrome).

Histopathologic stains, namely Gomori-methenamine-silver nitrate and Periodic acid-Schiff stains can be used to demonstrate fungi in tissues.

d. Cultivation

Since it is a challenging task to identify some fungi, it is required to culture them on a primary culture medium, e.g., Sabouraud's dextrose agar (SDA).

Sabouraud's dextrose agar medium is whitish and semi-transparent in appearance. In addition to this, it is a semi-synthetic and selective medium. It is an excellent medium to grow human pathogenic fungi. Its composition is:

Peptone	1 g
Dextrose (glucose)	4 g
Agar-agar powder	2 g
Distilled water	100 mL
Adjust pH to	5.6

1. Suspend the ingredients in distilled water.
2. Dissolve by heating to boiling.
3. Dispense approximately 20 mL amount in cotton-plugged (25x150 mm) pyrex test tubes (without lips) or screw-capped bottles as indicated.
4. Add antimicrobial agents after heating and before autoclaving the medium.
   (i) cycloheximide (250 mg dissolved in 5 mL acetone) inhibits saprophytic fungi, including *Cryptococcus neoformans*, some *Candida* spp. and some *Aspergillus* spp.
   (ii) chloramphenicol (25 mg dissolved in 5 mL of 95% ethanol) inhibits bacteria
5. Autoclave at 118°C for no longer than 10 minutes.
6. Slant the containers and allow them to harden and refrigerate.
7. Prepare plates too.

Following incubation at room temperature (25°-28°C) for 1-3 weeks, colony characteristics, namely shape, size, and color are recorded and a wet mount of colonial growth is examined under a light microscope by a technical expert. Both macroscopic and microscopic characteristics of some medically relevant fungi on Sabouraud's dextrose agar are listed in Table 43.9.

Table 43.9: Both macroscopic and microscopic characteristics of some medically relevant fungi on Sabouraud's dextrose agar

Fungus	Macroscopic findings	Microscopic findings
Aspergillus spp.	mycelial color varies from white to shades of green, black, yellow, brown, and gray	conidiophores, conidia, vesicles, and phialides
Fusarium spp.*	cottony growth, producing lavender or yellow pigment	canoe-shaped macroconidia
Penicillium spp.	mycelial color greenish-blue with a powdery or velvet texture	conidiophores, conidia, and phialides
Rhizopus spp.	mycelial appearance cottony and white initially and then becomes dotted with black dots	rhizoids, sporangiophores, sporangia, columellae, and sporangiospores
Rhodotorula spp.	mycelia are soft and pink to coral in color	budding cells (round or oval)
Scopulariopsis spp.	mycelial color ranges from light tan to dull gray	Conidiophores and chains of thick-walled conidia
Coccidioides immitis	mycelial color white and cottony	barrel-shaped arthroconidia
Sporotrichum (Sporothrix) schenckii	mycelial color white and powdery	flower-like arrangement of the oval conidia
Trichophyton rubrum	red to purplish pigment on the undersurface	macroconidia
Candida albicans	cream-colored and moist colonies	oval-shaped yeast form
Histoplasma capsulatum	filamentous white colony	chlamydospores
Cryptococcus neoformans	cream-colored convex colonies	large capsules (India-ink preparation)

*It is necessary to employ brain heart infusion (BHI) agar and blood agar to culture fastidious mycotic agents. It can cause life-threatening infections in cancer patients.

In many instances, it is required to subculture the unknown clinical isolate on specialized media, namely chromogenic media (e.g., CHROMagar™ Candida) and morphology agar (e.g., corn meal agar and rice extract/Tween 80) to promote the formation of chlamydospores or other fungal structures to complete the definitive identification. The best temperature for the incubation of fungal cultures is 30°C. If a special incubator is unavailable, plates can be incubated at room temperature (25°C). Additionally, plates should be sealed to reduce evaporation but allow air exchange. Plates should be examined every few days for four weeks before reporting them as negative. In most cases, yeasts grow within a few days (e.g., 3 days for *C. tropicalis*) to one week. For molds, it may take days to weeks. Though this conventional approach is reliable for definitive identification, the health care provider has to wait too long to treat the patient. The development of colored colonies by various *Candida* spp. on CHROMagar™ Candida is shown in Table 43.10.

Table 43.10: Colored colonies of various *Candida* spp. on CHROMagar™ Candida

Species	Color developed
Candida albicans	apple green
Candida parapsilosis	cream to pale pink
Candida glabrata	pale pink to purple
Candida krusei	pale pink with matt surface
*Candida tropicalis**	blue
Candida guilliermondii	pink to purple

*Virulent in patients with leukemia or similar malignancies (e.g., vaginitis or bronchopulmonary candidiasis).

B. Biochemical tests: Rapid comprehensive commercial kits are available for the identification of yeasts. For example, API 20C AUX, Yeast (bioMerieux) contains 19 carbon assimilation tests that are incubated at 30°C. After 48-72 hour long incubation, the reactions are read for turbidity.

Accurate identification of yeasts to the species level is of paramount importance for successful therapy. Various commercial key rapid test kits (e.g., Remel, Clinical Standards Laboratories, Inc.) are available for presumptive identification of *Candida albicans*. Some of those rapid test kits (5-30 minutes at 37°C) are highly specific and sensitive. These rapid test kits are based on β–galactosaminidase/L-proline aminopeptidase activity. Similarly, rapid test kits (3-24 hours at 42°C) are used for the presumptive identification of *C. glabrata*. Thus, rapid test kits enable screening for species (e.g., *C. glabrata*) associated with resistance to antifungal agents.

C. Proteomics-based approach: In recent years, matrix-assisted laser desorption ionization-time of flight mass spectrometry (MALDI-TOF-MS) has exceptionally emerged as a powerful tool in the identification of fungi. Considering its short analysis time, cost-effectiveness, and technical ease of performance, the technique has been implemented in clinical microbiology laboratories worldwide. Undoubtedly, MALDI-TOF-MS has contributed to the improved laboratory diagnosis of fungal infections by shortening the turnaround time (TAT).

For yeasts, a few colonies from a primary culture medium are deposited on a target slide followed by the addition of 0.5 µL of 25% formic acid and 1 µL of α–cyano-4-hydroxy cinnamic acid (CHCA) matrix solution. The spots are allowed to dry after each step of reagent addition. Sample preparation of molds involves suspending 1- 2 cm of mold growth using a wet swab from an agar plate in a 2 mL tube carrying 900 µL of 70% ethanol and the subsequent centrifugation at a speed of 10,000-14,000 g to obtain a pellet. After discarding the supernatant, 40 µL of 70% formic acid followed by 40 µL of acetonitrile are added to the pellet and mixed well. Then, the mixture is centrifuged at 10,000-14,000 g. Finally, 1 µL of protein extract (supernatant) is spotted onto a target slide and allowed to dry before the addition of 1 µL of the CHCA matrix solution.

According to Cassagne et al. (2014), MALDI-TOF-MS seems to be an excellent alternative to phenotypic and genotypic methods in the identification of dermatophytes (i.e., *Epidermophyton*, *Microsporum*, and *Trichophyton*).

MALDI-TOF-MS has largely replaced conventional biochemical-based identification methods.

Two drawbacks to MALDI-TOF-MS to date include the availability of extended reference spectra databases and the technique can only be used on isolated colonies. Also, more work on antifungal susceptibility/resistance testing and fungal strain typing is needed.

D. Genotypic approach: Like genotypic bacterial identification by sequencing of the 16S ribosomal DNA (PCR-based assay), the genotypic identification of yeasts and molds involves sequencing regions of ribosomal DNA, namely 18S rDNA subunit, 5.8S rDNA subunit, or 26S rDNA subunit:

1. sequencing of the D2 region of the large subunit ribosomal DNA (D2LSU)
2. sequencing of either one or both of the internal transcribed spacer regions (i.e., ITS1 and ITS2)

Some of those available universal fungal primers representing highly conserved regions are listed in Table 43.11.

Table 43.11: Some universal fungal primers

Primer	Nucleotide sequence (5' to 3')	rDNA subunit
ITS1	TCC GTA GGT GAA CCT GCG G	18S
ITS2	GCT GCG TTC TTC ATC GAT GC	5.8S
ITS3	GCA TCG ATG AAG AAC GCA GC	5.8S
ITS4	TCC TCC GCT TAT TGA TAT GC	26S
ITS5	GGA AGC AAA AGT CGT AAC AAG G	18S
Uni-F	GCA TAT CAA TAA GCG GAG GAA AAA G	26S

The development of molecular techniques has improved the speed as well as the accuracy of fungal identification. Currently, molecular methods are the gold standard for the identification of fungi to the species level. However, they are expensive and need specialized equipment. Today, molecular methods are simply used as a reference method for phylogeny and taxonomic studies.

This area is developing rapidly for making the availability of validated databases of ITS sequences.

Conclusion

Opportunistic invasive fungal diseases (IFDs) are a significant cause of morbidity and mortality in immunocompromised patients. The most common causes of IFDs are *Aspergillus* and *Candida* species. On the contrary, normal healthy individuals are infected with fungal diseases such as fungal keratitis, tinea capitis, mycetoma pedis (Madura foot), chromoblastomycosis, and sporotrichosis. Over 300 million people are infected worldwide annually with a serious fungal infection. The Centers for disease control and prevention (CDC) estimates that approximately 25,000 cases of candidemia (invasive candidiasis) occur in the United States each year. Despite the availability of a spectrum of antifungal agents, the clinical and economic burden of IFDs remains high.

Candida auris (discovered in 2009) can cause life-threatening infections, particularly in hospital settings. It can affect the bloodstream, heart, or brain. It is a multidrug-resistant yeast that could be misidentified by conventional laboratory techniques, thus making the patient's management difficult.

Apart from conventional approaches (phenotypic and biochemical) that are laborious and lengthy, medical mycologists are now interested in making improvements in the performance of both MALDI-TOF-MS and PCR-based assays.

According to one study (Maurizio S. and Brunella P., 2016), molecular methods fail to discriminate between *Aspergillus flavus* and *A. oryzae*. Likewise, internal transcribed spacer (ITS) sequence analysis cannot discriminate between the closely related species, *Trichophyton mentagrophytes,* and *T. interdigitale*. In contrast, MALDI-TOF-MS can discriminate against these species. Thus, both MALDI-TOF-MS and PCR-based assay have their limitations and complement each other in intra-species identification.

Chapter 44

Human Pathogenic Parasites

Introduction

Parasites are organisms that depend upon their hosts for nourishment. Apart from the books on parasitology, the reader will simply find a brief description of the parasitic worms in this chapter. Since the diagrams of adult worms, larvae, or eggs are very useful in the laboratory diagnosis of these parasitic infestations, the author has made all the efforts to include them. Depending on their location on the host, parasites are described as:

a. Ectoparasite:
- They inhabit the surface of the host's body without penetrating the tissues.
- They are important vectors that transmit the pathogenic microbes.
- The infection caused by these parasites is called infestation.

b. Endoparasite:
- They live within the body of the host. The endoparasites are further categorized as under:
  (i) *Obligate parasites:* They cannot exist without a parasitic life in the host.
  (ii) *Facultative parasites:* They can live a parasitic life or free-living life when the opportunity arises.
  (iii) *Accidental parasites:* They infect an unusual host.
  (iv) *Aberrant or wandering parasites:* They infect a host where they cannot live or develop further.

The parasites are classified into two main classes:

A. Helminths
B. Protozoa

A. Helminths (worms)

Helminths are multicellular animals. A few of them parasitize humans. The adult and larval stages of parasitic helminths are found in the definitive host and the intermediate host, respectively. Helminths can be monoecious (hermaphrodite) or dioecious. Helminths, in turn, are divided into three major groups as shown in Table 44.1.

Table 44.1: Comparative features among nematodes, cestodes, and trematodes

Feature	Nematodes (roundworms)	Cestodes (tapeworms)	Trematodes (flukes)
Shape	cylindrical	tape-like	leaf-like, flat
Suckers	absent	present	present
Hooklets	absent	mostly present	absent
Digestive canal	present	absent	present (incomplete)
Sex organs	separate	present in the same worm	present in the same worm

a. Nematodes

1. Trichinella spiralis: (see Fig. 44.1)
- Causes trichinellosis (also called trichinosis) which is a zoonotic infection acquired from domestic pigs or other carnivores
- Natural hosts: rodents, bears, dogs, and horses
- Man is an accidental host and acts as a dead end
- Transmitted by the consumption of undercooked meat, e.g., pork or pork products infected with pathogenic encysted larvae
- The severity of infection is dependent on the number of larvae ingested
- No symptoms, early symptoms associated with the digestive system (abdominal pains, nausea vomiting, and diarrhea), or late symptoms (fever, muscle pain, swelling of affected tissues)
- Serological tests, namely latex agglutination, and indirect immunofluorescence
- The most accurate laboratory diagnosis is done by muscle biopsies (17-24 days)

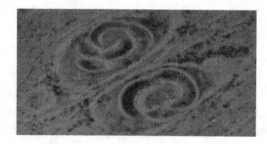

Fig. 44.1: *Trichinella spiralis* larvae encysted in a muscle.

2. Wuchereria bancrofti: (see Fig. 44.2)
- Transmitted by many blood-sucking mosquitoes
- The infective form called filariform larvae (third stage) are found in the proboscis of the mosquito
- Permanent enlargement of legs called elephantiasis
- Adult worms are located in the lymphatic vessels and lymph nodes
- Presence of microfilariae in a blood smear prepared at night

- Pathogenic *W. bancrofti* is found to be infected with a Rickettsia group of bacteria called *Wolbachia* and maintain an endosymbiotic relationship
- It is proved that this symbiotic relationship is essential for the survival of parasite, fertility, and larval development

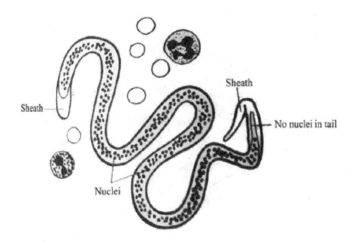

Fig. 44.2: Microfilaria of *Wuchereria bancrofti*.

3. Brugia malayi: (see Fig. 44.3)
- Very similar to *W. bancrofti*
- Transmitted by a mosquito
- Causes elephantiasis (filariasis)

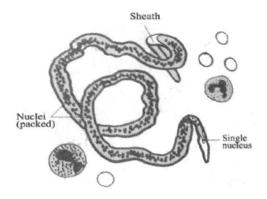

Fig. 44.3: Microfilaria of *Brugia malayi*.

4. Loa loa: (see Fig. 44.4)
- Also called African eye worm
- Transmitted by mango flies
- Adult worms migrate in subcutaneous tissues, including the eye
- Diagnosis is based on finding sheathed microfilariae

• Presence of microfilariae in a thick blood smear (10 AM-2 PM)

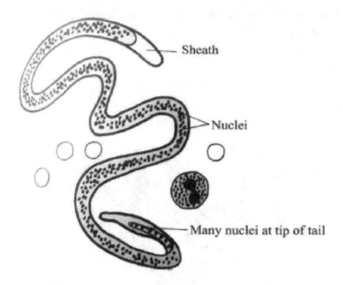

Fig. 44.4: *Loa loa* can be seen near the surface of the eye.

5. *Onchocerca volvulus:* (see Fig. 44.5)
   • Causes river blindness
   • Transmitted by black flies
   • Manifestations include dermatitis, subcutaneous fibrous nodule (onchocercoma), lymphadenitis, and ocular changes
   • Diagnosis is based on finding microfilariae in skin specimens

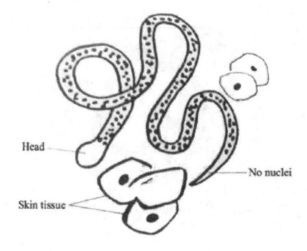

Fig. 44.5: Microfilaria of *Onchocerca volvulus.*

6. *Ancylostoma duodenale:* (see Fig. 54.1; # 15)
   • Acquired by contact with contaminated soil containing infective larvae
   • The hookworm has the ability to suck blood from the intestinal vessels

- Hookworm larvae of cats and dogs may penetrate human skin, causing cutaneous larva migrans
- Symptoms are abdominal pain, diarrhea, eosinophilia, and anemia
- The presence of ova and/or larvae in a stool specimen confirm the diagnosis
- It is postulated that hookworm infection can protect the individual from asthma and malaria but predispose to human immunodeficiency virus (HIV), tuberculosis, and other intestinal helminthic infections

Note: *Necator americanus* resembles *Ancylostoma duodenale* except mouthparts of ova, i.e., *A. duodenale* possesses pairs of teeth whereas *N. americanus* has cutting plates.

7. Enterobius vermicularis: (Fig. 54.1; # 16)
- Also called pinworm or threadworm
- Acquired by the ingestion of ova from non-living objects, e.g., toys or by inhalation
- Usually, asymptomatic (may cause itching around the vagina and anus, depending upon the migratory course of pinworms)
- Presence of ova in a cellulose tape (applied to the perianal area in the morning) constitutes the diagnosis

8. Trichuris trichiura (whipworm): (see Fig. 54.1; #18)
- Very common intestinal infection worldwide
- Transmitted via fecal-oral transmission
- Symptoms include abdominal pain, bloody diarrhea, nausea, vomiting, headache, sudden weight loss, and fecal incontinence
- Presence of ova in the stool specimen confirms the diagnosis

9. Ascaris lumbricoides: (see Fig. 54.1; #19)
- Is commonly called roundworm
- Acquired by the ingestion of ova in contaminated water or food
- Symptoms include abdominal pain and diarrhea, including obstruction
- Extraintestinal complications: Larger worms can enter and occlude the biliary tree, causing biliary colic, cholecystitis, and pancreatitis. Wandering worms may migrate to the pharynx and can cause respiratory obstruction or may block the eustachian tube
- Finding ova in a stool specimen confirms the diagnosis

10. Strongyloides stercoralis
- Initially known as military worm
- Strongyloidiasis is a worldwide infection
- Contracted by direct contact with soil carrying infective larvae
- Mild to moderate worm load: Adult worms and larvae traversing the upper small bowel mucosa may produce epigastric pain (resembling peptic ulcer), nausea, diarrhea, and blood loss
- Heavy larval load: Hyperinfection syndrome and disseminated strongyloidiasis are the important complications
- Finding larvae in a stool sample or other specimens confirm the diagnosis

b. Cestodes

1. Echinococcus granulosus: (see Fig. 44.6)
- Known as dog tapeworm
- Transmitted through the ingestion of ova from contaminated animal feces, e.g., dog (definitive host) and sheep, goats, and cattle (intermediate host). Man acts as an accidental intermediate host (dead end)
- Causes hydatid cyst
- Blockage and interference in the functions of organs, e.g., liver, lungs, and brain
- Diagnosis based on surgical removal of cysts and finding tapeworms and hooklets

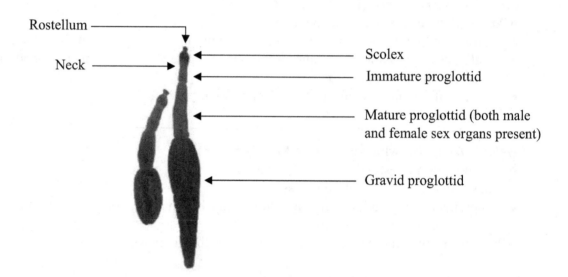

Rostellum

Neck

Scolex

Immature proglottid

Mature proglottid (both male and female sex organs present)

Gravid proglottid

Fig. 44.6: An adult *Echinococcus granulosus* having three proglottids.

2. Diphyllobothrium latum (fish or broad tapeworm)
- Widely distributed in the lake areas of Europe, Finland, the Far East, and Uganda
- Commonly called fish tapeworm is very long (up to 10 meters) with approximately 3,000-4,000 segments
- Transmitted by the ingestion of raw or undercooked freshwater fish (e.g. salmon, trout, perch, and pike) loaded with plerocercoid larvae
- Causes intestinal obstruction and gallbladder disease
- May interfere with vitamin B_{12} absorption, causing megaloblastic anemia
- Finding eggs or typical proglottids in stool specimen confirms the diagnosis

3. Taenia solium (pork tapeworm)
- 3-7 meters with less than 1,000 proglottids (segments)
- Causes both intestinal taeniasis and cysticercosis in man
- Acquired through the ingestion of raw or undercooked pork containing the cyst
- Also transmitted by food or water contaminated with feces from humans infected by the adult worms (cysticercosis)
- Symptoms include loss of appetite and weight, including digestive disorders

- Finding segments (13 mm in length and 8 mm in width) in stool confirms the diagnosis

4. Taenia saginata (beef tapeworm)
- Measures up to 10 meters in length with approximately 2,000 segments
- Men and cattle serve as the definitive host and the intermediate host, respectively
- Causes intestinal taeniasis in man
- Taeniasis is contracted by eating raw or insufficiently cooked beef containing the infective larvae
- Symptoms are similar to that of *Taenia solium*
- Presence of eggs or segments in a specimen ensures the diagnosis

Note:
1. The eggs of both *Taenia solium* and *T. saginata* are identical.
2. *Taenia asiatica* (Asian tapeworm) is limited to the Republic of Korea, China, Taiwan, Indonesia, and Thailand

c. Trematodes

All members except schistosomes have both sex organs within the same worm, i.e., hermaphroditic. They have a minimum of two hosts. Tail-bearing larvae discharged from the snail host infect the susceptible host. Laboratory diagnosis of almost all infections by trematodes in humans is based on the finding of ova in stool specimens. Therefore, the reader of this book is advised to refer to chapter 54 for the short details about trematodes.

B. Protozoa

Trophozoite, a motile and feeding form, is a common stage in several protozoan species. Mostly, trophozoites are found in fresh water bodies. Some protozoa can be seen in a cyst stage that offers protection against unfavorable environmental conditions, e.g., temperature and pH. Some protozoa show movement by using flagella, cilia, or pseudopodia. The stages and structures are important in the detection of protozoan diseases (i.e., laboratory diagnosis). They are grouped into three categories:

a. Amoebae
b. Blood and tissue protozoa
c. Malarial parasites

a. Amoebae

Generally, amoebae are found in two forms: free-living amoeba and cyst. Clinically significant amoebae are discussed in chapter 54.

b. Blood and tissue protozoa

- These protozoa are hemoflagellates, i.e., flagellated protozoa
- Found in peripheral blood circulation
- They complete their life cycle in two hosts, namely vertebrate host and insect vector. This is the reason why they are called digenetic or heteroxenous parasites

These protozoa have a single nucleus, a kinetoplast, and a single flagellum arising from kinetoplast. Based upon the arrangement of the flagellum, they exist in four different morphological stages:

1. *Amastigote:* Round- to oval-shaped and characterized by not having visible external flagella. The intracellular phase in the life-cycle of *Leishmania* species and *Trypanosoma cruzi* found in the human (reticuloendothelial cells) and reservoir hosts.

2. *Promastigote:* Lanceolate-shaped and has kinetoplast anterior to nucleus (antenuclear kinetoplast), characterized by prominent anterior flagellum. The extracellular form of *Leishmania* species found in the sandfly gut. This is the infective stage of *Leishmania* to man.

3. *Epimastigote:* Elongated and has kinetoplast placed close to the nucleus (juxtanuclear kinetoplast). It is characterized by the location of the flagellum being anterior of the nucleus, and in connection with the cell body by a short undulating membrane. This is the phase in unicellular life-cycle, typically of trypanosomes in insect vector.

4. *Trypomastigote:* Elongated and spindle-shaped with central nucleus. The kinetoplast lies near the posterior end and is characterized by the location of the flagellum being posterior of the nucleus, and in connection to the cell body by a long undulating membrane. It is the infective stage of *Trypanosoma* found in insect vector and peripheral blood of humans.

Except for amastigote, all the other three forms are motile because each one has a flagellum.

1. Leishmania donovani: {see Fig. 44.7 (a), (b)}
- Transmitted through the infected female sandfly vector
- Only two forms: amastigote (obligate intracellular form and the infective stage to vector, sand fly) and promastigote (extracellular form, infective stage to humans) are found
- Causes kala-azar (black sickness), affecting spleen, liver, and immune system

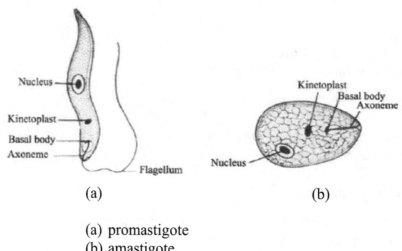

(a) promastigote
(b) amastigote

Fig. 44.7: *Leishmania donovani.*

2. Leishmania tropica: {see Fig. 44.8 (a), (b)}
- Transmitted through the sandfly vector
- Only amastigote and promastigote forms found
- Causes a cutaneous infection known as Delhi boil or Oriental sore

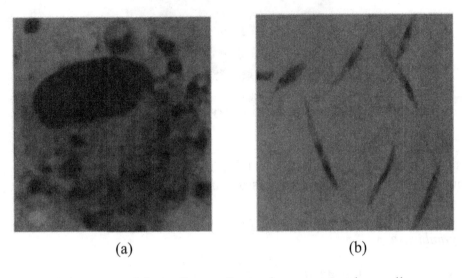

(a)   (b)

(a) small amastigotes in a mononuclear cell
(b) promastigotes

Fig. 44.8: *Leishmania tropica.*

Other species include *L. braziliensis* (Espundia) and *L. mexicana* (Chiclero's disease).

3. Trypanosoma brucei gambiense: (see Fig. 44.9)
- Causes human African trypanosomiasis (sleeping sickness) in West Africa
- Transmitted by the bite of tsetse fly (obligate parasite)
- Symptoms include fever, headache, and enlarged lymph glands in the early stages of the disease (a systemic and central nervous system infection)
- In humans, only the trypomastigote form (slender and spindle-shaped with an undulating membrane) is found
- The trypomastigotes undergo periodic antigenic variation that leads to frequent changes in the antigenic nature of variable surface glycoprotein (VSG) antigens present on their surface. This antigenic variation is the key mechanism of parasite for evading host immune response
- Laboratory diagnosis depends on the demonstration of trypanosomes in blood and lymph node samples in the early stages of the disease and serological tests, e.g., immunofluorescence

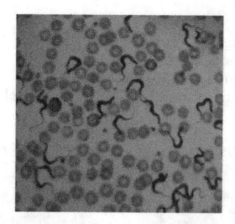

Fig. 44.9: Blood smear showing *Trypanosoma brucei gambiense.*

4. Trypanosoma brucei rhodesiense
- Causes human African trypanosomiasis (sleeping sickness) in East Africa
- Runs an acute course with rapid progression and early death as compared to *Trypanosoma brucei gambiense*
- Transmission, symptoms, and laboratory diagnosis are similar to that of *Trypanosoma brucei gambiense*

5. Trypanosoma cruzi: (see Fig. 44.10)
- Causes Chagas disease (American trypanosomiasis)
- Transmitted by the feces of blood-sucking triatomine bugs ("kissing" bugs), including blood transfusion, organ transplant, and transplacentally (mother-to-baby)
- Risk factors include: (i) have been exposed to blood products or received organs from a donor infected with Chagas disease (ii) have visited or traveled in rural Central or South America
- Symptoms may be acute (mild flu-like symptoms, rash, swelling or a sore near the eye or other infected site, loss of appetite, diarrhea, vomiting, and enlarged glands) or chronic (heart failure, multi-organ involvement difficulty in eating and passing stool)
- Laboratory diagnosis includes: (i) microscopic examination of thick and thin blood smears in the early stages of the disease (ii) serological, e.g., ELISA (iii) molecular tests, e.g., PCR and Western blot

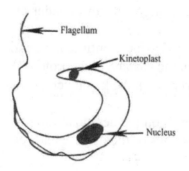

Fig. 44.10: *Trypanosoma cruzi* with a flagellum.

6. *Babesia microti*
- Most commonly seen species in the United States
- Over 100 known species of genus *Babesia*
- Transmitted by a tick-bite (*Ixodes dammini*) and blood transfusions with infected blood
- Tiny protozoan parasites infect red blood cells, causing hemolytic anemia
- Life-threatening infections in elderly and immunocompromised individuals
- Presence of four pear-shaped infective units (Maltese cross) confirms babesiosis

7. *Toxoplasma gondii*
- Causes worldwide toxoplasmosis (zoonosis)
- Is an obligate intracellular parasite
- Definitive host: cat; secondary host: human
- Exists in three morphological forms: (i) two asexual forms (tachyzoite and tissue cyst) and (ii) a sexual form (oocyst)
- *T. gondii* is unique among the protozoa as all three morphological forms can transmit the infection
- Directly transmitted by ingestion of fecal oocysts from infected cats or indirectly by ingestion of poorly cooked cyst-containing meats
- Other means of transmission include organ transplantation, congenital, transfusion with contaminated blood
- Laboratory diagnosis by serological assays

8. *Cryptosporidium parvum*
- Infects the epithelial cells lining the digestive tract in humans, causing diarrhea
- Acquired through ingestion of oocysts from contaminated water, infected lower animals
- May cause long-lasting cholera-like diarrhea in immunosuppressed individuals
- Laboratory diagnosis by a modified acid-fast technique, immunofluorescent methods, and gene sequencing

9. *Isospora belli*
- Causes long-lasting diarrhea, especially in immunocompromised patients, e.g., AIDS
- Contracted by ingestion of oocysts
- Laboratory diagnosis includes the detection of oocysts in stool samples and performance of a modified acid-fast stain of the material

c. Malarial parasites

Malaria is one of the most serious and widespread infections in man. It affects millions of people throughout Africa, Central and South America, and Asia. It causes about 20 million deaths worldwide per year. Over a million people die of malaria every year only in India.

Causative agents: There are five species of *Plasmodium* that cause malaria in humans:

1. *Plasmodium falciparum*: causes severe malaria called malignant tertian malaria (periodicity of fever is once in 48 hours, i.e., recurs every third day).
2. *P. malariae:* causes benign quartan malaria (periodicity of fever is once in 72 hours, i.e., recurs every fourth day).

3. *P. vivax*: causes benign tertian malaria (periodicity of fever is once in 48 hours, i.e. recurs every third day).
4. *P. ovale:* causes ovale tertian malaria (periodicity of fever is once in 48 hours, i.e., recurs every third day).
5. *P. knowlesi:* causes quotidian malaria (periodicity of fever is once in 24 hours, i.e., recurs every day). It is a parasite of monkey but can also affect humans. Many cases affecting man have been reported from Asia.

P. falciparum occurs mainly in the tropical countries (e.g., India) whereas *P. vivax* causes infection in a wider area. *P. ovale* is the least frequent malaria, with most cases in the West coast of Africa. It should be noted that a mixed infection by two malarial parasites may also occur. It is interesting to note that the Fy (a⁻b⁻) genotype appears to confer resistance to penetration by *P. vivax*.

Transmission: Malarial parasites are transmitted by the bite of an infected female *Anopheles* mosquito.

Life cycle: Malarial parasite has the following two hosts (see Fig. 44.11).

A. *Anopheles* mosquito (the definitive host): The malarial parasite multiplies sexually (sporogony).
B. Man (the intermediate host): The malarial parasite multiplies asexually (schizogony).

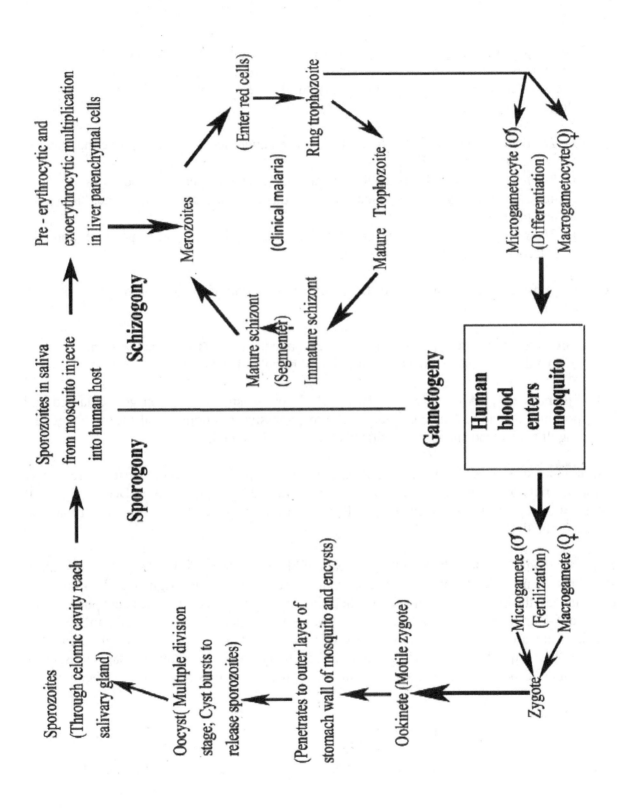

Fig. 44.11: Life cycle of the malaria parasites.

Clinical features of benign malaria: It is characterized by a triad of febrile paroxysm, anemia, and splenomegaly.

1. **Febrile paroxysm:** Fever develops intermittently depending on the species. Paroxysm corresponds to the release of the successive broods of merozoites into the bloodstream at the end of erythrocytic cycle. Each paroxysm of fever is comprised of three stages listed below:

   (i)   *The cold stage* (lasts for 15-60 minutes): The patient feels cold with shivering, nausea, vomiting, and headache.
   (ii) *The fever (febrile) stage* (lasts for several hours): The temperature reaches its peak, i.e., 40°C or more. Symptoms associated with this stage are severe headache, back pain, and joint pain.
   (iii) *The sweating stage*: There is a rapid fall in temperature. The patient perspires and falls asleep and later awakes feeling well.

   The classical paroxysm may not be always present due to maturation of generations of parasites at different times.

2. **Anemia:** After a few paroxysms of fever, patient develops normocytic normochromic anemia due to parasite induced destruction of red blood cells.

3. **Splenomegaly:** After a few weeks of febrile paroxysms, the spleen gets enlarged and becomes palpable. This condition is due to a massive proliferation of macrophages that engulf parasitized and non-parasitized coated red blood cells.

Out of the four species of *Plasmodium,* malaria caused by *P. falciparum* is the most severe. It may develop a variety of complications, e.g., cerebral malaria and black-water fever. Death may occur in cases of heavy and untreated infections. Relapses may occur due to the survival of malarial parasites in the liver.

Laboratory diagnosis: Both thick and thin smears of blood are prepared for diagnostic laboratory tests. Films are made from micropuncture or from a tube of EDTA anticoagulated blood. In most circumstances, the blood specimen to be studied should be collected during the acute phase of the disease, at 6-8 hr. intervals. It is not necessary to wait until the patient has fever and chills. Stained thick films are used to scan for the presence of parasites. Stained thin films are necessary for studying the morphology of parasites and infected erythrocytes, allowing parasite species differentiation. Blood films can be stained with one of the Romanowsky stains given below:

A. Giemsa's stain
B. Field's stain (for a thin smear)

Giemsa's staining method is widely used to stain blood films containing malarial parasites.

Staining procedure:

1. Fix the thick smear by passing the slide (smear facing upwards) three times through a bunsen burner flame
2. Dehemoglobinize the thick smear by washing it with distilled water
3. Fix the thin smear with methanol for 30 seconds
4. Allow both smears to air-dry
5. Place the smears in a staining jar of freshly prepared working Giemsa's stain for 20-30 minutes
6. Wash off with tap water
7. Allow the smears to air-dry in a draining rack
8. Examine the smears under oil-immersion lens

Note: One should examine the smear for 30 minutes before reporting negative.

It is advisable to make use of the information given in Fig. 44.12 while examining a stained smear.

Developmental stage	P. falciparum	P.vivax*	P. malariae	P. ovale
Rings	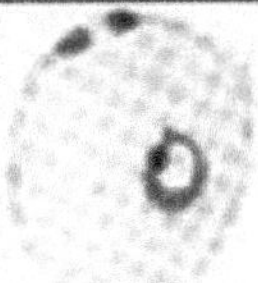	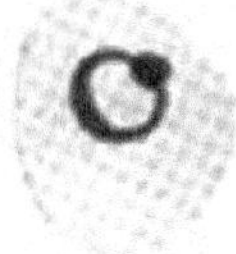	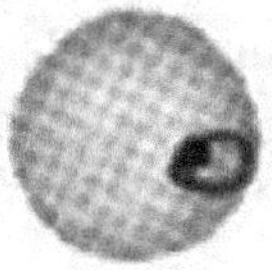	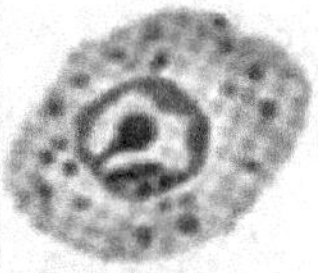
Schizonts	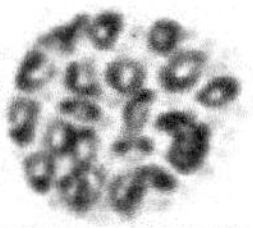	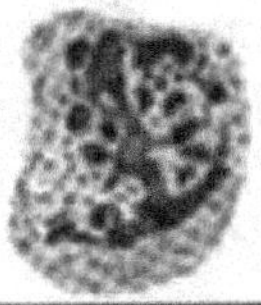	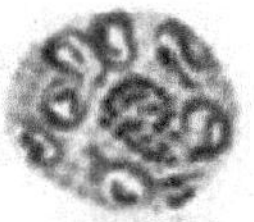	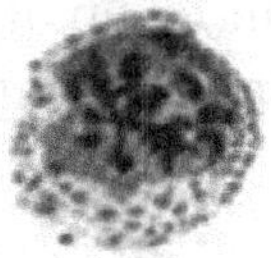
Gametocytes	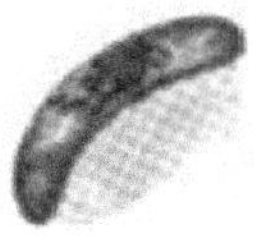	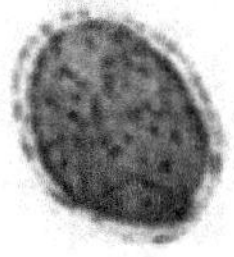	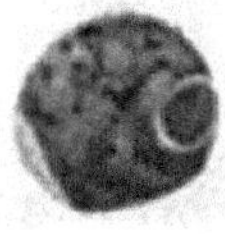	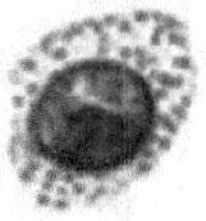

*The cell may contain Schuffner's stippling.

Fig. 44.12: Various stages of development in malarial parasites.

Chapter 45

Human Pathogenic Viruses

Introduction

Dmitri Ivanovsky (1892), the founder of virology, characterized the infectious agent of tobacco mosaic disease as filtrable through a porcelain Chamberland filter. In 1898, M. Beijerinck differentiated these tiny particles from bacteria and designated contagium vivum fluidum. Later, Wendell Stanley (1935) crystallized tobacco mosaic virus (TMV) in the laboratory and described protein and RNA as its constituents.

Despite the existence of many types of viruses (animal, plant, and bacterial), this chapter is strictly limited to clinically significant animal viruses. It briefly discusses their chemical composition, structure, replication, cultivation, transmission, and classification. Also, viral diseases in humans and their laboratory diagnostic tests are highlighted. It is very important to note that modern molecular tests play a vital role in the laboratory diagnosis of many viral diseases. Furthermore, some sophisticated techniques (e.g., electron microscopy and X-ray diffraction) have contributed a lot in understanding these ultramicroscopic particles.

When viruses are grown on susceptible cells, they develop clear areas on the monolayer of cells due to lysis of cells. Such patches are called plaques.

Structure

The virions are made up of basic components, namely genome and capsid. General outline of the structure of an animal and bacterial viruses is shown in {Fig. 45.1 (a), (b)}.

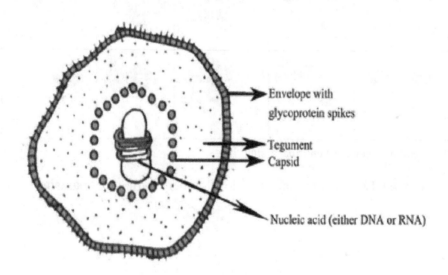

(a) Animal virus

Fig. 45.1: Structure of viruses.

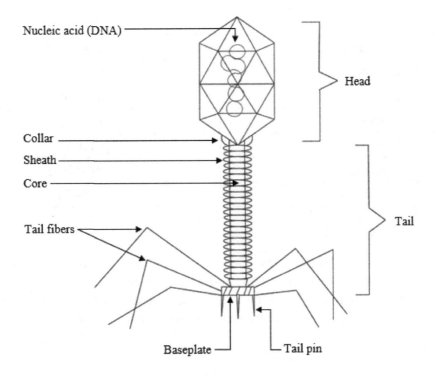

Nucleic acid (DNA)

Head

Collar

Sheath

Core

Tail

Tail fibers

Baseplate

Tail pin

(b) T4 bacteriophage

Fig. 45.1: Structure of viruses.

The genome consists of either DNA or RNA but never both. The nucleic acid may be single-stranded or double-stranded. In addition to this, the genome may be linear, e.g., Parvovirus or circular, e.g., Papillomavirus. The genome remains protected by a protein-made protective shell called a capsid. This capsid is made up of repeating subunits of polypeptides known as capsomeres. The symmetry of these structural subunits together is either helical or icosahedral (30 edges and 20 equilateral triangle faces with five meetings at each of its 12 vertices). In addition to a nucleoprotein, some viruses do have a lipid bilayer known as an envelope acquired from the host cell membrane. So-called enveloped viruses are susceptible to environmental conditions, e.g., pH, temperature, and dryness. On the other hand, those virions deprived of an envelope are labeled as naked viruses and are resistant to environmental conditions.

The size of filterable viruses ranges from 30 nm[33] in diameter (e.g., poxviruses) to 440 nm (e.g., mega virus chilensis). Techniques used in the determination of the size of viruses include ultrafiltration, ultracentrifugation, and electron microscopy. Most of the animal viruses are spheres in shape. However, some other shapes are also seen in animal viruses. This can be exemplified as shown in Table 45.1.

---

[33] Nanometer: 10^{-9} meters $= 10A^0 = 0.001$ microns.

Table 45.1: Appearance of some viruses

Virus	Appearance
Rotavirus	wheel-like
Rabies Virus	bullet-like
Astrovirus	star-like
Coronavirus	petal-like
Poxvirus	brick-like
Pandoravirus	oval-like

Lytic cycle: (see Fig. 45.2)

Viruses are obligate intracellular parasites. This means that they fail to grow on artificial culture media. They form a link between the living and nonliving organisms. Therefore, tissue (cell) culture, embryonated chicken egg, or animal host is used for the successful cultivation of virions. A normal infection cycle of a virus particle in a susceptible host involves the following steps:

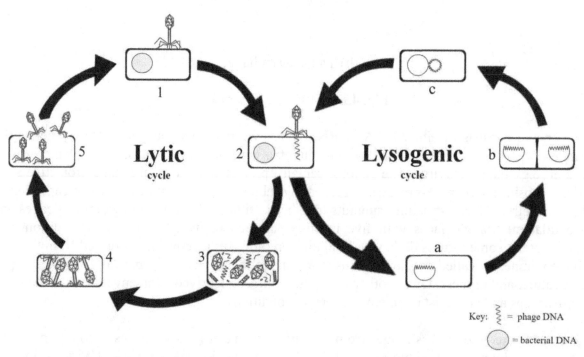

1. Attachment (adsorption)
2. Penetration
3. Replication (synthesis)
4. Assembly and maturation
5. Release (burst)

a. Integration
b. Normal cell division
c. Induction and excision

Fig. 45.2: Lytic and Lysogenic cycles.

Following the penetration of a virus particle, the viral nucleic acid takes control over an infected host cell. Then, the viral genome guides the host cell to make many replicas of its own and structural polypeptide subunits called capsomeres. Finally, many thousands of new virus particles are produced in the infected host cell. Many factors can influence this host-virus interaction, e.g., type of the host involved and environmental factors. Because viruses lack many enzymes needed for its replication cycle, virus particles are fully dependent on the host, making use of the host's complex cell machinery. In other words, the replication of virus particles takes place at the cost of the host.

Lysogenic cycle: (see Fig.45.2)

Unlike the lytic cycle, phage DNA is inserted into the bacterial genome after its penetration. In a normal cell division, bacterial genome and added phage DNA (prophage) undergo replication.

Therefore, the daughter cells do carry phage DNA as well and remain unharmed. Phages capable of entering a lysogenic cycle are called temperate phages.

The prophage expresses its genes during lysogenic cycle. This is how the host bacterium acquires new properties (e.g., virulence factors) and the phenomenon is called lysogenic conversion. The lysogenic conversion is mediated by a mechanism of gene transfer by a specific bacteriophage from the donor bacterium to the recipient bacterium called transduction. Some virulence factors that are encoded by a prophage are listed in Table 45.2.

Table 45.2: Some virulence factors encoded by a prophage

Host bacterium	Virulence factor
Streptococcus pyogenes	Erythrogenic toxin
Escherichia coli	Shiga-like toxin
Staphylococcus aureus	Enterotoxins A, D, E, staphylokinase, Toxic shock syndrome toxin-1
Clostridium botulinum	Neurotoxins C, D, E
Corynebacterium diphtheriae	Diphtheria toxin

Occasionally, prophage separates from a bacterial genome following the induction and enters a lytic cycle.

Cultivation

Unlike bacteria, viruses need living cells to support their growth. Cultivation of viruses uses one of the following methods:

1. Cell (tissue) culture
  a. Primary cell culture, e.g., monkey kidney cell culture and human amnion cell culture
  b. Semi-continuous cell lines (diploid cell culture), e.g., human embryonic lung strain

c. Continuous cell lines (heteroploid cell culture), e.g., HeLa (Human carcinoma of cervix cell line and HEP-2 (Human epithelioma of larynx cell line)

The choice of a method depends upon the purpose of propagation of viruses, e.g., identification, production of vaccines, and research. Many types of cell cultures are used to cultivate viruses. Primary cultures make use of cells taken from normal fetal, embryonic, and adult animal tissues. Such cultures are limited in the number of times they can be subcultured. Unlike primary cultures, the semi-continuous cell lines can be subcultured as many as 50 times. The continuous cultures, derived from the cancerous cells, allow subculturing indefinitely.

Cells are nourished by a defined growth medium. Antibiotics need to be added to reduce the problems of contamination by bacteria and fungi as well. Moreover, trypsin is also added to free cells to facilitate the formation of a monolayer. These cells are transferred to appropriate containers, e.g., Petri dishes and tubes. Such monolayer cultures permit their examination macroscopically and microscopically.

During viral growth, there appear lesions called cytopathic effects (CPEs) on tissue culture cells. Such lesions provide clues about the characteristics of virus particles. A variety of CPEs produced during viral cultivation include:

1. formation of inclusion bodies
2. formation of giant cells (syncytium)
3. abnormal cellular rounding and detachment
4. cellular necrosis

2. Embryonated egg (e.g., chicken, duck, and turkey)
Viruses can also be cultivated using an embryonated egg. Different tissues of an egg, e.g., amniotic sac, yolk sac, chorioallantoic membrane (CAM), or allantoic cavity can be used for propagating the viruses. The site of inoculation selected depends upon the type of a virus in question. For example, Herpes simplex virus and Poxvirus are inoculated in the chorioallantoic membrane. At the end of incubation, localized damage of the membrane occurs with the formation of typical pocks (opaque lesions). Such inoculation techniques in the embryonated chicken egg are shown in Fig. 45.3(a), (b).

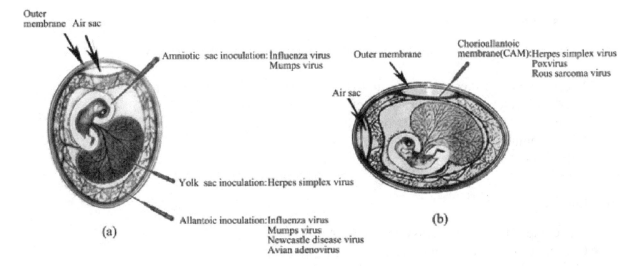

(a) Amniotic sac, yolk sac, and allantoic inoculations
(b) Chorioallantoic membrane inoculation

Fig. 45.3: Different sites of inoculation in the embryonated chicken egg.

3. Laboratory animals (e.g., mice, rats, hamsters, and guinea pigs)
Laboratory animals can also be used for the cultivation of viruses. For instance, the production of vaccines.

Classification

Classification of viruses is based on the key taxonomic criteria listed below:

1. Type of a nucleic acid
2. The symmetry of capsid, e.g., helical, or icosahedral
3. Type of host, e.g., bacteriophages, plant viruses, and animal viruses
4. Size of a virus particle
5. Presence or absence of an envelope
6. Presence or absence of some key enzymes, e.g., reverse transcriptase

Animal viruses are sub-grouped based on tissue tropism:

a. dermotropic (if skin infected)
b. neurotropic (if nerve tissue infected)
c. viscerotropic (if digestive tract infected)
d. pneumotropic (if respiratory tract infected)

Viruses are classified into orders, families, and genera. One should keep in mind that a plentiful amount of information will get accumulated about the properties of viruses in the days to come. This, in turn, will impact on the taxonomy of viruses. So, the author of this title considers the current classification simply a tentative one.

Transmission of viruses

Like bacteria, viruses are transmitted by different means as listed below:

1. Droplets, e.g., influenza, severe acute respiratory syndrome coronavirus 2 (SARS-CoV-2)
2. Food and water, e.g., Norovirus infection (stomach Flu), hepatitis A
3. Vector, e.g., West Nile virus (from birds), rabies (from rodents)
4. Direct contact, e.g., hepatitis B, HIV
5. Indirect contact, e.g., small-pox, molluscum

Risk factors

- The compromised immune system, e.g., AIDS
- Chronic diseases, e.g., tuberculosis, asthma, and diabetes
- Malnourishment
- Smoking
- Poor hygienic practices
- Crowded populations
- Stress and other mental health problems
- Unsafe sex
- Advanced age and young age

Representative viruses

This section is highlighted to familiarize the selected viral infections in humans. This can best be summarized in Table 45.3 (a), (b).

Table 45.3 (a): Representative RNA viruses

Nucleic acid	Single-stranded or Double-stranded	Enveloped or Naked	*Capsid*: Helical or Icosahedral	Virus(es)	Disease(s) caused
RNA ⟷	single-stranded ⟷	enveloped ⟷	helical ⟷	Rabies virus	rabies
				Rubella virus	mild rash
				Coronavirus	common cold
				Influenzaviruses	influenza
				RSV*	respiratory infection
				Arboviruses	yellow fewer, dengue
				Paramyxoviruses	croup in children
				HIV**	AIDS
				Calicivirus	enteritis
				Echovirus	febrile disease
				Rhinovirus	common cold
				Poliovirus	poliomyelitis
				Hepatitis A	hepatitis A
			cone-shaped	Coxsackievirus	febrile disease
		naked ⟷	icosahedral ⟷		
	double-stranded	naked	icosahedral	Rotavirus	diarrhea

* Respiratory Syncytial Virus.
** Human Immunodeficiency Virus.

405

Table 45.3 (b): Representative DNA viruses

Nucleic acid	Single-stranded or Double-stranded	Enveloped or Naked	*Capsid*: Helical or Icosahedral	Virus(es)	Disease(s) caused
DNA	double-stranded	enveloped	icosahedral	Varicella-Zoster virus	chicken pox and shingles
				Epstein-Barr virus	Burkitt's lymphoma, Infectious mononucleosis, and nasopharyngeal carcinoma
				Cytomegalovirus	IM* – like illness and interstitial pneumonia
				Herpes-simplex virus 1	cold sores
				Herpes-simplex virus 2	genital herpes
				Human herpes virus 6	roseola
				Human herpes virus 7 and 8	both infect AIDS patients
				Poxviruses	small-pox and cow-pox
		naked	icosahedral	Adenovirus	infects intestinal tract, eye, and respiratory tract
				Papillomavirus	STD**
	partial double-stranded	naked	icosahedral	Hepatitis B	severe hepatitis
	single-stranded	naked	icosahedral	Parvovirus B19	Erythema infectiosum (fifth disease)

* Infectious mononucleosis.
** Sexually transmitted disease.

Laboratory diagnosis

Before the listing of the diagnostic methods for the detection of viral agents, the collection and care of a representative specimen are of prime importance in the success and accuracy of the method engaged in the detection. It is required that a valid specimen is collected from the right site at the right time followed by transportation to the diagnostic facility without any delay and drying.

Some techniques (e.g., monolayer cell culture inoculation) are expensive and time-consuming. Serological and molecular methods are more convenient to perform and straightforward to interpret. Methods used for the detection of viral agents are categorized into four major groups as under:

a. Microscopic methods: Examination of clinical specimens to reveal the morphology of viruses (e.g., electron microscopy) is a direct approach. Also, fluorescent microscopy is a valuable tool in examining the virus-infected cells that have undergone treatment with a fluorescein-labeled antibody. However, these tools are not routinely used in a diagnostic facility because clinical specimens usually contain a few virus particles along with some debris, obscuring their existence.

b. Serological procedures: e.g., enzyme-linked immunosorbent assay (ELISA), complement fixation test (CFT), and radioimmunoassay (RIA). These methods aid in the detection of IgM in the early phase of an acute infection, a rise in IgG titer during a convalescent-phase, and the detection of viral antigens, e.g., P24.

c. Inoculation techniques: e.g., cell (tissue) culture. Different animal viral agents produce specific cytopathic effects.

d. Molecular assays: e.g., nucleic acid hybridization (DNA and RNA probes available) and polymerase chain reaction. These assays are very sensitive.

Viroids are the smallest infectious particles composed of a short strand of a single-stranded circular RNA. Unlike virions (whole virus particles), viroids lack a protein coat. These subviral particles are inhabitants of higher plants.

Prions are misfolded proteins capable of causing fatal progressive neurodegenerative diseases in animals (e.g., "mad cow disease") and humans (e.g., Creutzfeldt-Jakob disease). Unlike viroids, prions lack the genome for genetic information.

Very little information is available for both infectious entities to date.

Coronaviruses

There are various types of human coronaviruses. Some of them cause only mild symptoms of the upper respiratory tract. SARS-CoV-2 (a novel virus), first identified in Wuhan; Province of Hubei, China, has been disseminating in many parts of the world. It is a positive-sense RNA virus that caused coronavirus disease, COVID-19 pandemic. It is an enveloped virus with club-like spikes as shown in Fig. 45.4.

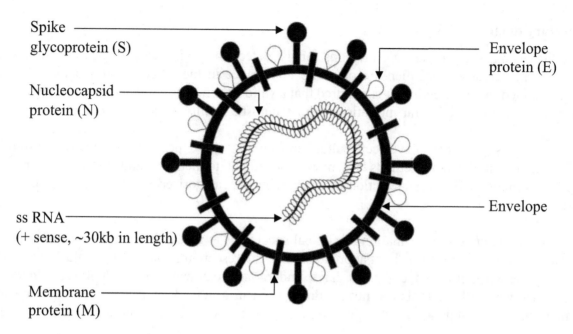

Fig. 45.4: Schematic structure of SARS-CoV-2.

It is transmitted by airborne droplets that are generated during coughing, sneezing, or talking. Infected persons develop symptoms such as fever, dry cough, and shortness of breath within 2-14 days (i.e., incubation period).

Laboratory diagnosis
The first real-time reverse transcription-PCR (RT-PCR) test was developed by Dr.Victor Corman and his associates (Berlin, Germany) in January 2020. Unlike DNA viruses, RNA viruses require an additional specific step called reverse transcription prior to the amplification. The transcription of RNA into DNA is catalyzed by reverse transcriptase. The SARS-CoV-2, RNA virus, consists of about 30,000 base pairs as opposed to more than 3 billion base pairs in human genome. Interestingly, the RT-PCR test detects some specific fragments (i.e., gene sequences) and not the whole viral genome.

Sample
Collecting the appropriate respiratory tract specimen at the right time from the right anatomic site is essential for accurate molecular diagnosis of COVID-19. The preferred site for sampling is the nasopharyngeal approach using a fiber plastic shaft swab. When collection with a nasopharyngeal swab is impossible, oropharyngeal swabs, nasal mid-turbinate swabs, or anterior nares (nasal) swabs are also acceptable alternatives. After collection, swabs should be placed into sterile tubes containing about 3 mL of a viral transport medium to preserve viral integrity. Specimens can be stored at 2°-8°C for up to 72 hours. In cases of delayed testing or shipping, specimens should be stored at -70°C or below.

Once the specimen arrives at the testing facility, the assays procedures should be performed without delay in a biosafety cabinet of class II or higher. Care should be taken to minimize aerosol generation during specimen processing.

Principle
Highlighting the RNA sequences present in three genes of the SARS-CoV-2:

1. Envelope protein gene (E)
2. RNA-dependent RNA polymerase gene (RdRp)
3. Nucleocapsid protein gene (N)

Working
To know the presence of the sequences of these genes in the sample, it is required to amplify the sequences of these genes to obtain a signal sufficient for its detection and quantification.

Cycle 1: target x 2 (2 copies)
Cycle 2: target x 4 (4 copies)
Cycle 3: target x 8 (8 copies)
Cycle 4: target x 16 (16 copies)
Cycle 5: target x 32 (32 copies)
Cycle 6: target x 64 (64 copies)
and so on till 40 to 60 cycles.

When a person states that the Cycle Time or Cycle Threshold or RT-PCR positivity threshold (Ct) is equal to 40, it means that the testing facility has used 40 amplification cycles to obtain 2^{40} copies. This is what underlies the sensitivity of the RT-PCR assay.

Interpretation
Many authorities consider RT-PCR test to be a gold standard for viral infections, including SARS-CoV-2. However, the level of Cycle Threshold (Ct) largely influences the interpretation of the result. It is very difficult to culture the virus in case of Ct levels above 30. For example, the probability of culturing the virus decreases by 8% in samples with Ct levels greater than 35. Therefore, the reported binary result (positive /negative) without a chosen Ct may be misleading. In the past, many diagnostic laboratories across the globe have reported as positives without mentioning the Ct level used for asymptomatic persons. According to experts, use of a maximum Ct of 30 is recommended to avoid false positives.

Advantages
1. Specificity and sensitivity
2. Short turnaround time

Disadvantages
1. False positives if an appropriate threshold of positivity is not chosen
2. Mutations in the virus invalidate certain primers
3. Expensive
4. Possible cross-reactivity, e.g., benign cold coronaviruses

Review Questions:

1. Name the etiological agent of whooping cough.
2. Name the causative agent of Hansen's disease.
3. Name the most important pathogen responsible for gas gangrene.
4. Name the predominant causative agent of aspergillosis.
5. Name the etiologic agent of Q (Query) fever.
6. Which equipment is used to sterilize heat-labile substances (e.g., egg white)?
7. Which is the best preferred specimen for the isolation of *Brucella abortus*?
8. Give two names of bacterial species that cannot be cultivated on an artificial cell-free media.
9. Name the selective medium routinely employed for the isolation of *Neisseria gonorrhoeae*?
10. Name the flagella staining technique most commonly used in clinical laboratories?
11. Which chemical reagent is used in wet mount preparations to examine the fungi?
12. Which agar medium is employed for the cultivation of most fungi?
13. Which enzyme is detected to distinguish between *Staphylococcus aureus* from *S. epidermidis*?
14. Which reagent is used to detect the presence of capsules?
15. Which dye is used in the preparation of the TSI agar medium to indicate carbohydrate fermentation?
16. Which dye is used to observe unstained yeasts in pus, sputum, or exudates?
17. Which enteric species produces an acid butt, an alkaline slant, a slight blackening of the butt, and no gas in a TSI agar slant?
18. Which *Clostridium* species has the following characteristics?
    Cells are large, Gram-positive thick rods; oval spores which may be located centrally or subterminally; colonies are translucent with a granular surface, irregular or circular; shows hemolysis on blood agar.
19. Which test is employed to differentiate between late lactose fermenters and lactose non-fermenters?
20. Which agar medium is most frequently used for susceptibility testing?
21. Give three examples of zoonotic infections.
22. Name the causative agent of chancroid.
23. Name the etiological agent that causes a peptic ulcer in humans.
24. List the name of a Gram-negative bacterial species that needs cysteine or cysteine for growth and is also associated with tularemia.
25. What is the name of a causative agent for Legionnaires' disease?
26. Mention three names of microbes that can be identified by polymerase chain reaction (PCR).
27. Which gas is used to sterilize steam-sensitive hospital instruments?
28. Mention the name of an anticoagulant used in blood cultures.
29. Mention any two bacterial genera that belong to the fastidious group.
30. List any two culture media that are selective for Gram-positive bacteria.

31-35 Questions: True (mark as A) and False (mark as B):

31. Viruses are obligate intracellular parasites that contain either DNA or RNA _____.
32. Both cytopathic effect (CPE) and immunofluorescence can be used to detect viral agents _____.
33. Koplik spots are peculiar lesions seen in measles infection_____.
34. Viral infections namely, measles, mumps, parainfluenza, and respiratory syncytial produce multinucleated giant cells in tissue culture and become helpful in making a rapid presumptive diagnosis possible_____.
35. Rabid animals produce demonstrable Negri bodies in the brain tissue_____.

36. Which of the following infectious diseases is caused by rickettsial organisms?
    A. Epidemic typhus
    B. Endemic typhus
    C. Scrub typhus
    D. Rocky Mountain spotted fever
    E. All of the above
37. Which of the following infectious diseases can be diagnosed by the Weil-Felix agglutination reaction?
    A. Typhus fever
    B. Mumps
    C. Influenza
    D. Rubella
    E. None of the above
38. Which of the following rickettsial infections is caused by *Rickettsia prowazekii*?
    A. Endemic typhus fever
    B. Epidemic typhus fever
    C. Scrub typhus fever
    D. Rocky Mountain spotted fever
    E. None of the above
39. Which of the following rickettsial infections is the most severe and the most frequently reported in the United States?
    A. Endemic typhus
    B. Scrub typhus fever
    C. Epidemic typhus fever
    D. Rocky Mountain spotted fever
    E. None of the above
40. Rickettsiae are now reclassified with bacteria because of the following characteristics *except:*
    A. Binary fission as a mode of multiplication
    B. Susceptible to antibiotics
    C. Possess both DNA and RNA
    D. Contain many metabolic enzymes
    E. Cultivation on artificial culture media

Answers:

1. *Bordetella pertussis*
2. *Mycobacterium leprae*
3. *Clostridium welchii (Cl. perfringens)*
4. *Aspergillus fumigatus*
5. *Coxiella burnetii*
6. Inspissator
7. Blood
8. *Mycobacterium leprae* and *Treponema pallidum*
9. Thayer and Martin medium
10. Leifson
11. 10% potassium (or sodium) hydroxide
12. Sabouraud's glucose agar medium
13. Coagulase
14. 'Omni-serum'
15. Phenol red
16. India ink
17. *Salmonella typhi*
18. *Clostridium botulinum*
19. O.N.P.G. (ortho-nitrophenyl-Beta-D-galactopyranoside) test
20. Mueller-Hinton agar medium
21. Lyme disease, brucellosis, and plague
22. *Haemophilus ducreyi*
23. *Helicobacter pylori*
24. *Francisella tularensis*
25. *Legionella pneumophila*
26. *Neisseria gonorrhoeae, Chlamydia trachomatis,* and human immunodeficiency virus (HIV)
27. Ethylene oxide (C_2H_4O)
28. Sodium polyanethole sulfonate (SPS)
29. *Haemophilus* and *Neisseria*
30. Phenylethyl alcohol (PEA) agar and colistin nalidixic acid (CAN) agar
31. A
32. A
33. A
34. A
35. A
36. E
37. A
38. B
39. D
40. E

Section V: Blood Banking/Immunohematology

Chapter 46

ABO and Rhesus Blood Group Systems

Introduction

The blood bank is an independent division of a clinical laboratory in a hospital setting. Unlike other areas of a laboratory, human blood and blood products are processed and stored at appropriate temperatures for patients' use. Technically, blood products must be promptly and safely transfused to patients. Thus, a blood bank professional plays a direct role in the treatment of a patient. Therefore, a blood bank technologist has to work with great responsibility. A blood bank technologist should be knowledgeable and well-organized in his/her work. A technologist intending to work in a blood bank should take working experience in the presence of another trained technologist.

Nowadays, automated blood bank instruments have made the job easier compared to about 15 years ago. Today, we look at the blood bank with its transformed facet because almost all manual tests, namely ABO grouping, Rh typing, and antibody screening are now fully automated. Also, it has been very productive in that one can successfully manage the workflow of a busy blood bank with a limited staff. For the sake of a better understanding of the concept, the author will include the discussion based on a "test-tube" method. Also, the discussion will include the patient's plasma as a specimen of choice for reverse grouping, detection, and identification of antibodies. One should bear the following points in mind while performing the blood bank-related tests:

1. Use clean and dry glasswares for testing
2. Use reagent antisera and reagent red cells from a standard manufacturer, e.g., Ortho Clinical Diagnostics and Immucor, Inc.
3. Use an acceptable patient's blood specimen (pink top) labeled with complete and accurate details, e.g., the full name of a patient, date of collection, and a valid initial of a phlebotomist
4. Include both reagent controls and procedural controls to ensure the expected reactivity and appropriate test conditions (e.g., temperature and centrifugation), respectively
5. Consult the blood bank officer/director On-call (24/7) for questions or concerns
6. Enter the test results immediately in the laboratory information system or designated register to keep an up-to-date record of test results
7. Store patient's specimen at 4°-6°C after testing for future use

ABO Blood Group System

Genotypes and phenotypes

This aspect explains how different blood groups are inherited from parents to offspring. There are 46 chromosomes (i.e., 23 pairs) in the nucleus of human body cells. Out of these 23 pairs, there are 22 pairs of autosomes and a pair of sex chromosomes (XX in the female; XY in the male). Crossing over occurs during meiosis, thus allowing homologous chromosomes to exchange pieces of genetic material. This is how each chromosome entering the gamete includes variable amounts of paternal and maternal genetic material. A zygote (a diploid cell) is produced as a result of the fusion of an ovum and a sperm, each having one-half of the genetic material (i.e., haploid).

Many genes are found on each chromosome. These genes control different physical characteristics, e.g., blood group, the color of skin, the color of hair, etc. Alleles of the ABO group system are present on chromosome number 9. Each gene occupies its site along the length of a chromosome termed locus. But, some inherited characteristics are represented by a group of genes and only one of these genes occupies the locus. Such genes governing inherited traits are called alleles or allelomorphic genes. The genetic makeup for a particular inherited characteristic is called a genotype. The expressed inherited characteristic is termed phenotype. There are three allele-morphic genes listed below:

1. Gene A
2. Gene B
3. Gene O

The child may be homozygous or heterozygous. If similar genes are inherited from mother and father, the child is said to be homozygous. On the other hand, the child is said to be heterozygous if inherited genes are different. This is exemplified as under:

1. *Homozygous*

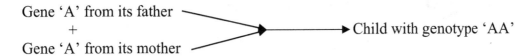

Gene 'A' from its father
        +
Gene 'A' from its mother → Child with genotype 'AA'

2. *Heterozygous*

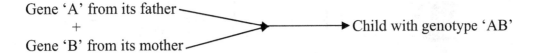

Gene 'A' from its father
        +
Gene 'B' from its mother → Child with genotype 'AB'

Also, a gene may be dominant or recessive. The dominant gene is expressed if there is a pair of dominant and recessive genes. A recessive gene is expressed only when a pair of recessive genes exist (i.e., the absence of a dominant gene). In the case of the ABO blood group system, *A* and *B* genes are dominant over the *O* gene. Also, both *A* and *B* genes are codominant, enabling them for simultaneous expression (i.e., AB blood group). According to this rule, if an offspring receives *A* and *O* genes from parents, it will belong to group A. But, the blood group of an offspring is O if it receives *O* genes from parents as mentioned in Table 46.1.

Table 46.1: Relationship between ABO genotypes and phenotypes

Genotype	Phenotype
AA *AO*	A
BB *BO*	B
AB	AB
OO	O

ABO antigens and secretory substances

Chemically, **H**, **A**, and **B** red cell antigens (agglutinogens) are glycolipids. The enzymatic synthesis of these red cell antigens has been precisely known as illustrated in Fig. 46.1.

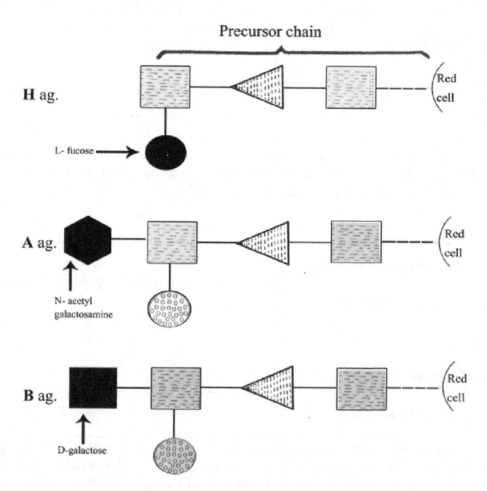

Fig. 46.1: Schematic illustration of the oligosaccharide structures of the H, A, and B antigens.
(Courtesy of Ortho Diagnostic Systems Inc.; Raritan, N. J.)

1. **H** *antigen:* The formation of **H** antigen occurs by adding an immunodominant sugar named L-fucose, primarily to type 2 (β-1,4 linkage) precursor chains. The addition of L-fucose is catalyzed by the *H* gene specified L-fucosyl transferase:

Oligosaccharide + L-fucose $\xrightarrow{\text{L-fucosyltransferase}}$ Oligosaccharide-L-fucose
(red cell membrane)   (**H** antigen)

2. **A** *antigen:* The formation of **A** red cell antigen takes place by incorporating N-acetyl-D-galactosamine (GalNAc) to **H** antigen (precursor) through a catalytic effect of N-acetylgalactosaminyltransferase (*A* gene specified) as under:

$$\text{H antigen} + \text{N-acetyl-D-galactosamine} \xrightarrow{\text{N-acetyl-D-galactosyltransferase}} \text{H antigen-N-acetyl-D-galactosamine}$$

(precursor)   (**A** antigen)

3. **B** *antigen:* The biosynthesis of **B** antigen results following the attachment of D-galactose moiety to **H** antigen, serving as a precursor. This reaction is catalyzed by D-galactosyl transferase ((*B* gene specified) as shown below:

$$\text{H antigen} + \text{D-galactose} \xrightarrow{\text{D-galactosyl transferase}} \text{H antigen-D-galactose}$$

(precursor)   (**B** antigen)

Unlike the **H, A,** and **B** red cell antigens, blood group substances are glycoproteins and secreted in body fluids, e.g., saliva. Moreover, these blood group substances are predominantly synthesized on type 1 (β-1,3 linkage) precursor chains. To secrete **H, A,** and **B** substances, the inheritance of at least one *Se* gene is essential as a regulator gene. Studies indicate that genes located at the ABO and secretory loci are inherited independently. Approximately 80% of Caucasians are "secretors". In other words, these persons do possess either *Se/Se* or *Se/se* genotype as opposed to "non-secretors" who possess *se/se* (homozygous) genotype. Since the *se* gene is an amorph, it remains unexpressed (i.e., no gene product).

The ABH substances found in the saliva of "secretors" are listed in Table 46.2.

Table 46.2: The ABH substances present in the saliva of "secretors"

Blood group	Substances in saliva		
	A	B	H
A	++	-	+
B	-	++	+
A,B	++	++	+
O	-	-	++

Key: - = absent, + and ++ denote the concentration

Saliva tests are valuable in cases of irregularities encountered during ABO testing, e.g., resolution of the genetic makeup of a person having an unusual blood type and determination of a subgroup.

ABO antibodies

a. Naturally occurring: These alloantibodies (isoagglutinins) of the ABO system predominantly belong to the IgM class of immunoglobulins that react best at room temperature or lower. Other immunoglobulins, namely IgG and IgA may be found in negligible amounts if present.

It is believed that naturally occurring antibodies develop from the widespread distribution of antigens in the environment (e.g., plants, animals, and microbes) because they are closely related to the blood group antigens. The levels of ABO isoagglutinins are too low to detect until a newborn infant turns about four months of age. There occurs a gradual rise in titers, peaking at 5-10 years of age. Also, the titers of antibodies decline gradually in the elderly population (> 65 years). This explains why the results of reverse grouping fail to agree with the results of forward grouping in some individuals. Besides, decreased levels of ABO antibodies may be attributed to diseases (e.g., leukemia) and immunosuppressive drugs.

Unlike IgG, IgM is the largest pentameric molecule that cannot cross the placenta. Importantly, IgM is a potent activator of the classical pathway of complement, causing intravascular hemolysis.

b. Immune: These antibodies predominantly belong to the IgG class of immunoglobulins. IgG molecules are monomers that can cross the placenta. Unlike naturally occurring antibodies, immune antibodies are formed following exposure to foreign red cell antigens through blood transfusion or pregnancy. For example, O group individuals produce anti-A, anti-B, and anti-A,B. Most cases of ABO incompatibility lead to HDFN with mild symptoms. Indirectly, this indicates the presence of IgG fraction in anti-A,B, anti-A, and anti-B produced.

Hemagglutination

Hemagglutination is a clumping reaction, involving erythrocytes. The reader is requested to refer to chapter 33 for a better understanding of hemagglutination. It is necessary to understand the blood group antigens and antibodies. Important variables affecting hemagglutination are listed below:

1. Ionic strength
2. pH
3. Temperature
4. Incubation time
5. Antigen-antibody ratio
6. Centrifugation
7. Potentiator, e.g., Low ionic-strength saline (LISS), polyethylene glycol (PeG), and albumin

Direct antihuman globulin test (Coombs)

Procedure
1. Take 1 volume of 2-5% suspension of the red cells in a tube.
2. Wash the cells carefully three times in clean saline to remove all the surrounding globulin from the cells.
3. Add 1 volume of a fresh and broad-spectrum antihuman globulin reagent to 1 volume of the 2-5% cell suspension deposit immediately.

4. Mix the contents of the tube and centrifuge at 1,000 rpm for one minute.
5. Shake the tube gently to dislodge the cell button and examine the red cells under the low power of the microscope for agglutination.

Results
Agglutination of the red cells suggests a positive direct antiglobulin (Coombs) test.

Applications
   a. Diagnosis of hemolytic disease of the fetus and newborn (HDFN)
   b. Diagnosis of autoimmune hemolytic anemias
   c. Investigation of drug-induced red cell sensitization
   d. Investigation of hemolytic transfusion reactions (HTRs)

Indirect antihuman globulin test (Coombs)

Procedure
   1. Take 2 drops of the patient's fresh plasma in a tube.
   2. Add 1 drop of 4-5% suspension of washed red cells (usually O-positive cells).
   3. Mix and incubate at 37°C for 30-60 minutes.
   4. Centrifuge at 1,000 rpm for one minute.
   5. Examine for hemolysis and/or agglutination under the microscope. Agglutination at this stage indicates the presence of saline reacting (complete) antibodies.

If agglutination is not seen, proceed as under:
   6. Wash the red cells three times in clean saline, and decant supernatant completely.
   7. Add 1-2 drops of antihuman globulin (Coombs) reagent.
   8. Mix and centrifuge at 1,000 rpm for one minute.
   9. Shake the tube gently to dislodge the button, and examine for agglutination under the low-power of the microscope.

Results
   • Agglutination indicates a positive test
   • No agglutination at either stage suggests a negative test

Applications
   a. Detection of incomplete antibodies and complement-fixing antibodies
   b. Screening and detection of unexpected antibodies in the plasma
   c. Detection of red cell antigens (e.g., Fy^a, Fy^b, Le^a, etc.) by other techniques
   d. Compatibility testing

False-positive Coombs test may be due to over centrifugation, Wharton's jelly, and Aldomet. False-negative Coombs test may be due to inadequate washing procedure, cell suspensions, inactive antiglobulin serum, and under centrifugation.

Determination of ABO blood group (Tube method)

The ABO blood group system was discovered by Karl Landsteiner (1900). It is the most significant of all blood group systems in transfusion medicine. This is to say that transfusion of ABO-incompatible blood could be fatal.

Landsteiner was the first person to perform both forward and reverse groupings. This pioneering work led him to describe blood groups, namely A, B, and O. Later, Sturle and Von Descatello described the AB blood group. Landsteiner generalized that a specific blood group antigen and its corresponding antibody cannot coexist in one person as depicted in Table 46.3.

Table 46.3: The ABO blood group antigens and antibodies present in humans

Blood group	Red cell antigen(s)	Plasma antibody(ies)
A	A	Anti-B
B	B	Anti-A
AB	A and B	No Anti-A and Anti-B
O	Neither A nor B antigen	Anti-A and Anti-B

Routinely, forward grouping (patient's red cells) and reverse grouping (patient's plasma/serum) are performed by using diagnostic antisera and reagent red cells, respectively.

a. Forward (cell) grouping
b. Reverse (plasma) grouping

a. Forward (cell) grouping
Red cells are tested to know whether A, B, or AB antigens present. For this purpose, ready-made known anti-A serum (blue) and anti-B serum (yellow) are used from a standard manufacturer.

Tube method

1. Prepare a 2-5 percent suspension of red cells in normal saline
2. Label two clean and dry glass tubes (10x75mm) as anti-A and anti-B. It is advisable to include anti-A,B in the procedure to confirm group O blood specimens
3. After arranging tubes in a test-tube rack, add one drop of anti-A in a tube labeled as anti-A and one drop of anti-B in another tube marked as anti-B
4. Add one drop of the red cell suspension to each tube
5. Mix the contents of both tubes by tapping them gently with the finger and allow them to stand for five minutes at room temperature
6. Centrifuge both tubes at a speed of 1000 rpm for one minute
7. Take the tubes out from the centrifuge machine and read the results after tapping each tube gently
8. Examine the contents of tubes microscopically on a glass slide under low power, if no agglutinate is seen with the naked eye
9. Record the results in the laboratory information system (LIS)/designated register immediately

The expected test results of forward grouping are shown in Table 46.4.

Table 46.4: Expected test results of forward grouping

Red cells of unknown blood	Reaction with anti-A serum	Reaction with anti-B serum	Interpretation (blood group)
X.........	-	-	O
X.........	+	-	A
X.........	-	+	B
X.........	+	+	AB

Key: + = agglutination; - = no agglutination

The ABO blood group (phenotype) frequencies vary from race to race as shown in Table 46.5.

Table 46.5: Frequencies of ABO blood group in the United States

Blood group	Whites, %	Blacks, %	Mexicans, %	Asians, %
O	45	49	56	43
A_1	33	19	22	27
A_2	8	8	6	Rare
B	10	19	13	25
A_1B	3	3	4	5
A_2B	1	1	Rare	Rare

Except for rare Bombay (Oh) blood group red cells, all remaining blood groups demonstrate decreasing reactivity to anti-H in the order shown below:

$$O > A_2 > B > A_2B > A_1 > A_1B$$

Thus, red cells of O blood group contain the most H substance as opposed to A_1B cells with the least amount of H substance.

b. Reverse (plasma) grouping
Reverse grouping is an inevitable test in routine blood banking because:

1. It confirms the blood group accurately
2. Individuals having blood group A2 or A2B are not erroneously included as blood group O or B, respectively
3. It detects anti-A1 in persons having either blood group A2 or A2B
4. It avoids any errors developing from patients with an abnormal protein profile

Reverse grouping can be carried out by the 'tube method'. It differs from forward grouping only like reactants used in the test. In other words, reverse grouping makes use of unknown plasma of a patient and known A1 and B reagent red cells. The expected test results of reverse grouping are shown in Table 46.6.

Table 46.6: Expected test results of reverse grouping

Patient's unknown plasma	Reaction with reagent A₁ red cells	Reaction with reagent B red cells	Antibody detected	Interpretation (blood group)
x......	-	+	Anti-B	A
x......	+	-	Anti-A	B
x......	+	+	Anti-A and Anti-B	O
x......	-	-	No Anti-A and Anti-B	AB

Key: + = agglutination; - = no agglutination

ABO discrepancies

There are instances in which forward grouping and reverse grouping do not correlate. These problems must be identified and resolved. The cause of discrepant results may be:

   a. Technical
   b. Red cells
   c. Plasma/serum

a. Technical
The ABO discrepancies are primarily caused by technical errors listed below:

1. Failure to use correct and active reagent antisera (forward grouping) and reagent red cells (reverse grouping)
2. Failure to follow the directions of the manufacturer of reagents
3. Failure to use clean and dry glasswares
4. Improper labeling of a patient's blood specimen (misidentification of a patient)
5. Improper labeling of ABO grouping-related test tubes
6. Failure to add reagent antisera and/or reagent red cells incorrectly labeled test tubes
7. Use of patient's red cell suspension either too heavy or too light
8. Bacterial contamination
9. Conducting the ABO grouping test at temperatures above 22°C
10. Carelessness in reading the test results
11. Mistakes made in recording the test results in the laboratory information system (LIS)/designated register

Technical errors can be resolved by repeating the test as per SOP in place.

b. Red cells
Rare blood types can cause ABO discrepancies:

1. Subgroups of A: These are usually associated with ABO grouping discrepancies. There are several subgroups of A, namely A_1, A_2, A_3, Ax, and Am. A_1 and A_2 are significant since they comprise about 99% of all A group individuals. Approximately 80% of A group individuals belong to A_1 alone. The remaining 20% A individuals can have largely A_2 or weaker phenotypes, e.g., Ax and Am. Subgroups of A weaker than A_2 are rare (about 1%) and therefore are of academic interest only. Anti-A_1 lectin (*Dolichos biflorus*) is used to differentiate A_1 from A_2. A_1 red cells react readily with anti-A_1 lectin whereas A_2 red cells do not. Also, naturally occurring anti-A_1 is found in the plasma of A_2 (1-8%) and A_2B (22-35%) individuals.

Red cells of A_3 individuals exhibit a classical mixed-field agglutination with anti-A and anti-A,B reagent sera. Anti-A_1 can be detected in the serum of A_3 persons.

2. Subgroups of B: These are very rare compared to subgroups of A. They include B, B_3, Bx, Bm, and Bel. Anti-B and anti-A,B reagent sera can be used in the detection of weak subgroups of B. Red cells of B_3 individuals show a mixed-field agglutination with anti-B and anti-A,B reagent sera.

3. Bombay (Oh) group: is the rarest blood group. It is called the Bombay blood group because it was discovered in a Bombay-based patient by Bhende and his associates in 1952. The Bombay group individuals lack all three antigens, namely A, B, and H on their red cells. Therefore, the Bombay group individuals can produce all three corresponding alloantibodies, namely anti-A, anti-B, and anti-H. Fortunately, these persons do not suffer any deleterious effects.

Strongly reacting anti-H is produced in the serum of the Bombay group individuals. The Bombay group individuals must receive blood only from the Bombay blood group donor. Interestingly, there are four hundred registered donors of the Bombay blood group in India to date. Red cells of the Bombay group persons do not react with anti-H lectin (*Ulex europaeus*).

4. Acquired B *antigen*: Occasionally, a weak reaction of reagent anti-B with patient's red cells (forward grouping) is encountered in some group A persons. However, test results on reverse grouping are as per expectation for group A individuals (i.e., only reagent B cells react but not reagent A_1 cells). The weak reaction between the reagent anti-B and the patient's red cells is due to a B-like antigen called acquired B antigen (not a true B antigen). This acquired B antigen is linked to some disorders (e.g., carcinoma of the colon or rectum and infection by Gram-negative bacteria) in group A persons. Acquired B antigen-associated discrepancy can be resolved by the use of a monoclonal anti-B reagent or acidified serum.

5. Polyagglutination: means red cells (forward grouping) demonstrate agglutination by almost all human sera from adults but not by sera from newborns and autologous serum. It may be transient or persistent. Exposure of cryptantigens (hidden antigens) on red cells is caused by an infection or mutation, e.g., T and Tk. Such exposed antigens can then react with their corresponding antibodies (i.e., anti-T and anti-Tk) because these antibodies are normally present in anti-A and anti-B grouping sera.

Lectins can be used in resolving the suspected cases of polyagglutination. Some classic reaction patterns with some lectins are shown in Table 46.7.

Table 46.7: Some polyagglutinable cells and their reactions with lectins

Lectin	T	Th	Tn	HEMPAS*	Cad
Arachis hypogea	+	+	0	0	0
Glycine max (soja)	+	0	+	0	0
Salvia sclarea	0	0	+	0	0
Salvia horminum	0	0	+	0	+
Dolichos biflorus	0	0	+	0	+

*Hereditary erythroblastic multinuclearity with positive acidified serum.

6. Chimerism: means the presence of two cell populations in a person, showing a mixed-field reaction. Chimeras may occur in circumstances, namely blood transfusions (e.g., O red cells received by A or B person), exchange transfusions, fetal-maternal bleeding, and transplanted bone marrow. True chimerism is rarely encountered in twins.

c. Plasma/serum

1. Rouleaux formation: also called pseudoagglutination, may cause red cells to appear agglutinated in the absence of true agglutination. It occurs when levels of globulin are elevated (e.g., multiple myeloma, Waldenstrom's macroglobulinemia). Other causes include increased levels of fibrinogen, plasma expanders (e.g., dextran), and Wharton's jelly. It can also be observed if whole blood is used instead of saline washed cells in the test.

Rouleaux described as a stacked coin-like appearance (see Fig. 46.2), can easily be differentiated from true clumping by microscopic examination. It disappears in 1-2 minutes following the addition of saline to the cells. In contrast, red cells remain clumped in the presence of saline if it is a true agglutination.

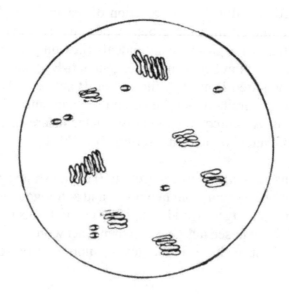

Fig. 46.2: Rouleaux formation.

2. ABO alloantibodies: are predominantly IgM. Weak and negative reactions of reverse grouping are due to decreased levels and absence of ABO isoagglutinins, respectively. This is frequently encountered while testing newborns and elderly persons. Also, some disorders cause hypogammaglobulinemia or agammaglobulinemia. They include leukemias (e.g., CLL), lymphomas (e.g., malignant lymphomas), immunosuppressive drugs-related hypogammaglobulinemia, and congenital agammaglobulinemia. Weakly reacting serum-cell mixtures may be incubated at room temperature or 4°C for about 20 minutes to enhance the antigen-antibody reaction.

3. Cold antibodies: There are two types of cold antibodies, namely allo- and auto-antibodies. If cold autoantibodies (e.g., anti-I) are suspected, the reagent red cells and plasma can be prewarmed at 37°C before performing reverse grouping. Sometimes, autoadsorption is performed to remove the interfering cold autoantibody from the plasma sample followed by reverse grouping on auto adsorbed plasma. For forward grouping, the patient's cells can be washed using prewarmed saline before typing.

4. Warm autoantibodies: If warm autoantibodies are involved, a heat elution (45°C) can be performed on the patient's cells to remove the bound immunoglobulins. Then, the patient's cells can successfully be retyped.

5. Unexpected alloantibodies: There are instances where discrepancies in ABO grouping occur due to the presence of some unexpected alloantibodies present in a patient's plasma, e.g., anti-M, anti-P_1, anti-A_1, and anti-Lewis. This can easily be convinced from the reactivity pattern of screening cells and by performing some additional tests, e.g., use of anti-A_1 lectin in case of group A/AB person to determine a subgroup, if any.

Some examples of ABO discrepancies are shown in Table 46.8.

Table 46.8: Some examples of ABO discrepancies

Forward grouping (red cell grouping)		Reverse grouping (plasma grouping)		Additional tests needed	Possible interpretation
Reagent antisera		*Reagent red cells*			
Anti-A	Anti-B	A_1	B		
3+	0	1+	4+	Anti-A_1 lectin; reagent A_2 cells	A_2 with Anti-A_1
0	0	4+	4+	Anti-H lectin; reagent O cells	Bombay (*Oh*) group with Anti-H
4+	1+	0	4+	Anti-A_1 lectin; reagent A_2 cells	A_1 with acquired B antigen
0	4+	4+	3+	Antibody identification	B with unexpected alloantibody

Rhesus Blood Group System

It is next in importance to the ABO system in the priority list in transfusion practice. The existence of this system was indicated by Prof. Philip Levine (1900-1987) and Stetson in 1939. They published their results on the serum of a female patient with O blood group. She suffered a transfusion reaction after receiving the blood of her husband having the same blood group.

In 1940, Landsteiner and Wiener produced antibodies by introducing red blood cells from *Macacus rhesus* monkeys into rabbits and guinea-pigs. This antibody reacted with the red cells of about 85 percent of the white population (called Rh-positive individuals). In contrast, red cells of about 15 percent of the white population did not react with the antibody so produced (called Rh-negative individuals). The determinant was called the Rh factor because it was present on red blood cells of all rhesus monkeys. This Rh factor (D antigen) is present in about 95% of Indians (i.e., Rh-positive).

Nomenclature

Fisher named six genes, namely *C*, *c*, *D*, *d*, *E*, and *e*. They occur in pairs as alleles. They occupy three loci on a chromosome. Thus, each locus is occupied by a specific gene or its allele. For example, one locus is occupied by either gene *C* or its allele *c*. Except for the amorph *d*, all remaining genes produce the respective antigens on the red cells.

If a child inherits one chromosome from each parent, e.g., *CDe* and *cDE*, the most probable genotype could be *CDe/cDE*. The most common gene complex found in blacks is *Dce*.

Wiener, on the other hand, described that the Rh system has only one gene with many alleles occupying only one locus. Wiener called these alleles as Rh^0, Rh^1, Rh^2, Rh^z, *rh*, *rh'*, *rh"*, and rh^y. He assigned different names to antigens produced by corresponding alleles. For example, Rh_0 antigen is produced by Rh^0 allele.

Wiener also added in his description that all those antigens are made up of antigen factors. For example, Rh_0 antigen is composed of Rh_0, hr', and hr" factors.

Different notations were used by different biologists while postulating their theories for the inheritance of the Rh system. Notations used by Fisher-Race and Wiener are compared as shown in Table 46.9.

Table 46.9: Comparison of the Fisher-Race and Wiener notations

Fisher-Race		Wiener	
Gene complex	Antigens	Gene	Antigen
Dce	D, c, e	Rh^0	Rh_0
DCe	D, C, e	Rh^1	Rh_1
DcE	D, c, E	Rh^2	Rh_2
DCE	D, C, E	Rh^Z	Rh_z
dce	c, e	*rh*	rh
dCe	C, e	*rh'*	rh'
dcE	c, E	*rh''*	rh''
dCE	C, E	rh^y	rh_y

Rh antigens

The Rh system consists of several antigens. However, antigen D (Fisher) or antigen Rh_0 (Wiener) is the most important one. Therefore, it is routinely tested in individuals. Antisera to test the remaining antigens are available. Characteristics of antigen D (Rh_0) are:

1. present on the red blood cell: The number of D antigen sites on the red cell is about a hundred times less than the number of ABO antigen sites.
2. proteinic
3. a strong immunogen (i.e., D > c > E > C > e)
4. readily inactivated by phospholipase A2 and C
5. molecular weight of 170,000 to 300,000 daltons
6. not found in body fluids or natural substances

In some individuals, antigen D is weaker than normal antigen D. Such D antigen is called D^u. This antigen has been found in about 10% of Africans. The donor type D^u must donate blood as an Rh-positive donor but receive blood as an Rh-negative individual.

Determination of Rh type

Rh factor can be detected by a modified tube method:
1. Add one volume of anti-D (anti-Rho) serum in a clean and dry tube (8 x 50 mm)
2. Add one volume of an approximately 5% suspension of the patient's red cells in normal saline
3. Mix the contents of the tube and centrifuge at 1,000 rpm for one minute
4. Remove the tube and shake it gently to disturb the button formed of the red cells at the bottom
5. Observe the results microscopically in case of negative macroscopic results

Note
1. The user of anti-D (anti-Rho) serum should follow the manufacturer's directions supplied with each reagent. (Please note that manufacturers change directions from time to time)
2. One should include a negative control (patient's cells + saline)

Results
1. If agglutination occurs: Rh-positive person
2. If no agglutination (smooth suspension): Rh-negative person

D" (weak D) phenotype

If the test result is Rh-negative, red cells are re-tested by indirect antihuman globulin (Coombs) test to rule out the possibility of the presence of D^u.

Procedure
1. Prepare an approximately 5% suspension of red blood cells under test in normal saline
2. Place one drop of 5% suspension of red blood cells in a tube (8 x 50 mm)
3. Add one drop of anti-D (anti-Rho) serum
4. Mix the contents of the tube and incubate at 37°C for 15 minutes (for the sensitization of the red cells by anti-D)
5. Centrifuge the tubes at 1,000 rpm for 1 minute
6. Discard the supernatant and wash the cells 4 times with normal saline
7. Add one drop of Coombs serum to the cells
8. Centrifuge at 1,000 rpm for 1 minute immediately after the addition of Coombs serum
9. Observe the results of the tubes macroscopically and microscopically for evidence of agglutination

Note

It is necessary to setup a negative control (patient's cells + saline) along with the test.

Results
1. Agglutination indicates the presence of D^u antigen (Rh-positive)
2. The absence of agglutination suggests the absence of D^u antigen (Rh-negative)

Partial D: is different from D^u (weak D) because the partial D phenotype is due to an alteration in D epitopes. In other words, the partial D phenotype is qualitatively different from normal D antigen-positive individuals. In the case of D^u, there is a reduced number of D antigens compared to that of the normal D antigen-positive individuals (quantitative difference). Because individuals with partial D phenotype may produce an anti-D if alloimmunized, they should be labeled as D positive (while donating) and should be labeled as D negative (while receiving). Earlier, partial D was called the 'D mosaic' or 'D variant'.

Rh_null phenotype: means red blood cells without Rh antigens. Rh_null red cells not only lack antigens (e.g., LW and Fy5) but also show weak expression of antigens, namely S, s, and U. Only 44 individuals have been reported globally to have Rh_null phenotype. Such red cells are structurally abnormal (e.g., stomatocytosis) and defective in their cell membrane.

Rh-antibodies

These antibodies are also called 'incomplete' or 'coating' antibodies since they require a protein medium (albumin or serum) for the agglutination to occur. Most Rh antibodies are IgG immunoglobulins. These IgG immunoglobulins are reactive in albumin, with enzymes, and by antihuman globulin tests. They do not bind complement but cause extravascular hemolysis. Sometimes IgM immunoglobulins are detected. IgM immunoglobulins are saline-reactive antibodies. Anti-D (anti-Rho) reacts best at 37°C.

Clinical significance

As discussed above, only Rh antigen present on red cells can stimulate the formation of anti-Rh in Rh-negative persons. There are two possible ways of exposing Rh-negative persons against Rh antigen:

a. Transfusion of Rh-positive blood to Rh-negative recipients. Usually, this occurs due to clerical or technical errors. About 50-70 percent of Rh-negative persons develop anti-D if transfused with Rh-positive blood.

b. In the case of an Rh-negative mother, Rh-positive red cells may pass from fetal circulation to maternal circulation through the placenta during her pregnancy, resulting in the formation of anti-D. The anti-D so formed enters into the fetal circulation, causing *erythroblastosis fetalis*. This almost always occurs, to some extent, at delivery and occasionally in the advanced stage of pregnancy. Only 20 percent of Rh-negative mothers develop anti-D after harboring an Rh-positive fetus. Immunosuppressive therapy (e.g., RhoGAM) is used in such circumstances.

Titration of Rh-antibody

Assay of anti-D (anti-Rho) is a valuable test for Rh-negative mothers during pregnancy. It is very simple to carry out by two-fold (doubling) dilutions (e.g. 1:2, 1:4, 1:8, 1:16, 1:32, etc.) of the patient's serum using normal saline as a diluent.

Other antigens and their corresponding antibodies of the Rh system are discussed in chapter 47.

Chapter 47

Blood Group Systems other than ABO

Introduction

In addition to the ABO blood group system, there are more major blood group systems, namely Rh, Lewis, Kidd, MNSs, P, Kell, Duffy, Lutheran, Colton, Xgᵃ, Diego, Ii, Dombrock, and Cartwright. These are sometimes important in cross-matching of blood. Most of them have been summarized in this chapter.

Key characteristics of the Rhesus (Rh-hr) system are outlined in Table 47.1.

Table 47.1: The Rhesus (Rh-hr) system

Blood group system	Antibodies produced	Characteristics of antibodies	Clinical significance	Geographical distribution
Rhesus (Rh-hr)	Anti-D	-Immune -Usually IgG class -Often occurs with anti-C	-May cause HTR -May cause severe HDFN	*D antigen-positive:* -85% of whites -92% of blacks
	Anti-C	-Immune -Usually IgG class -Often occurs with anti-D, anti-e, or anti-Cʷ	-May cause HTR -May cause HDFN	*C antigen-positive:* -70% of whites -33% of blacks
	Anti-E	-Usually immune, occasionally naturally occurring -Usually IgG class, occasionally IgM class -Often occurs with anti-c	-May cause HTR -May cause HDFN	*E antigen-positive:* -30% of whites -21% of blacks
	Anti-c	-Immune -Usually IgG class -Often occurs with anti-E	-May cause HTR -May cause HDFN	*c antigen-positive:* -80% of whites -97% of blacks
	Anti-e	-Immune -IgG class -Often occurs with anti-C	-May cause HTR -May cause HDFN	*e antigen-positive:* -98% of whites -99% of blacks

Table 47.1 (cont.)**:** The Rhesus (Rh-hr) system

Blood group system	Antibodies produced	Characteristics of antibodies	Clinical significance	Geographical distribution
Rhesus (Rh-hr)	Anti-C^w	-Usually immune, occasionally naturally occurring -Usually IgG class, occasionally IgM class -Low frequency -Often occurs with anti-C	-May cause HTR -May cause HDFN	*C^w antigen-positive:* - 1% of whites - <1% of blacks

Note:
1. Rh genes are located on chromosome number 1. The Rh-hr system comprises 50 antigens.
2. Immunogenicity: D > c > E > C > e.
3. All antigens of the Rh-hr system are expressed strongly at birth.
4. All antibodies of the Rh-hr system react best at 37°C and the AHG phase.
5. Except for anti-D, the rest of the antibodies of the Rh-hr system demonstrate dosage.
6. All antibodies of the Rh-hr system exhibit enhanced reactivity with enzyme-treated red blood cells.
7. All antibodies of the Rh-hr system do not bind complement and cause extravascular hemolysis.
8. Patients with anti-C^w should receive red cell units that are cross-matched compatible at the AHG phase. Additionally, patients with sickle cell disease who developed anti-C^w should receive C^w-negative red cell units.

Abbreviations:
IgG = immunoglobulin G; IgM = immunoglobulin M; AHG = anti-human globulin;
HTR = hemolytic transfusion reaction; HDFN = hemolytic disease of the fetus and newborn

Key characteristics of the Lewis system are outlined in Table 47.2.

Table 47.2: The Lewis system

Blood group system	Antibodies produced	Characteristics of antibodies	Clinical significance	Geographical distribution
Lewis	Anti-Le^a	-Naturally occurring, occasionally immune -IgM class, rarely IgG class	-Rarely causes HTR	*Le^a antigen-positive:* -22% of whites -23% of blacks
	Anti-Le^b	-Naturally occurring -IgM class	-Clinically insignificant	*Le^b antigen-positive:* -72% of whites -55% of blacks

Note:
1. Frequently detected in prenatal sera and often found together in individuals with Le(a- b-) phenotype.
2. Anti-Le^a and anti-Le^b react best at RT.
3. The reactivity of both anti-Le^a and anti-Le^b is enhanced by enzyme-treated red cells.
4. Anti-Le^a and anti-Le^b demonstrate **no** dosage.
5. Anti-Le^a and anti-Le^b can be neutralized by a Lewis substance.

Abbreviations:
IgG = immunoglobulin G; IgM = immunoglobulin M; RT = room temperature
HTR = hemolytic transfusion reaction; HDFN = hemolytic disease of the fetus and newborn

Key characteristics of the Kidd system are outlined in Table 47.3.

Table 47.3: The Kidd system

Blood group system	Antibodies produced	Characteristics of antibodies	Clinical significance	Geographical distribution
Kidd	Anti-Jk^a	-Immune -IgG class -Deteriorates rapidly in vivo and in vitro	-May cause delayed HTR -May cause mild HDFN	*Jk^a antigen-positive:* -77% of whites -91% of blacks
	Anti-Jk^b	-Immune -IgG class	-May cause delayed HTR -May cause mild HDFN	*Jk^b antigen-positive:* -73% of whites -43% of blacks

Note:
1. Both anti-Jk^a and anti-Jk^b react best at the AHG phase
2. Antibodies of the Kidd system may bind complement and some antibodies may exhibit dosage.
3. The reactivity of the antibodies of the Kidd system is enhanced with enzyme-treated red blood cells.
4. Both anti-Jk^a and anti-Jk^b are "tricky" as well as inconsistent in their reactivity.
5. Usually, they occur with other antibodies. Anti-Jk^a is more common than anti-Jk^b.
6. Advisable to collect a patient's antibody history on his/her from previously admitted hospital(s).

Abbreviations:
IgG = immunoglobulin G; IgM = immunoglobulin M; AHG = anti-human globulin;
HTR = hemolytic transfusion reaction; HDFN = hemolytic disease of the fetus and newborn

Key characteristics of the MNSs system are outlined in Table 47.4.

Table 47.4: The MNSs system

Blood group system	Antibodies produced	Characteristics of antibodies	Clinical significance	Geographical Distribution
MNSs	Anti-M	-Naturally occurring, occasionally immune -Usually IgM class, occasionally IgG class -Reacts best at RT and acidic pH	-Rarely causes HTR -Rarely causes HDFN	*M antigen-positive:* -78% of whites -70% of blacks
	Anti-N	-Naturally occurring -Usually IgM class -Reacts best at RT -Induced by formaldehyde e.g., dialysis patients	-Clinically insignificant	*N antigen-positive:* -72% of whites -74% of blacks
	Anti-S	-Immune, occasionally naturally occurring -IgG class, occasionally IgM class -Reacts best at AHG phase	-May cause HTR -May cause HDFN	*S antigen-positive:* -55% of whites -31% of blacks
	Anti-s	-Immune -IgG class, occasionally IgM class -Reacts best at AHG phase	-May cause HTR -May cause HDFN	*s antigen-positive:* -89% of whites -93% of blacks
	Anti-U	-Immune -IgG class -Reacts best at AHG phase	-May cause HTR -May cause HDFN	*U antigen-positive:* -100% of whites -99% of blacks

Note:
1. Except for anti-U, the rest of the antibodies of the MNSs system demonstrate dosage and diminished reactivity with enzyme-treated red cells.
2. Lectins for anti-M and anti-N are *Iberis amara* and *Vicia graminea*, respectively.
3. Most U- red cells are S- s-.

Abbreviations:
IgG = immunoglobulin G; IgM = immunoglobulin M; RT = room temperature ; AHG = anti-human globulin; HTR = hemolytic transfusion reaction; HDFN = hemolytic disease of the fetus and newborn

Key characteristics of the P system are outlined in Table 47.5.

Table 47.5: The P system

Blood group system	Antibodies produced	Characteristics of antibodies	Clinical significance	Geographical distribution
P	Anti-P$_1$	-Naturally occurring -Predominantly IgM class -Reacts best at RT -Neutralized by hydatid cyst fluid -Increased reactivity with enzyme-treated cells	-Clinically insignificant	*P$_1$ antigen-positive:* -79% of whites -94% of blacks *P$_2$ antigen-positive:* -20% of whites -5% of blacks
	Anti-P	-Naturally occurring -Usually IgM class, rarely IgG class -Found in P^k individuals -Usually IgM class	-May cause HTR	*P antigen-positive:* -100% of whites -100% of blacks
	Anti-PP$_1$P^k	-Naturally occurring -IgM class -Composed of anti-P, anti-P$_1$, and anti-P^k -Complete hemolysis in serum	-May cause delayed HTR -May cause HDFN -Associated with early spontaneous abortions	*PP$_1$P^k antigen-positive:* -100% of whites -100% of blacks
	Auto anti-P (Donath-Landsteiner)	-IgG class -A biphasic hemolysin	-Associated with paroxysmal cold hemoglobinuria (PCH)	

Note:
1. Very strong anti-PP$_1$P^k is produced in individuals with rare P phenotype (i.e., absence of P antigens).
2. Auto anti-P antibodies escape detection during routine testing. The Donath-Landsteiner test (incubation at 4°C and 37°C) can be performed.
3. Because P$_1$ antigen expression is variable and fades during storage, it causes inconsistent reactivity patterns in the panel.

Abbreviations:
IgG = immunoglobulin G; IgM = immunoglobulin M; RT = room temperature; AHG = anti-human globulin; HTR = hemolytic transfusion reaction; HDFN = hemolytic disease of the fetus and newborn

Key characteristics of the Kell system are outlined in Table 47.6.

Table 47.6: The Kell system

Blood group system	Antibodies produced	Characteristics of antibodies	Clinical significance	Geographical distribution
Kell	Anti-K	-Immune -IgG class -Reacts optimally at AHG phase -Most common (next to anti-D)	-May cause severe HTR -May cause HDFN	*K(1) antigen-positive:* -9% of whites -2% of blacks
	Anti-k	-Immune -IgG class -Reacts optimally at AHG phase -Very rare	-May cause severe HTR -May cause HDFN	*k(K2) antigen-positive:* -99.8% of whites - >99.9% of blacks

Note:
1. Other antigens of the Kell system include Js^a, Js^b, Kp^a, and Kp^b.
2. Antigens of the Kell system remain unaffected by proteolytic enzymes. However, most antigens are denatured by dithiothreitol (DTT).
3. Kell null (K_0) phenotype lacks Kell antigens with increased Kx.
4. McLeod phenotype lacks Kx with decreased Kell antigens. This phenotype is associated with X-linked chronic granulomatous disease (CGD) and acanthocytic hemolytic anemia.

Abbreviations:
IgG = immunoglobulin G; IgM = immunoglobulin M; AHG = anti-human globulin;
HTR = hemolytic transfusion reaction; HDFN = hemolytic disease of the fetus and newborn

Key characteristics of the Duffy system are outlined in Table 47.7.

Table 47.7: The Duffy system

Blood group system	Antibodies produced	Characteristics of antibodies	Clinical significance	Geographical distribution
Duffy	Anti-Fy^a	-Immune -IgG class - Reacts best at AHG phase	-Causes HTR -Causes HDFN	*Fy^a antigen-positive:* -65% of whites -10% of blacks
	Anti-Fy^b	-Immune -IgG class -Reacts optimally at AHG phase	-Causes HTR -May cause HDFN	*Fy^b antigen-positive:* -80% of whites -23% of blacks

Note:

1. Though the antigens of the Duffy blood group system are well-developed at birth, they are weakly immunogenic (Fy^a > Fy^b).
2. The antigens of the Duffy blood group system tend to get eluted off the red cells in an acidic medium.
3. The Fy (a- b-) phenotype (68% blacks) is linked to resistance by malarial parasites, namely *Plasmodium vivax* and *P. knowlesi.*
4. Both anti-Fy^a and anti-Fy^b demonstrate diminished reactivity with enzyme-treated cells.
5. Both anti-Fy^a and anti-Fy^b may show dosage. Anti-Fy^b, a very rare antibody, is often accompanied by other more common antibodies, e.g., anti-K in patients with a sickle cell disease.

Abbreviations:
IgG = immunoglobulin G; IgM = immunoglobulin M; AHG = anti-human globulin;
HTR = hemolytic transfusion reaction; HDFN = hemolytic disease of the fetus and newborn

Key characteristics of the Lutheran system are outlined in Table 47.8.

Table 47.8: The Lutheran system

Blood group system	Antibodies produced	Characteristics of antibodies	Clinical significance	Geographical distribution
Lutheran	Anti-Lu^a	-Naturally occurring or immune - Most often IgM class - Occasionally IgG class - Reacts best at RT	- Clinically insignificant	*Lu^a antigen-positive:* -7.6% of whites -5.3% of blacks
	Anti-Lu^b	-Immune -Mainly IgG class -Reacts best at AHG phase	-May cause HTR -May cause mild HDFN	*Lu^b antigen-positive:* -99.8% of whites -99.9% of blacks

Note:
1. Lu(a- b-) phenotype is very rare.
2. Both antigens (Lu^a and Lu^b) are weakly expressed at birth. Also, they are expressed by allelic codominant genes.
3. Lu^a antigen can be destroyed by trypsin and chymotrypsin.
4. Both anti-Lu^a and anti-Lu^b demonstrate dosage and a classical loose mixed-field agglutination.

Abbreviations:
IgG = immunoglobulin G; IgM = immunoglobulin M; RT = room temperature; AHG = anti-human globulin; HTR = hemolytic transfusion reaction; HDFN = hemolytic disease of the fetus and newborn

Key characteristics of the Colton system are outlined in Table 47.9.

Table 47.9: The Colton system

Blood group system	Antibodies produced	Characteristics of antibodies	Clinical significance	Geographical distribution
Colton	Anti-Co^a	-Immune -IgG class, occasionally IgM class	-May cause HTR -May cause HDFN	*Co^a antigen-positive:* -99.7% of whites
	Anti-Co^b	-Immune -IgG class	-May cause HTR -May cause mild HDFN	*Co^b antigen-positive:* -10% of whites
Note: 1. Both anti-Co^a and anti-Co^b react at the AHG phase. 2. Reactivity of both anti-Co^a and anti-Co^b is enhanced with enzyme-treated red cells.				

Abbreviations:
IgG = immunoglobulin G; IgM = immunoglobulin M; RT = room temperature; AHG = anti-human globulin; HTR = hemolytic transfusion reaction; HDFN = hemolytic disease of the fetus and newborn

Key characteristics of the Xg system are outlined in Table 47.10.

Table 47.10: The Xg system

Blood group system	Antibodies produced	Characteristics of antibodies	Clinical significance	Geographical distribution
Xg	Anti-Xg^a	-Immune -IgG class	-Clinically insignificant	*Xg^a antigen-positive:* -88.7% of white females -65.6% of white males
Note: 1. Inherited by an X-linked gene. 2. Reacts best at the AHG phase. 3. Reactivity of anti-Xg^a is diminished with enzyme-treated red cells. 4. Binds complement.				

Abbreviations:
IgG = immunoglobulin G; IgM = immunoglobulin M; RT = room temperature; AHG = anti-human globulin; HTR = hemolytic transfusion reaction; HDFN = hemolytic disease of the fetus and newborn

Low-incidence antigens

Low-incidence antigens occur in less than 1% of the population. Therefore, they are usually absent on screening and antibody panel red cells. This explains why antibodies directed against low-frequency antigens go undetected while performing antibody workup. Also, they cause incompatible cross-match, especially at the AHG phase. It is very easy to find antigen-negative donor red cell units for cross-matching purposes. Examples of low-incidence antigens include C^w, V, Js^a, and kp^a.

High-incidence antigens

High-incidence antigens occur in greater than 99% of the population. Therefore, antibodies directed against high-frequency antigens display uniform positive reactivity (i.e., same strength and at the same phase) with all screening and antibody panel cells. However, auto control turns out negative. Also, it is difficult to find antigen-negative donor red cell units to cross-match. Examples of high-frequency antigens are k, Js^b, kp^b, and Lu^b.

According to the International Society of Blood Transfusion (ISBT), there are 33 blood group systems recognized to date. A total of about 300 blood group antigens have been discovered so far and more are being added to the list over time.

High titer low avidity (HTLA) antibodies

High titer low avidity antibodies occur in high titer with poor reactivity (e.g., 1+) with their corresponding antigens, e.g., anti-Ch^a and anti-Rg^a.

All HTLA antibodies are produced due to exposure to antigens (i.e., immune). In addition, the HTLA antibodies react optimally at the antihuman globulin (AHG) phase because they belong to the IgG class. Fortunately, most HTLA antibodies are clinically insignificant.

Miscellaneous blood group systems

Also, antigens possessed by red blood cells, leukocytes, platelets, and tissue cells also harbor some antigens. Dr. Dausset discovered the HLA (human leukocyte antigen) system in 1958 and was awarded the Nobel Prize in 1980. The nucleated cells of the HLA system possess the strongest antigens. These HLA antigens are valuable in organ transplant survival. So, organ transplantation will require compatibility testing of HLA antigen between the donor and the recipient.

The author of this manual prefers to exclude the discussion on characteristics of antibodies that still require exhaustive research.

Chapter 48

Detection and Identification of Plasma Antibodies, and Cross-matching

Introduction

Detection and identification of clinically significant plasma antibodies from a prospective recipient is most crucial in transfusion medicine. Sometimes, it takes longer than expected time, causing a delay in blood transfusion or cancellation of elective surgeries. In rare cases, specimens are sent out to a reference laboratory for the follow-up test.

Antibody Screening (gel technique)

This is a key test in immunohematology. It involves 2 or 3 screening cells for the test. The screening cells licensed by the food and drug administration (FDA) are O group with specific profiles for the antigens which are listed below:

D, C, E, c, e, K, k, Fy^a, Fy^b, Jk^a, Jk^b, M, N, S, s, P_1, Le^a, Le^b, Lu^a, and Lu^b

If one or more of these screening cells show agglutination (positive) as shown in Fig.48.1 (a), (b), it may suggest the presence of an antibody or multiple antibodies in the plasma. The "Coombs control" cells are added to all those negative screening cells to ensure the inclusion of an active antihuman globulin (AHG) reagent in the test (tube method only). Then, it is required to identify antibodies from the plasma, if any. It is very important to collect information about the patients, namely age, clinical diagnosis, history of a recent blood transfusion, and pregnancy.

The lot numbers on the printed antigram and vials of screening cells must be the same because antigen profiles of screening cells vary with each lot number. The frequency of the positive antibody screen is 0.3-2% of the general population. This can be understood from the following two case studies given in Fig. 48.1 (a), (b).

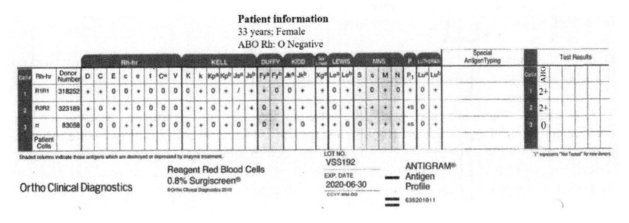

(a) Case study #1

Fig. 48.1: Antibody screening results (gel technique).
(Reproduced ANTIGRAM® with permission from Ortho Clinical Diagnostics, Raritan, N.J.)

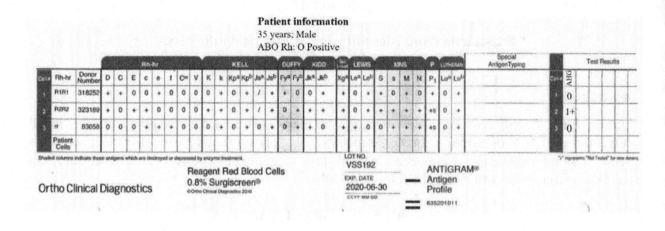

Patient information
35 years; Male
ABO Rh: O Positive

Cell	Rh-hr	Donor Number	Rh-hr									KELL					DUFFY		KIDD			LEWIS		MNS				P	LUTHERAN		Special Antigen Typing	Cell	AHG	Test Results
			D	C	E	c	e	f	Cʷ	V	K	k	Kpª	Kpᵇ	Jsª	Jsᵇ	Fyª	Fyᵇ	Jkª	Jkᵇ	Xgª	Leª	Leᵇ	S	s	M	N	P₁	Luª	Luᵇ				
1	R1R1	318252	+	+	0	0	+	0	0	0	0	+	0	+	/	+	+	0	0	+	+	0	+	+	0	+	0	+	0	+		1	0	
2	R2R2	323189	+	0	+	+	0	0	0	0	+	+	0	+	/	+	0	+	+	+	+	0	+	+	+	+	+	+s	0	+		2	1+	
3	rr	83058	0	0	0	+	+	+	0	0	0	+	0	+	0	+	0	+	0	+	+	0	0	+	+	+	+s	0	+		3	0	
	Patient Cells																																		

Shaded columns indicate those antigens which are destroyed or depressed by enzyme treatment.   "/" represents "Not Tested" for new donors.

Ortho Clinical Diagnostics

Reagent Red Blood Cells
0.8% Surgiscreen®
©Ortho Clinical Diagnostics 2010

LOT NO.
VSS192
EXP. DATE
2020-06-30
CCYY-MM-DD

ANTIGRAM®
Antigen
Profile
635201011

(b) Case study #2

Fig. 48.1: Antibody screening results (gel technique).
(Reproduced ANTIGRAM® with permission from Ortho Clinical Diagnostics, Raritan, N.J.)

Antibody Identification (gel technique)

Usually, it is an easy task to do antibody identification from plasma specimens containing one kind of antibody and negative auto control. This test involves a panel of 8 or more cells and one additional tube for auto control (patient's cells + patient's plasma) as shown in Fig. 48.1 (a), (b). Reactions are read and recorded at the antihuman globulin (AHG)[34] phase. Finally, it needs to rule out the possible antigens using homozygous cells in the panel showing only negative reactions at the antihuman globulin (AHG) phase. Some key points need to be addressed before undertaking the identification of an antibody(ies). They are:

a. Quantity of acceptable patient's specimen
b. Allowable time, e.g., emergency
c. Availability of reagents, e.g., rare antisera
d. Expertise

Once all the above-listed needs are fulfilled, one may proceed step-by-step for antibody workup to gather the facts to justify the identity of an antibody(ies):

1. Auto control: There are cases where the patient's red cells are agglutinated as evidenced by positive auto control and direct antiglobulin test results. Besides, all cells of the panel are reactive, thereby making the problem more complex in determining the specificity of underlying alloantibody(ies), if any. For example, the following alloantibodies in their descending order can be detected in approximately 15-40% of patients with autoimmune hemolytic anemia (AIHA):

anti-E, anti-K, anti-C, anti-Fyª, anti-Jkª, and anti-c

---

[34] Different phases, namely immediate spin, 37°C, and antihuman globulin are included in traditional tube testing.

The warm-reactive autoantibody is a frequent cause of the problem. Therefore, warm auto-adsorption is performed to prepare autoantibody-free plasma before repeating the panel. This is how a better pattern of reactivity of an underlying alloantibody develops. However, the warm autoadsorption procedure is not useful in patients who have been transfused within the past 30 days. This may be overcome by adapting allogeneic adsorption.

2. Ruling out (exclusion): This is an important step of a careful exclusion of antibody(ies) based on a negative reaction of the panel red cells which are positive for corresponding antigens. Some blood group antibodies demonstrate a stronger agglutination of red cells with a homozygous expression of an antigen (double dose) as opposed to the red cells having a heterozygous expression (single dose) of the same antigen. This characteristic of the antibody is called a dosage effect. Therefore, poorly-reacting heterozygous red cells may not be agglutinated in the presence of weak antibodies. This is how antibodies may go undetected. Therefore, it may be wise to rule out with panel red cells that display only a homozygous expression of an antigen. Antibodies directed against antigens of the following blood group systems demonstrate dosage:

- Rhesus (except D)
- Kidd
- Duffy
- MNSs

3. Absolute exclusion: It is necessary to perfectly exclude all clinically significant antibodies. There are instances where primary panel cells lack certain phenotypes needed for this purpose. So, it is necessary to include selected cells from other panels. The following antibodies are usually recognized as clinically significant antibodies:

ABO, Rh, Kell, Kidd, Duffy, S, s, U, and Vel

Antibodies that are usually encountered in the patient's plasma include:

- anti-A, -B
- anti-D, -E, -c
- anti-K
- anti-Jk^a, -Jk^b
- anti-Fy^a, -Fy^b
- anti-M
- anti-P_1
- anti-Le^a, -Le^b
- autoanti-I

Usually, anti-I is benign. However, a high titer (1000 >) can be detected in cold agglutinin syndrome (CAS). It has a high thermal amplitude that favors the hemolytic anemia. Therefore, a blood warmer is recommended during transfusion. Fortunately, it is not associated with HDFN as well as HTR.

A few antibodies, namely anti-Jk^a, anti-Jk^b, anti-c, and anti-C are notorious for causing severe immediate transfusion reactions with intravenous hemolysis and should be treated with the same caution as an ABO incompatibility.

4. Rule of 3: Honoring a rule of 3 means a given antibody shows positive reactions and negative reactions with three antigen-positive and three antigen-negative red cells, respectively. This gives a probability (P) value of 0.05. In other words, the findings are correct 95 percent of the time.

5. Phenotyping: Once the antibody(ies) is identified, the last step is to do antigen typing of the patient's red cells. The antigen(s) corresponding to the identified antibody(ies) must be absent from the patient's red cells. It is a very useful datum to reason the true identity of an alloantibody. Since phenotyping of a patient's cells provides a significant clue to support the claimed antibody, it is prudent that antigen typing is performed accurately. This explains why extended phenotyping is usually performed in patients who undergo frequent red cell transfusions, e.g., sickle cell disease (SCD) and thalassemia to avoid false-positives. Also, sickle cell disease patients are prone to alloimmunization, thus complicating transfusion therapy.

Case studies

Routinely, health care providers request a test "type and screen" for those patients who require blood transfusion and pregnant women. Pre-transfusion testing of a patient requires the processing of the patient's blood to determine ABO and Rh types along with an antibody screen. The antibody screen helps detect antibody(ies) from the patient's plasma/serum if present. In most cases, antibody screen results turn out negative. If the antibody screen result turns out positive, it is indicative of the possibility of an antibody(ies) in a patient's plasma/serum. One or more of the screening cells showing a positive reaction, irrespective of the strength of a reaction and/or phase of a reaction, constitutes a positive antibody screen as shown in two case studies {Fig. 48.1 (a), (b)}. A positive antibody screen warrants a follow-up test called "antibody identification". Identifying an antibody or multiple antibodies in a patient's plasma/serum is sometimes challenging. This is why it necessitates the involvement of a well-experienced blood bank professional to resolve such issues accurately on time.

The following two case studies depicted in Fig. 48.2 and Fig 48.3 will be helpful to understand the antibody identification.

Case study #1 (see Fig. 48.2)

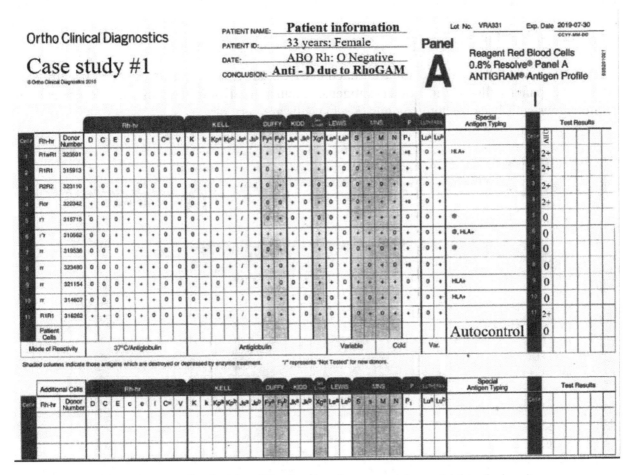

Fig. 48.2: Antibody identification in plasma specimen (gel technique).
(Reproduced ANTIGRAM® with permission from Ortho Clinical Diagnostics, Raritan, N.J.)

1. Ruling out: An accurate ruling is required to watch out for "dosage effect". This means a homozygous, e.g., Jk (a+ b-) cell shows a stronger reaction than a heterozygous Jk(a+ b+) cell. Thus, the patient's plasma/serum reacts with reagent red cells of a panel Nos. 1, 2, 3, 4, and 11 at the antihuman globulin (AHG) phase. On the other hand, the patient's plasma/serum fails to react with reagent cells of a panel Nos. 5, 6, 7, 8, 9, and 10. Upon completion of ruling out, the resulting pattern of reactions is matched against the pattern of antigen profile displayed on the antigram. Auto control (patient's cells + patient's serum) is negative, thus eliminating the probability of a positive direct antiglobulin test (DAT) and/or free autoantibody in the patient's plasma/serum. It reveals the presence of anti-D. To ensure that no antibody other than the anti-D present, crossing out of the antigens present on panel cells is necessary. For example, cell No. 5 is non-reactive with the patient's plasma/serum and available antigens are C, c, e, k, Fy^b, Jk^b, Le^b, S, s, M, N, and Lu^b. However, C, c, S, s, M, and N cannot be crossed out because they are not homozygous. Furthermore, cells Nos. 6, 7, 8, 9, and 10 are used in crossing out more antigens.

2. Phenotyping: Once the preliminary identification of an antibody is completed, the patient's cells are phenotyped to confirm the identity of a corresponding antibody, i.e., anti-D. Because the

patient's cells are negative for D antigen, the phenotyping result is supportive to the identity of anti-D in the patient's plasma/serum.

Case study #2 (see Fig. 48.3)

The reader should follow all directions outlined in case study #1 while crossing out of the antigens present on panel cells. Unlike other antigens, exclusion of anti-K is usually dependent on heterozygous cells because homozygous (K+ k-) cells are very rare.

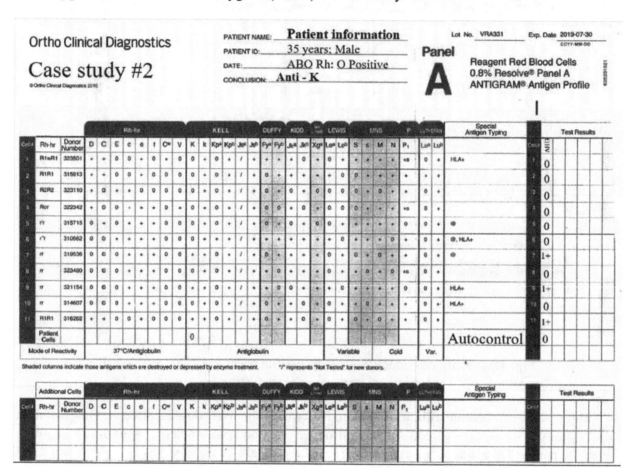

Fig. 48.3: Antibody identification in plasma specimen (gel technique).
(Reproduced ANTIGRAM® with permission from Ortho Clinical Diagnostics, Rariten, N.J.)

In this scenario, anti-K is present in the patient's plasma/serum because:

(i) Having ruled out all clinically significant antibodies, it creates a perfectly fitting reactivity pattern of anti-K

(ii) Patient's cells are Kell negative

Therefore, there is no likelihood of the presence of the antibody(ies) other than anti-K in the patient's plasma/serum.

In most cases, the identification of a single antibody is straightforward. In some complicated cases (e.g., multiple antibodies, false-positive results, cold reactive autoantibodies, and warm autoantibodies), specimens are sent out to a reference laboratory (operates 24/7) for further workup identification. This is quite understandable because small-scale laboratories lack resources and expertise.

Special techniques

Sometimes, it is a very difficult and time-consuming process to resolve the antibody identification problem. Knowledge about the nature of various clinically significant antibodies is very helpful in the case of multiple antibodies e.g., presence of anti-C and anti-D and the occurrence of anti-E and anti-c together. To resolve these problems, one has to perform additional tests.

A blood bank technologist must be well-versed with the basic principles of techniques used in the detection and identification of an antibody, particularly complex problems (e.g., multiple antibodies). Usually, the techniques discussed below help resolve the antibody-related problems:

1. Adsorption
2. Elution
3. Prewarming
4. Use of chemical agents
5. Titration

1. Adsorption
Adsorption is a surface-related phenomenon as opposed to a volume-related process called absorption. This is to say that adsorption is limited to the surface layer of an adsorbent, e.g., red cells and activated charcoal. The technique is used to remove the interfering antibody(ies) from a plasma specimen. The antibody can be auto- and/or alloantibody. The resulting plasma, "adsorbed plasma", is a better specimen to use in the determination of the specificity of an underlying antibody(ies).

In autoadsorption, the patient's plasma is incubated with the patient's red cells to remove the autoantibody (i.e., cold and warm). The incubation temperatures used for cold autoadsorption and warm autoadsorption are 4°C and 37°C, respectively. Alloadsorption requires incubation of the patient's plasma with red cells carrying antigen corresponding to the antibody of interest to eliminate. For example, the elimination of anti-S from plasma can be affected by using S+ red cells.

2. Elution
Elution is a process by which the adhering antibody from the surface of sensitized red cells (in vivo) is carefully recovered for further testing. Different methods, namely the cold, warm, or chemical method may be used to obtain an eluate. Out of these three methods, the chemical method (e.g., acid elution) is widely used to prepare an eluate. In a digitonin-based acid elution method, the sensitized red cells (i.e., positive DATs) are treated with an acidic reagent to lower the pH (about 3), dissociating the antibody from the surface of red cells. So-called an acid eluate is then gradually mixed with a buffer to bring the pH near neutrality before testing. Like a plasma specimen, the eluate is tested to determine the identity of an antibody, if present.

Chloroquine diphosphate is used to perform an elution on sensitized red cells (positive DATs) because it does not damage the red cell membrane. Such intact red cells are suitable for phenotyping. ZZAP (a mixture of dithiothreitol and cysteine-activated papain) is another chemical agent to carry out an elution on sensitized red cells, although these red cells are suitable simply for autoadsorption use. The technique is tedious and time-consuming.

3. Prewarming

Prewarming is a technique to avoid interference by a cold-reactive antibody, e.g., anti-I. It is required to incubate the patient's plasma, reagent red cells, and saline separately before mixing and the subsequent incubation. However, there are some cold-reactive antibodies (e.g., anti-Vel) with a wide thermal range and may cause severe and acute hemolytic transfusion reactions. Therefore, cold-reactive antibodies with demonstrable reactivity at AHG (Coombs) phase must not be overlooked.

4. Use of chemical agents

Several biological or chemical agents may be used in antibody work-up:

(i) Proteolytic enzymes: The proteolytic enzymes, namely ficin, papain, and bromelin are successfully used to alter the antigenic expression on reagent red cells. In other words, some red cell antigens show the enhanced effect as opposed to the diminished effect on other red cell antigens as depicted in Table 48.1.

Table 48.1: Effect of proteolytic enzymes on several red cell antigens

Antigen	Ficin	Papain	Bromelin
H, A, B	+	+	+
D, C, E	+	+	+
Jk^a, Jk^b	+	+	+
Le^a, Le^b	+	+	+
Fy^a, Fy^b	-	-	-
M, N, S	-	-	-
K	0	0	0

Key: + = enhanced; - = destroyed; 0 = unaffected

Enzyme-treated red cells may be used either to confirm the presence of an antibody or to detect additional antibodies. Besides, reference laboratories use the other proteolytic enzymes, namely neuraminidase, trypsin, and chymotrypsin.

(ii) Neutralizing substances: A limited number of antibodies can be inhibited by the use of substances containing soluble antigens. For example, commercial preparations of Lewis and P_1 substances are available to neutralize anti-Lewis and anti-P_1, respectively. The patient's plasma suspected for a specific antibody and its corresponding neutralizing substance (i.e., antigen) are mixed and incubated at room temperature. The antigen from the substance brings about the neutralization of the antibody by occupying the antigen-binding sites. The resulting neutralized plasma fails to agglutinate the reagent red cells, a phenomenon called 'hemagglutination inhibition'. It is necessary to run a parallel control (plasma + saline), making sure that the antibody was not diluted out with accompanying loss of reactivity.

The technique is valuable either in the confirmation of the identity of an antibody or exclusion of an antibody in problems with multiple antibodies.

(iii) Hypotonic solution: Unfortunately, the microhematocrit cell separation method is not effective in a sickle cell patient with transfused red cells. Sickle cells (Hb SS or Hb SC) remain intact compared to transfused red cells (Hb AA) if suspended in 0.3% NaCl (hypotonic) solution. About six washes may be sufficient to selectively lyse the transfused red cells. Thus, autologous sickle cells are saved from hemolysis due to increased cell permeability. This means that autologous red cells of SCD patients are resistant to hemolysis. Finally, autologous sickle cells are washed twice with 0.9% NaCl to restore tonicity and suspended in 0.9% NaCl for additional testing, e.g., phenotyping, DAT studies, or autoadsorption procedures.

(iv) 2-Aminoethylisothiouronium bromide (AET): inactivates some red cell antigens, e.g., Lu^b and Kell blood group antigens except Kx. Such phenotypically altered K_0K_0 cells can be used in the determination of the identity of antibodies of the Kell system.

(v) Use of sulfhydryl compounds: Sulfhydryl compounds, namely dithiothreitol (DTT) and 2-mercaptoethanol (2-ME), selectively inactivate IgM through cleavage of disulfide bonds. There is no adverse effect of these reagents on IgG. For example, a plasma specimen containing both cold autoantibody (IgM) and alloantibody (IgG) can be treated with one of the sulfhydryl reagents to denature only IgM. Then, IgM-free plasma specimens can be tested for IgG alloantibody, if present.

Alternatively, IgM can be eliminated by ion-exchange chromatography.

(vi) Lectins: discussed in chapter 46

(vii) Drug-induced positive DATs: The most common cause of a positive DAT and the subsequent immune hemolytic anemia is the formation of red cell autoantibodies to drugs, e.g., penicillin. They can cause irregularities in both ABO and Rh types and antibody screens. There are different types of mechanisms, depending on the nature of the medication involved.

Daratumumab is an anti-cancer drug indicated for the treatment of adult patients with multiple myeloma. It binds to CD38, a transmembrane glycoprotein, on red cells. Such binding results in a positive indirect antiglobulin test (IAT) in both antibody screening and cross-matching procedures. However, it has no adverse effects on ABO and Rh grouping procedures. It is highly recommended that typing and screening are performed before starting daratumumab treatment, thus eliminating pan-reactive serologic reactions in all IAT tests.

5. Titration

It is necessary to monitor antibody titers in pregnant women because the rising titers of a maternal antibody indicate the presence of a corresponding antigen on fetal red cells. This means that the child is at a risk for HDFN. The method called "serial dilution" to measure the antibody titer from plasma is outlined in chapter 33 (Fig. 33.3).

Cross-matching

The single most important aspect of cross-matching or compatibility testing of blood is absolute patient identification. Also, it serves the following two purposes:

1. It detects some errors of ABO grouping.
2. It detects unusual antibodies in the patient's serum e.g., antibodies developed during multiple blood transfusions.

Therefore, there is no substitute for a cross-matching test. It is performed with knowledge, care, and accuracy. It is desirable to transfuse the blood of the patient's blood group. The selection of blood donors should be done as indicated in Table 48.2.

Table 48.2: Selection of blood donors

Patient's blood group	Priority of donor's blood
A	(i) A (ii) O
B	(i) B (ii) O
O	O
AB	(i) AB (ii) A (iii) B (iv) O

Thus, individuals belonging to group 'O' are 'universal donors' because their red blood cells do not possess antigens A or B. On the other hand, individuals belonging to group 'AB' are 'universal recipients' since recipients' plasma does not contain anti-A as well as anti-B.

Cross-matching tests (tube method)

Cross-matching of blood requires testing the patient's plasma against donor's cells (major cross-match) and patient's red cells against donor's plasma (minor cross-match). However, only the major cross-match is routinely performed.

It is necessary to understand the following factors that affect the cross-matching of blood:

1. Concentrations of antigen and antibody

2. Surrounding medium as a potentiator
3. Temperature
4. Time of incubation
5. Centrifugation
6. Drugs (e.g., L-dopa, keflin, penicillin, and Lasix) causing incompatibilities in the major cross-match

The patient's plasma should be allowed to react with the donor's red cells in three different potentiating media for safe cross-matching:

1. Saline (detection of complete antibodies usually of IgM type)
2. Albumin (detection of incomplete antibodies usually of IgG type)
3. Antihuman globulin reagent also called Coombs serum (detection of immune antibodies, e.g., anti-Rho)

After exhaustive research and accumulation of a good amount of experience in areas, namely ABO blood group system, Rh system, and other clinically significant blood group systems, regulatory agencies have established guidelines for cross-matching of red blood cells by one of those four methods based on circumstances and patient's antibody screen result:

1. Immediate spin cross-match: involves the mixing of the patient's plasma (2 drops) and donor's red blood cells (1 drop of 3-5% suspension) followed by centrifugation and examination for agglutination and/or hemolysis. It may be performed if the patient's plasma has a negative antibody screen. It is also a preliminary test of an extended (full) cross-match procedure.

2. Extended cross-match: is performed in case of the presence of a clinically significant antibody. The first and the most important step is to find a donor unit of red cells negative for a corresponding antigen. For example, a given patient has anti-K in his/her plasma. Therefore, a blood bank professional needs to find a donor unit of red blood cells negative for K-antigen. The so-called an extended cross-match involves all phases, namely immediate spin, albumin, and AHG (IAT). In the end, reactions are read macroscopically and microscopically for agglutination and/or hemolysis. If there is an absence of agglutination, a donor unit is said to be cross-matched compatible. This type of cross-match is performed by a tube method. In a gel card test, reactants (i.e., patient's plasma + donor's red blood cells) are added into a microtube followed by incubation (15 minutes at 37°C) and centrifugation before reading the reaction.

For patients having a clinically significant antibody(ies), the red cell donor units need to be screened for corresponding antigen(s) before cross-matching. It requires the following information:

1. How many red cell donor units are required for transfusion?
2. What is the frequency (%) of antigen(s) in question in the general population?

In the case of compatibility frequency, it is required to find what percentage of the population lack the antigen

Then, values are plugged in the formula given below:

$$\text{Number of red cell units to be tested } (?) = \frac{\text{Number of red cell units required}}{\%\ \text{Compatibility in general population}}$$

Examples

Problem #1: Find 2 red cell donor units that are c negative:

Solution:
The frequency of c antigen is 80%. In other words, 20% of the population is c negative (% compatible).

Now, plugging these in the above formula:

$$\text{Number of red cell donor units to be tested } (?) = \frac{2}{0.2}$$

$$= 10$$

Answer: 10 units are to be tested.

Problem #2: Find 2 red cell donor units that are E negative and c negative:

Solution:
Frequency of E antigen = 30%;
Frequency of c antigen = 80%

Therefore, E negative (i.e., % compatible) and c negative donor units (i.e., % compatible) are 70% and 20%, respectively.

In order to calculate the percentage of red cell units compatible, compatibility frequencies of each antigen are multiplied:
$$= 70\% \times 20\%$$
$$= 0.70 \times 0.20$$
$$= 0.14$$

Now, plugging values in the above formula:
We get,

$$\text{Number of red cell units to be tested } (?) = \frac{2}{0.14}$$

$$= 14.28$$
$$= 14 \text{ (after rounding up)}$$

Answer: 14 units are to be tested.

3. Emergency cross-match: In the case of extreme emergencies, blood is to be issued in a short time. Such a short time does not allow the blood bank technologist to perform a standard cross-match. So, an emergency cross-matches (desperate cross-match) is carried out. But, it is necessary to run a standard cross-match while transfusing the issued blood. If any abnormalities are indicated, the doctor monitoring the patient should be informed.

Procedure
Follow all steps of a standard cross-match. But, read the results at the end of 10 minutes instead of 30 minutes. In case of dire emergency, the blood of an O-negative donor can be transfused. It is necessary to put a label - 'emergency cross-match'. Also, complete details of the cross-match must be recorded in the register or laboratory information system.

Alternatively, O-positive red blood cells for male patients and O-negative red blood cells for female patients may be released to save the limited stock of O-negative units in inventory. To expedite the process of transfusion, some institutions install mini-refrigerators both in ER and OR to store red blood cells (e.g., 8 units of O-positive + 2 units of O-negative). The blood bank keeps control over the quality control of refrigerators and the maintenance of red cells' inventory.

4. Electronic cross-match: it may be performed on a patient having a negative antibody screen result. Also, there have to be at least two valid specimens drawn for ABO grouping and Rh typing within 72- hour time frame. The database software allows blood bank professionals to release group-specific or compatible red blood cell units, thus excluding the actual test performance.

Chapter 49

Blood Donation and Preparation of Components

Introduction

There are patients with varied disorders, requiring blood transfusion. For example, a patient with thalassemia major needs blood every 20 days. Furthermore, a satisfactory substitute for blood has not been made available to date. Thus, blood transfusion is a must for some patients. In addition to whole blood, there are some special conditions where only 1 or 2 components of the whole blood are needed for transfusion. Nowadays, it has become possible to obtain a desired component from the whole blood through the application of sophisticated separation techniques. A list of blood-derived components is given in Table 49.1.

Table 49.1: Blood derived components with their respective shelf life and uses

Blood component	Shelf life	Uses
Packed cells/Sedimented cells	4 hours or 1 day (if open)	-Anemias, liver, kidney, and cardiovascular diseases
Fresh frozen plasma (FFP)	1 year	-Severe burn cases, dehydration, protein deficiency, maintenance of blood volume, and clotting factors deficiency
Cryoprecipitate	1 year	-Hemophilia A, afibrinogenemia, and von Willebrand's disease
Leukocytes	1 day	-Agranulocytosis and granulocytopenia in certain leukemias
Platelets	5 days	-Thrombocytopenia, leukemic conditions, and platelet disorders
Gamma globulin (Ig) anti-D (anti-Rho)	3 years	-Prophylactic use in Rh-negative mothers to prevent erythroblastosis fetalis

Blood donors

As concluded, a blood donor is the sole source of whole blood or its components. Blood donors can be grouped into the following three categories:

    A. Volunteer donors
    B. Professional (paid) donors
    C. Replacement donors

Selection of blood donors

It is necessary to consider the resulting ill-effects in either the donor or the recipient (patient) while selecting the prospective blood donors. In other words, the collection as well as transfusion of blood should be safe and harmless for donors and recipients, respectively.

The World Health Organization (WHO) makes recommendations for blood donation. However, some countries do not follow. The criteria for blood donation vary from country to country, depending on the laws of an individual country and the policies of a collecting organization. In the United States, the food and drug administration (FDA) requires prospective donors to meet the following criteria for eligibility:

1. Age: between 17-76 years (must be healthy and feeling well)
2. Bodyweight: > 110 lbs for donating 450 mL of blood
3. Oral temperature: between 96°-99°F
4. Pregnancy: Pregnant women cannot donate blood
5. The interval between blood donations: (i) whole blood donation: 56 days
   (ii) power red donation: 112 days (up to 3 times/year)
   (iii) platelet donation: 7 days (up to 24 times/year)
   (iv) plasma donation: 28 days (up to 13 times/year)
6. Pulse: 50-100 beats per minute (optimum 73/minute) and regular
7. Blood pressure: systolic - 90-180 mm Hg (optimum 125 mm Hg)
   diastolic 50-100 mm Hg (optimum 75 mm Hg)
8. Hemoglobin: 13-20 g%
9. Hematocrit: >38%
10. Time of collection: Should be at least 3 hours after the meals
10. Chronic diseases: Prospective donor must not be suffering from any chronic diseases, e.g., asthma
11. Vaccinations: A vaccinated person cannot donate blood up to 3 weeks
12. Transmissible diseases through blood transfusion:
    a. AIDS
    b. Viral hepatitis
    c. Cytomegalovirus (CMV)
    d. Malaria (cannot donate blood for 1 year if traveled to malaria-endemic countries, e.g., India)
    e. Filariasis
    f. American trypanosomiasis and African trypanosomiasis.
    g. Kala-azar
    h. Syphilis and yaws

Note:
1. Blood from donors with G6PD deficiency and sickle cell trait can be used for ordinary blood transfusions.
2. Persons with babesiosis are deferred for their whole life.
3. Persons who lived in Europe from 1980 onwards are deferred from blood donation in the USA. As of 2018, a total of 231 cases of variant Creutzfeldt-Jakob disease (mad cow disease) have been reported throughout the world.

4. Individuals who have ever had an HIV-positive, viral hepatitis (B or C), certain forms of cancer, or hemophilia are deferred permanently.

The following are common reasons for temporary deferrals:

   a. Illness, e.g., 3 days after the disappearance of flu symptoms
   b. Medications, e.g., 7 days and 2 days after taking Coumadin and aspirin, respectively
   c. Low iron
   d. Travel outside of the United States: It depends upon the country and the length of stay, e.g., one-year deferral if visited malaria-endemic countries such as India.

Collection (see Fig. 49.1)

The room used to collect blood should be well-ventilated with pleasant surroundings. Also, the blood bank technologist should behave friendly with the donor. If the donor appears afraid of donating blood, he/she should be reassured by explaining the need for blood donation. The receptionist will collect information, including the name and address of a selected donor (i.e., registration of donor). The donor must be attended to during the withdrawal of blood. The total amount of blood routinely taken from a blood donor is 450 mL plus pilot tubes. Moreover, the blood container should be sterile, pyrogen-free, and transparent.

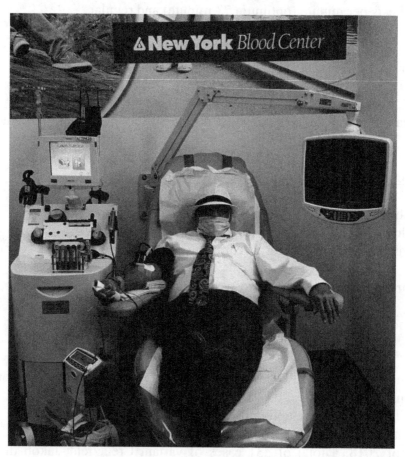

Fig. 49.1: Prof. Arvind H. Patel donates whole blood at New York Blood Center.
(Reproduced with permission from the New York Blood Center, New York, N.Y.)

The amount of blood allowed to donate can be calculated, using the following formula:

$$\frac{\text{Donor's weight}}{110} \times 450 = \text{Amount in mL allowed to donate}$$

Anticoagulants

The use of an anticoagulant is a must in blood collection procedures just to prevent the clotting of blood. They are summarized below:

a. AS-3 solution

Ingredient	Amount (g/100 mL)
Dextrose (anhydrous)	1.000
Sodium chloride	0.410
Adenine	0.030
Citric acid (monohydrate)	0.042
Sodium citrate (dihydrate)	0.588
Monobasic sodium phosphate (monohydrate)	0.276

AS-3 (Nutricel®) is an approved preservative solution for red cells in the United States. The shelf life of red cells is 42 days at 1-6°C. Other similar preservative solutions include AS-1(Adsol®) and AS-5(Optisol®) that contain mannitol as an additional ingredient.

The acid citrate prevents the caramelization of the dextrose while sterilizing the solution. Red blood cells are nourished by dextrose during blood storage.

The resulting solution is filtered and sterilized before its use.

b. CPD (Citrate Phosphate Dextrose) solution

Tri-sodium citrate	2.63 g
Citric acid	0.327 g
Dextrose	2.55 g
Monobasic sodium phosphate	0.222 g
Fresh distilled water	to 100 mL

The ratio of anticoagulant volume to 100 mL of whole blood   1:4

CPD anticoagulants have been shown to have a better post-transfusion survival of red blood cells.

c. CPD-1 (Citrate Phosphate Dextrose Adenine) solution
This preservative solution was developed in 1978. Adenine maintains the viability of red blood cells for 35 days through ATP regeneration.

d. Heparin solution

Heparin sodium	7,500 U
Fresh distilled water to	100 mL

Note: Blood collected in heparin solution must be used within 48 hours. EDTA is not used as an anticoagulant in the blood bank to collect blood because it is a strong chelating agent.

The proper amount of anticoagulant may be calculated by using the following formula:

$$\text{Adjusted anticoagulant volume} = \text{Normal anticoagulant volume} \times \frac{\text{Donated blood in mL}}{450}$$

Containers

Containers used for the collection of blood and blood components meant for blood transfusion therapy are disposable plastic bags.

They are light, unbreakable, disposable, and require less space. Furthermore, the chances of bacterial contamination are very rare. Therefore, they are ideal to prepare blood products.

The disposable plastic bags are used without any air-venting system during blood-taking or blood-giving because they inflate while collecting blood. In either case of containers, the user should follow the manufacturer's instructions.

Procedure
1. Apply a pressure cuff to the upper arm and inflate to between 80-100 mm Hg to make the veins more prominent. Select a large firmly attached vein for venipuncture.
2. Apply 70% methylated spirit to the intended site of venipuncture.
3. Do venipuncture immediately uncovering the sterile needle and tape the needle in place. Cover the venipuncture site with sterile gauze.
4. Decrease the pressure of the cuff between 40-60 mm Hg as soon as blood begins to flow. Ask the donor to squeeze a small object, e.g., a rubber ball to keep the donor's hand open and close.
5. When the level of blood has almost reached the desired mark, bring the pressure to zero and ask the patient to remove the object from the hand.
6. Seal the tubing 4-5 inches from the needle with the help of a metal clip.
7. Remove the pressure cuff.
8. Remove the needle from the vein, keeping cotton wool in place with pressure.
9. Ask the donor to bend the arm upwards, keeping cotton wool over the puncture site.

10. Collect pilot samples, including smears e.g., for malaria from the blood in the tubing.
11. Dispose of needle assembly into a special container.
12. Invert the plastic bag several times to mix the blood well with the anticoagulant. Do not shake it.
13. Put a label on the plastic bag, indicating the group, Rh factor, expiry date, and the anticoagulant used.
14. Check arm and apply bandages after bleeding stops.
15. Ask the donor to take a rest and provide a drink e.g., tea or orange juice to make up his fluid loss. Do not serve alcohol to the donor.
16. Thank the donor for blood donation and give him a certificate for the same.

It is necessary to take certain precautions to prevent slowing down of the flow of blood due to the following causes:

1. Blocking of the air outlet
2. A fall of the pressure in the cuff
3. A bend in the tubing of the donor set
4. Improper adjustment of the needle in the vein
5. Clotting of blood in one of the donor set needles

Moreover, if a donor feels unwell, (e.g., faint during or after blood collection) the donor is encouraged to remain to lie on the bed and a blood bank officer should be informed. It is also necessary to discontinue the blood collection.

Usually, blood donors remain anonymous. In other words, a blood component recipient is not aware of the identity of the donor whose blood component he/she is receiving. Occasionally, some recipients prefer to use blood component(s) from a known person as mentioned below:

(i) *Autologous donation:* is a kind of medical practice whereby a person donates blood, making its reservation for his/her use during a scheduled elective surgery to recover from a blood loss if needed.

(ii) *Directed (designated) donation:* is a kind of practice in medicine in which a given patient chooses a family member/friend to donate blood intended for that particular patient's use only, e.g., planned elective surgery with an anticipated blood transfusion.

Apheresis

Apheresis is a medical procedure whereby whole blood is withdrawn from the donor's or patient's arm and the desired component is separated for retention followed by subsequent reinfusion of the remaining blood components to the bloodstream of a patient or donor. One should be cautious not to mistakenly use a closely similar term "pheresis", the Greek origin, meaning "to take away". Apheresis, a widely practiced technique, uses the novel electronics-assisted apheresis system for different purposes. The whole blood passing through a sterile tubing is subjected to differential centrifugation, separating plasma (55%), platelets (1%), and red cells (44%).

1. Donor apheresis: Being a virtually risk-free technique, it is used for the collection of blood components for future use. The eligibility criteria for donor apheresis are almost the same as those for a whole blood donor. Depending on the desired component to be collected, the procedure is named as shown in Table 49.2.

Table 49.2: Different blood donation procedures

Apheresis	Component collected	Donation time (minutes)	Frequency of donation (days)
Erythrocytapheresis	double red cells	90	112
Plateletpheresis	platelets	90-120	7
Plasmapheresis	plasma	90	28

Rarely used apheresis donor techniques include leukapheresis and neo cytapheresis for granulocytes and neocytes, respectively.

2. Therapeutic apheresis: is a procedure in which a symptom-causing cellular or plasma component is removed using an automated centrifugation-equipped instrument. However, these procedures are very expensive and time-consuming. This can be exemplified as under:

(i) Platelet apheresis: is used in patients with an abnormally high platelet count, e.g., polycythemia vera. Using platelet apheresis, platelets are removed to bring the count to normal. It may require 3-5 procedures because one procedure decreases the count by approximately 1/2 of its initial count. It helps avoid platelet-related bleeding and thrombosis.

(ii) Plasmapheresis: helps eliminate some disease-provoking components present in the plasma e.g., antigen-antibody complexes in autoimmune diseases. It is a very effective therapy in hyperviscosity syndrome and many cancers as well.

(iii) Erythrocytapheresis: helps to get rid of sickle cells and replaces them with normal red cells, e.g., sickle cell disease with the crisis.

Generally, therapeutic apheresis is not performed on patients with certain conditions, e.g., unstable heart or lung conditions and bleeding tendency.

Storage

Blood is satisfactorily stored in an electric thermostatically controlled refrigerator at 4-6°C. It can be stored up to 21 days if collected in ACD or CPD solution. The storage period is 35 days when the CPD solution containing adenine is used. But, blood collected in heparin must be used within 48 hours.

The refrigerator should be equipped with the following accessories:

(i) a fan for circulation of air to maintain a uniform temperature throughout the refrigerator

(ii) the sensor for the temperature recording system

(iii) alarm system to indicate a change of temperature from 4°-6°C

The following precautions are to be taken for successful storage of blood:

1. The refrigerator should be used to store only blood and its components
2. The door of the refrigerator should not be opened too often
3. Blood should not be kept next to the freezing compartment to avoid hemolysis
4. Blood taken out of the refrigerator for more than 1 hour should not be restored for future use
5. Partly used blood is not to be restored and must be discarded. Changes occurring during the storage of blood are collectively called 'storage lesion'

Transportation

The temperature of blood to be controlled during the transportation is between 1°-10°C. For this purpose, the containers should be sturdy, well-insulated, and made up of cardboard or plastic.

Wet ice in waterproof containers is used as a refrigerant while transporting blood from one facility to another. It is necessary to avoid direct contact of blood with the ice. Both supercooled canned ice and dry ice cannot be used in transporting whole blood or red blood cells. If transportation of blood is to be made for long-distances or at high environmental temperatures, the ice should be at least twice the volume of blood.

It is necessary to control the temperature of blood in case of local transportation from the blood bank to other parts of the hospital. Blood should be used or returned within 30 minutes because blood stored at 1°-6°C exceeds 10°C at room temperature in approximately 30 minutes. An insulated paper bag precooled to 1°-6°C is used when transportation needs a slightly longer time.

Transportation of fresh frozen plasma requires the addition of enough dry ice to keep the temperature of plasma below minus 20°C.

Storage lesion

Storage lesion refers to the changes in blood components during storage. For example, it begins after about 2 weeks post hypothermic storage of red cells. Once the whole blood leaves the donor's body, both the survival and the function of blood components are adversely affected. Some biochemical changes play a major role in a deleterious effect on blood components. More research work is still to be undertaken in understanding storage lesions.

a. Red cell storage lesion

1. Depletion of ATP due to a decreased rate of glycolysis, leading to the formation of irreversible spheroechinocytes
2. Decrease in 2,3-diphosphoglycerate (2,3-DPG) levels, causing an increased affinity of hemoglobin to oxygen and a subsequent decline in the efficiency of red cells to release oxygen into tissues
3. Lysis of red blood cells

4. Elevated levels of potassium
5. A reduction in antioxidant defense system, protein oxidation, and lipid peroxidation altogether cause membrane vesiculation and loss of red cell deformability
6. Reduced tissue perfusion due to decreased bioavailability of nitric oxide (NO)

b. Platelet storage lesion

1. Conformational changes of platelet glycoprotein complex GPIIb/IIIa
2. Elevated levels of phosphatidylserine cause lysis of the membrane
3. Release of lactate dehydrogenase (LDH) and metabolic failure lead to apoptosis

c. Plasma storage lesion

1. Damage to plasma proteins (e.g., cleavage of protein backbone) by proteases released by lysed neutrophils and mononuclear phagocytes
2. Plasma has an innate ability to counteract the proteases by under protease inhibitors, namely α-1-protease inhibitor, tissue inhibitor of metalloprotease, α-2-macroglobulin (α2M), and plasminogen activator inhibitor-1 (antioxidant defense system)
3. Both lipid peroxidation and advanced glycation occur during storage

Conclusion

The author, an experienced blood bank professional, strongly believes that there will be no replacement for blood and its components for transfusion therapy. So, donating blood or its components serves as a precious gift for needy patients. It should be remembered that red cells and/or blood components can save more lives if used wisely with an appropriate diagnostic strategy. To learn more about the eligibility criteria for blood donation, please visit the website www.NYBC.org. The phone number for donors to call is 1-800-933-BLOOD (2566).

Chapter 50

Blood Component Therapy

Introduction

In 1818, a British obstetrician named James Blundell successfully transfused human blood to a patient having a hemorrhage during the delivery. Coincidentally, World War II attracted researchers and medical professionals to develop techniques of blood preservation and blood transfusion. Thus, the value of blood transfusion was demonstrated as a life-saving procedure for wounded soldiers. The pioneering work of Dr. Charles Drew led to the establishment of blood banks globally.

Blood transfusion can be a life-saving therapy for patients with a variety of medical and surgical conditions. Advances in the use of blood components have made whole blood transfusions rarely necessary. However, whole blood is used for exchange transfusion and to replace the loss of both red cell mass and plasma volume. Blood component therapy provides better treatment for the patient by transfusing only the specific component needed. Such therapy helps to conserve blood resources because components from one unit of whole blood can be used to treat several patients.

A. Red blood cells (RBCs)

Red blood cell transfusions increase oxygen-carrying capacity in anemic patients. Transfusing one unit of RBCs will usually increase the hemoglobin (Hb) by 1g/dL and the hematocrit (Hct) by 3% in an average 70 kg adult. Also, hemoglobin present in red blood cells plays an important role in the removal of CO_2 from blood to the lungs. A red blood cell transfusion is a very common practice for treating patients in all hospital settings. There may be one of those two major reasons behind a red blood cell transfusion, namely loss of blood (e.g., trauma and surgery) or anemia (e.g., iron deficiency anemia and vitamin B_{12} deficiency anemia).

Adequate oxygen-carrying capacity can be met by a hemoglobin value of 7g/dL (a hematocrit value of approximately 21%) or even less when the intravascular volume is adequate for perfusion. In deciding whether to transfuse a specific patient, the physician should consider the person's age, etiology, degree of anemia, hemodynamic stability, and presence of coexisting cardiac, pulmonary, or vascular conditions. To meet oxygen needs, some patients may require RBC transfusions at higher hemoglobin levels.

Some patients (e.g., newborns and leukemic) undergoing blood transfusion have special requirements for blood products as mentioned below:

(i) CMV-negative: Patients such as neonates and transplant recipients are transfused with CMV-negative red blood cells because they are at high risk. Sometimes patients are transfused with leukocyte-depleted red blood cells and/ or "single donor" platelets as "CMV-reduced-risk" if CMV-negative products are in short supply. Leukocyte-reduced red blood cells and "single donor" platelets are prepared by the removal of leukocytes at a time of phlebotomy using high-grade filters or immediately before storage. More than 80% of packed red blood cells and almost all apheresis "single donor" platelets in the United States are leuko-depleted.

(ii) Irradiated: Irradiated red blood cells are transfused to patients at risk from transfusion-associated graft-versus-host disease (GVHD). The GVHD, a rare but deadly disease, is primarily caused by viable T lymphocytes. T lymphocytes trigger an immune response in patients by engrafting in the marrow, attacking the patient's tissues. Patients at risk from GVHD include selected immunocompromised or immunocompetent recipients, recipients undergoing marrow transplantation, recipients of platelets selected for HLA-matched platelets, fetuses undergoing intrauterine transfusion, etc. Irradiation of red blood cells helps stop the proliferation of T lymphocytes. However, the process of irradiation harms the survival of red blood cells, thus reducing the overall viability of red blood cells. This explains why the expiration of an irradiated blood unit is modified. Platelets are also irradiated for some patients.

(iii) Hemoglobin S negative: Sickle cell disease patients tend to develop antibodies against antigens from donor's red blood cells. Therefore, a sickle cell disease patient is phenotyped for antigens, namely Rh antigens (i.e., C, c, E, and e) and Kell antigen. This ensures that the patient receives a transfusion of red blood cells negative for those antigens displaying negative on the patient's phenotype. For example, if a sickle cell disease patient's cells are c negative, E negative, and K negative with a negative antibody screen, it is necessary to use donor red blood cells that are c negative, E negative, and K negative. Hemoglobin S negative blood is indicated for patients with sickle cell disease and infants less than four months old.

(iv) Washed red blood cells: (free from plasma and leukocytes) and frozen deglycerolized red blood cells (free from plasma, platelets, and leukocytes) are used interchangeably. The shelf life of frozen deglycerolized red blood cells is ten years or more. These products are helpful to prevent urticarial as well as febrile transfusion reactions. Also, they are used for IgA deficient patients (rare) with anti-IgA.

(v) Neocytes: are transfused in preference to red blood cells to patients undergoing frequent red blood cell transfusions, e.g., thalassemia major. This benefits the patient in decreasing the frequency of transfusions and reducing the problem of iron accumulation. However, the continuous flow hemapheresis technique for obtaining neocytes is time-consuming and very expensive to practice.

When a treatable cause of anemia can be identified, a specific replacement therapy (e.g., vitamin B_{12}, iron, and folate) should always be used before RBC transfusion is considered. If volume expanders are indicated, fluids such as crystalloid or non-blood colloid solutions should be administered. RBC transfusions are often used inappropriately as volume expanders.

Red blood cell transfusion is NOT used

1. for volume expansion
2. in place of a hematinic
3. to enhance wound healing
4. to improve general "well-being"

B. Platelet products

Platelet transfusions are administered to control or prevent bleeding associated with deficiencies in platelet number or function. Platelets from plateletpheresis are called "single donor" contain 3.0 x 10^{10} platelets per unit and have less hepatitis risk. One unit of platelet concentrate called "random donor" should increase the platelet count in an average 70 kg adult recipient by at least 5,000 platelets/μL. Both "single donor" as well as "random donor" units are stored at room temperature (RT) with continuous rotation with a shelf life of 5 days. There has to be a sufficient plasma volume to maintain a minimum pH of 6.0 to keep the platelets viable. Unlike the red blood cells, the transfusion of platelets does not need the ABO match.

Prophylactic platelet transfusion may be indicated to prevent bleeding in patients with severe thrombocytopenia. For the clinically stable patient with an intact vascular system and normal platelet function, prophylactic platelet transfusions may be indicated for platelet counts of <10,000-20,000/μL. A patient undergoing an operation or other invasive procedure is unlikely to benefit from prophylactic platelet transfusions if the platelet count is at least 50,000/μL and thrombocytopenia is the sole abnormality. Platelet transfusions at higher platelet counts may be required for patients with systemic bleeding and patients at a higher risk of bleeding because of additional coagulation defects, sepsis, or platelet dysfunction related to medication or disease.

There are instances where patients are transfused with human leukocyte antigen (HLA) matched platelets. These patients are either at risk of producing or have produced antibodies against HLA antigens. The HLA antibodies are produced in response to alloimmunization through transfusion, pregnancy, or transplantation. The presence of HLA antibodies may lead to failure in achieving satisfactory responses in patients receiving platelets from random donors called platelet refractoriness. Approximately 20% of platelet refractoriness occurs in patients with HLA antibodies. In preparation for HLA matched platelets, HLA Class I antigen typing and detection of HLA antibodies are performed. The detection of HLA antibodies can be performed by techniques such as ELISA or flow cytometry. Clinical indications for HLA matched platelets include:

(i) Patients with platelet refractoriness due to HLA antibodies
(ii) Patients with congenital disorders, e.g., Bernard-Soulier syndrome, Glanzmann's thrombasthenia
(iii) Patients undergoing stem cell transplantation using donor's stem cells without a full HLA compatibility

Platelets are NOT transfused

(i) to patients with immune thrombocytopenic purpura (unless there is life-threatening bleeding)
(ii) prophylactically with massive blood transfusion
(iii) prophylactically following a cardiopulmonary bypass

C. Plasma products

Fresh frozen plasma (FFP) transfusion should be considered only to increase the level of clotting factors in patients with a demonstrated deficiency. Laboratory tests should be used to monitor the patient with a suspected clotting disorder. If prothrombin time (PT) and partial thromboplastin time (PTT) are <1.5 times normal, FFP transfusion is rarely indicated. The fresh frozen plasma contains all coagulation factors, including labile V and VIII.

Patients who have been administered with anticoagulant warfarin sodium become deficient in vitamin k-dependent coagulation factors II, VII, IX, and X. If these patients bleed or require emergency surgery, they may be candidates for FFP transfusion to achieve immediate hemostasis when the time does not permit warfarin reversal by stopping the drug or administering vitamin K. Patients with rare conditions such as antithrombin III deficiency and thrombotic thrombocytopenic purpura may be benefited from FFP transfusion and often in conjunction with plasma exchange.

Other indications of FFP include replacement of labile plasma clotting factors during cardiac bypass surgery, liver disorders, massive loss of blood, or acute disseminated intravascular coagulation (DIC) with active bleeding in conjunction with abnormal coagulation test results.

The size of a given patient and the existing clinical situation are the major determining factors for the volume of FFP to be transfused. However, assays of coagulation function are considered as guidelines in determining the dosage. Generally, the patients are transfused with 10-15 mL/kg per dose.

Like cryoprecipitate, entry ports of the plasma unit are protected from water contamination while thawing in a water bath at 30°-37°C. Therefore, a frozen plasma unit is wrapped around a plastic bag that serves as a protective layer. Once the unit is thawed, the expiration date is changed on the unit, making it good for 24 hours at 1°-6°C.

Fresh frozen plasma is NOT transfused

  (i) for volume expansion
 (ii) as a nutritional supplement
(iii) prophylactically with massive blood transfusion
(iv) prophylactically following a cardiopulmonary bypass

D. Cryoprecipitate

Cryoprecipitate is a cold-precipitated concentration of Factor VIII. To make cryoprecipitate, Fresh Frozen Plasma (FFP) is allowed to thaw slowly at 4°C. This product contains fibrinogen, fibronectin, Factor VIII-C, Factor VIII-vWF, and Factor XIII. While making this product from FFP, conditions are strictly controlled so that a minimum of 80 IU of Factor VIII is present per bag in the final product. After completion of the separation step, cryoprecipitate is refrozen within one hour of its preparation and stored at -18°C or lower for up to one year from the date of phlebotomy.

Thawing of cryoprecipitate is carried out in a water bath maintained at temperatures between 30°-37°C. Like fresh frozen plasma (FFP), individual cryoprecipitate units are wrapped around fresh plastic bags to protect the openings during thawing. The thawed units can be stored at room temperature (20°-24°C) for up to six hours. Typically, clinicians request a "pooled" cryoprecipitate, meaning multiple individual units (usually 10) are combined in one bag under aseptic conditions. The unique number is assigned to a newly "pooled" product by the facility, keeping a record of all those individual donor units. The expiration of the "pooled" cryoprecipitate is four hours and stored at room temperature. Thus, combining all individual random units into one bag simplifies the transfusion job.

Cryoprecipitate is used to treat classic hemophilia, hypofibrinogenemia, von Willebrand's disease, and Factor XIII deficiency. While considering cryoprecipitate for infusion, the blood type of donors and recipients do not matter as far as compatibility is concerned.

E. Granulocytes

Granulocytes are present in the "buffy coat" layer. They can be prepared using the 'apheresis' procedure. Granulocytes must be irradiated to prevent transfusion-associated graft-versus-host disease. They are stored at 20°-24°C without agitation and 24 hours expiry shelf-life.

Doses of at least $1x10^{10}$ granulocytes per transfusion seem to be required to prevent infection. Granulocytes should be transfused as soon as possible after collection. They should be infused into a patient, provided the absolute neutrophil count is below 500/μL i.e. neutropenia. Thus, the use of granulocytes is limited to patients in whom possible benefits outweigh the hazards and after antibiotics have failed.

Massive transfusion protocol (MTP)

Some trauma centers have implemented a massive transfusion protocol (MTP) system. The system is activated in case of a penetrating injury or uncontrolled bleed during a major surgery (e.g., liver transplant). The justification is made by an emergency physician at a trauma center in the emergency room (ER) or a surgeon/anesthesiologist in the operating room (OR), respectively. Time is a critical factor in saving the life of a patient with massive blood loss. This is an integration of many stakeholders who work efficiently, focusing on only one patient. The MTP protocol varies from hospital to hospital. The overall goal is to expedite the supply of red blood cells, fresh frozen plasma (FFP), platelets, and cryoprecipitate on time as per the protocol.

Red blood cells and FFPs are supplied in validated coolers appropriately labeled with the serial numbers (e.g., MTP 1 RBCS and MTP 1 FFPs) in the chain of supply. If an ordering physician wants to transfuse in less than 10 minutes without type and screen results, it requires the physician to sign a request form "emergency order for uncross-matched blood". This request allows the blood bank professional to issue 2 units of O negative red blood cells in a validated cooler with ice packs.

The RN is responsible for sending the patient's specimen (one full 6.0 mL pink top tube) as soon as possible. Specimens are collected for hematology (e.g., complete blood count), coagulation studies (e.g., PT, aPTT, fibrinogen, and platelets), and chemistry (e.g., pH, pCO_2, and electrolytes) as well.

Typically, a blood bank prepares 5 units of a group-specific or compatible red blood cell if the patient's type and screen results are available. The same applies to 5 units of a group-specific or compatible thawed plasma in a validated cooler and labeled with accurate and complete details.

At 15 minute intervals, red blood cells and FFPs are supplied promptly to the patient's bedside until MTP is called off. A "single donor" platelet and a bag of "pooled" cryoprecipitate are supplied (at room temperature) afterward as per the needs of an ordering physician. All unused blood products should be returned to the blood bank within 4 hours from the issue time. There are times where MTP is reactivated. The MTP system needs an efficient and cooperative team to make it successful.

The blood bank professional needs to perform post-cross-match on segments of transfused blood units and order more blood products from the supplier to maintain inventory.

It is very important that a blood bank professional documents all details (e.g., time of phone calls, pick up time of coolers by a runner) clearly in an MTP log sheet to avoid any confusion for the medical director in reviewing the episode. The medical director/designee may discuss the pitfalls to the transfusion committee for taking the corrective actions in improving the patient's care.

Risks common to all blood components

Infection and alloimmunization are the major complications associated with the transfusion of blood components. There is a relationship between these risks and the number of donor exposures. The risk of infection is geographically variable. Major risks associated with the blood component transfusion therapy are:

1. Hepatitis C virus can be transmitted by blood transfusion. With the recent introduction of a screening test to detect HCV in donated blood and the discarding of positive units, the risk of transfusion-related hepatitis C has been greatly lessened. However, the exact risk per unit transfused is not yet known.
2. The human immunodeficiency virus, presently, poses a relatively small hazard. The wide range of estimated risk (1:30,000 to 1:300,000) reflects geographic variance.
3. Other infectious diseases or agents may be transmitted via transfusion (e.g., hepatitis B, I/II, cytomegalovirus, and malarial parasites).
4. Fatal hemolytic transfusion reactions can take place. They are usually caused by an ABO incompatibility due to errors in patient identification at the bedside.
5. Recipients of any blood product may produce antibodies against donor antigens, i.e., alloimmunization. This condition can result in an inadequate response to transfusion.
6. Allergic reactions, febrile reactions, and circulatory overload may also occur.

Chapter 51

Transfusion Reactions and
Hemolytic Disease of the Fetus and Newborn

Introduction

Complications that develop in a recipient (patient) during or following a blood transfusion are called transfusion reactions. These reactions may be mild or fatal. It is reported that as high as 40-50% of hemolytic transfusion reactions are fatal. They are indicated by a rise in temperature, headache, chills, and pain in the lumbar region. The cause of the resulting reaction may be due to technical or clerical errors. About 90% of such reactions occur because of clerical errors. It is necessary to adhere to the following principles of blood transfusion:

1. It is important to know the exact ABO and Rh groups of the donor and the recipient.
2. The transfusion must always be group-specific or cross-matched compatible.
3. Knowledge about the presence or absence of antibodies in the sera of the recipient as well as donor is required.
4. The broad-spectrum compatibility testing at various phases, namely immediate spin, 37°C, or AHG (Coombs) rules out almost all possibilities of mismatched transfusion and transfusion reactions.
5. Strict sterile precautions are to be taken during blood collection, storage, transportation, and during the actual transfusion.

There should be a standard operating procedure (SOP) including the details for documentation, reporting, evaluation, and follow-up of all transfusion-related adverse reactions or events. Transfusion-associated adverse reactions can be categorized as immunological and non-immunological as shown in Table 51.1.

Table 51.1: Transfusion-associated adverse reactions categorized as immunological and non-immunological

A. Immunological	B. Non-immunological

1. Hemolytic transfusion reactions
  a. acute
  b. delayed
2. Febrile (non-hemolytic) reactions
3. Allergic reactions
  a.urticaria
  b.anaphylaxis
4. Post-transfusion purpura (PTP)
	1. Bacterial contamination (infections)
	2. Transfusion-associated circulatory overload (TACO)
	3. Transfusion-related acute lung injury (TRALI)
	4. Hypothermia
	5. Citrate toxicity
	6. Potassium effects
	7. Infectious disease transmission
	8. Transfusion-associated Graft-versus-host disease (Ta-GVHD)
	9. Coagulopathy

A. Immunological

1. Hemolytic transfusion reactions: Hemolytic transfusion reactions may be acute (immediate) or delayed. They are briefly summarized as under:

a. Acute hemolytic transfusion reactions (AHTRs): are antigen-antibody mediated reactions. They are almost always caused by potent complement-activating antibodies such as anti-A and anti-B. Therefore, it is apparent that ABO incompatibility can lead to acute hemolytic transfusion reactions. Mostly, transfusion of ABO-incompatible red blood cells may occur due to a clerical error, e.g., mislabeling of a patient's specimen for "type and screen". With the advent of automated instruments in immunohematology laboratories and strict guidelines (e.g., multiple checkpoints) by a regulatory agency, the probability of ABO-related clerical errors is extremely low.

Acute transfusion reactions may be severe to life-threatening and sometimes fatal. Symptoms such as disseminated intravascular coagulation (DIC) and renal failure are common following the reaction. The reaction can be triggered by as small as 1 mL of packed red blood cells. This explains why a nurse verifies the patient's information on a label of a donor unit with another nurse and transfuses slowly (i.e., 2mL/min for the first 15 minutes) in the beginning with continuous supervision of a patient.

In the case of intravascular, hemolysis occurs primarily in the bloodstream, developing the immediate clinical effect. These reactions are mediated by the activation of complement. Hemolysis occurs only if complement activation proceeds to completion. The sequence of attachment of complement factors to the sensitized red blood cells is C_1, C_2, C_3, and C_4. AHTRs and associated mortality occur at approximately 1 in 76,000 and 1 in 1.8 million units transfused, respectively.

Also, antibodies directed against Kell and Duffy antigens may cause AHTRs.

Expected laboratory findings are:

1. ABO discrepancy
   (i) Between the original (pre-transfusion) and repeat (post-transfusion) blood samples from a patient
   (ii) Between the pre-transfusion and repeat testing on segmented tubing of the donor unit
2. Usually cause a positive direct antiglobulin test (DAT), reflecting the presence of complement (C3d) as well as the patient's anti-A, anti-B, or anti-AB
3. Occasionally donor-derived IgG anti-A, anti-B, or anti-A,B detected on patient's circulating red cells
4. Significant increase of indirect bilirubin and lactate dehydrogenase (LDH) levels accompanied by a sharp drop in the patient's haptoglobin level
5. Formation of schistocytes and hemoglobinuria

b. Delayed hemolytic transfusion reactions (DHTRs): are also antigen-antibody mediated reactions. Unlike acute hemolytic transfusion reactions, delayed transfusion reactions are triggered by antibodies, namely anti-Fy^a, anti-Jk^a, anti-Jk^b, anti-K, anti-C, and anti-E. Since reactions occur 2-14 days or some weeks of post-transfusion, they are called delayed transfusion reactions. In other words, they occur as an anamnestic response due to previous exposure to the same antigen. They can be asymptomatic, mild, or severe and red blood cells are eliminated by extravascular hemolysis. In the case of extravascular hemolysis, an antibody to the red cell antigen opsonizes the red cells, leading to their sequestration and subsequent phagocytosis in the reticuloendothelial system (liver and spleen). In DHTRs, acute renal failure and DIC are not manifested.

The incidence of delayed hemolytic transfusion reactions (DHTRs) is estimated at approximately 1 in 6000 units transfused. The majority of DHTRs require no treatment since red cell destruction occurs gradually. However, patients with low hemoglobin can be transfused with antigen-negative packed RBCs.

Expected laboratory findings are:

1. Elevated LDH and bilirubin levels
2. Low haptoglobin
3. Presence of hemoglobin in the urine

Both acute and delayed forms of a hemolytic transfusion reaction are classical examples of a cytotoxic (Type II) hypersensitivity.

2. Febrile (non-hemolytic) reactions: Fever (a temperature rise of 1°C over 37°C) and chills are presumably caused by:

(i) Recipient-derived antibodies that react with leukocyte antigens or their fragments in the blood component. Multiparous women and multiply-transfused patients are vulnerable to this form of reaction.

(ii) Accumulated cytokines in the blood component during storage (e.g., platelets at warmer temperatures) are thought to be implicated with the syndrome. The frequency of fever by platelet and red cell transfusions is 10-30% and 1-2%, respectively. Differential diagnosis needs to be performed because fever may be the initial symptom, e.g., transfusion-related bacterial sepsis and acute hemolytic reaction. This explains why the pre-transfusion temperature is checked.

These reactions are commonly encountered in transfusion medicine and are treated with antipyretics, e.g., oral acetaminophen. Therefore, leuko-depleted red blood cells and leuko-depleted platelets are transfused to patients experiencing febrile reactions quite often. The pre-storage leukoreduction is useful and is more effective than bedside leukoreduction.

Expected laboratory findings are:

1. Negative DAT
2. No ABO discrepancy on retyping of patient's and donor unit red cells
3. Patient's plasma and urine samples have a normal appearance on visual inspection

3. Allergic reactions: are further divided into two types as below:

471

a. Urticaria: is believed to be associated with plasma proteins. Symptoms include hives and itching without fever and can last for hours or up to several days. More extensive cases may be accompanied by angioedema. The incidence is 1-3%. Patients experiencing urticarial reactions are transfused with minimal plasma. Antihistamines may be used for the treatment.

b. Anaphylaxis: is commonly seen in IgA-deficient recipients with anti-IgA. It has an incidence of 1:20,000-1:50,000 transfusions. Symptoms include severe hypotension, shock, and loss of consciousness. Though these fever-free reactions are very rare, they are triggered following the infusion of a few milliliters of red cells/plasma products. To prevent very severe reactions, patients are to be transfused with IgA-deficient red cells (e.g., washed or deglycerolized) and plasma collected from IgA-deficient donors.

4. Post-transfusion purpura (PTP): occurs usually 5-10 days after a platelet-containing blood component transfusion (e.g., whole blood, packed red cells, platelets, fresh plasma). Antibodies directed against platelet antigens, anti-human platelet antigen-1a (anti-HPA-1a) being the most common culprit, are implicated with rare but severe thrombocytopenia (< 10,000/μL). Petechiae develop on the chest and arms due to mucocutaneous bleeding. The condition is self-limiting, lasting for approximately 2 weeks.

Post-transfusion purpura is usually seen in multiparous women older than 40 years due to alloimmunization (transfusion or pregnancy). The incidence ranges from 1:24,000 to 1:50,000-1:100,000 transfusions with a mortality rate of >10%. The primary cause of mortality is intracranial hemorrhage. The best treatment options include intravenous immunoglobulin and plasmapheresis. Usually, platelet transfusions are ineffective in raising the platelet counts.

B. Non-immunological

1. Bacterial contamination (infections): occur following the transfusion of blood components rather than the whole blood. They are associated with endotoxins from contaminating Gram-negative bacteria. They are rare but fatal. Therefore, all aseptic steps from a donor to the patient receiving the transfusion are closely supervised to avoid the risk of infection to the blood product. Bacterial contamination of platelet products takes place due to a storage temperature of 22°C. The signs, namely clots, agglutinates, and abnormal color presumably reflects the bacterial contamination of blood products.

Signs and symptoms include hyperpyrexia, pain in limbs and chest, dyspnea, pallor, headache, low blood pressure, and rapid pulse.

2. Transfusion-associated circulatory overload (TACO): These reactions occur in patients undergoing multiple plasma transfusions. Patients at high risk are elderly patients, infants, patients with renal failure, congestive heart failure, having anemia, hypoalbuminemia, or fluid overload. It occurs if the plasma is transfused too quickly or in large volumes. For example, plasma is used as a replacement fluid during the plasma exchange procedure to treat myasthenia gravis or thrombotic thrombocytopenic purpura (TTP). According to a recent FDA report, 20% of deaths are linked to transfusion-associated circulatory overload (TACO) reactions. Signs and symptoms

include pulmonary edema (within 6 hours after blood transfusion), dyspnea, orthopnea, cyanosis, tachycardia headache, pedal edema, and heaviness in limbs.

Circulatory overload can be prevented by avoiding unnecessary fluids and optimizing the rate of infusion. Diuretics may be administered as needed.

3. Transfusion-related acute lung injury (TRALI): is caused by activated recipient neutrophils that adhere to the pulmonary endothelium, increasing the permeability and the resultant noncardiogenic pulmonary edema. The activation of neutrophils is effected by donor-derived antibodies, e.g., anti-human leukocyte antigen (anti-HLA) or anti-human neutrophil antigen (anti-HNA). The syndrome develops during or within 6 hours of transfusion without any underlying risk factors. The syndrome includes acute dyspnea, hypoxemia, fever, hypotension, and tachycardia. Chest radiography shows bilateral pulmonary infiltrates. According to the US food and drug administration (FDA), it is the leading cause of transfusion-related deaths. The incidence is approximately 1 in every 5000 blood component transfusions. The mortality rate is 5-24%.

All plasma-containing components, namely whole blood, packed RBCs, platelets, cryoprecipitate, and fresh frozen plasma, have been implicated in TRALI.

4. Hypothermia: is caused by rapid infusion of large volumes of stored blood, e.g., massive or exchange transfusion in infants. To prevent hypothermia, the use of blood warmers and the warming of other intravenous fluids are recommended.

5. Citrate toxicity: Citrate, an anticoagulant in blood products, is rapidly metabolized by the liver. Hypocalcemia and hypomagnesemia are caused due to the rapid infusion of large volumes of stored blood. Binding of citrate with calcium and magnesium occurs, lowering their levels in the recipient's blood. This, in turn, results in coagulopathy or myocardial depression. Patients at risk include neonates with immature liver function and patients with dysfunction of the liver. This can be managed by slowing or temporarily stopping the transfusion.

6. Potassium effects: is caused by potassium leakage from stored red cells during their storage. The rate of potassium leakage is enhanced by irradiation. Hyperkalemia may occur during the rapid administration of large volumes of older red cells in small infants. Hyperkalemia can be prevented by irradiating red cell units just before their use. Also, the red cell units less than 7 days old are used for rapid and massive transfusion in small infants, e.g., exchange transfusion and cardiac surgery.

7. Infectious disease transmission: Many infectious agents may be transmitted by transfusion, e.g., malaria and hepatitis B. Definitive diagnosis include:

(i) demonstration of recipient seroconversion
   or
(ii) a new infection in the patient and isolation of an infectious agent with genomic identity from both the patient and the implicated donor.

8. Transfusion-associated graft-versus-host disease (Ta-GVHD): occurs when donor T-lymphocytes engraft in a susceptible recipient. The donor lymphocytes undergo proliferation, damaging target tissues, namely bone marrow, liver, skin, and digestive tract. The syndrome comprises fever, maculopapular rash, pancytopenia, enterocolitis with watery diarrhea, and dysfunction of the liver. It manifests 8-10 days post-transfusion. Although rare in occurrence, the mortality rate is 90%.

Ta-GVHD can be prevented by transfusing irradiated cellular blood components (RBCs, platelets, and granulocytes), especially in patients at risk of Ta-GVHD.

9. Coagulopathy: is associated with massive transfusion, resulting in dilution of platelets and clotting factors. Consumption coagulopathy is an important factor too.

Investigation of transfusion reactions

Whenever a transfusion reaction is suspected, the attending medical personnel should discontinue the blood transfusion immediately and should inform the laboratory. Moreover, blood and cross-match labels should be sent to the laboratory.

It is advisable to check all the records of the pre-transfusion tests to confirm any clerical errors before an incompatible blood reaction is investigated. The procedure to follow the technical error is as under:
1. Collect 10 mL of venous blood from that recipient's arm not used for the blood transfusion. It is important to take precautions to avoid hemolysis as the resulting serum is to be examined for hemolysis.
2. Carry out the re-grouping of the recipient, using both pre-transfusion and post-transfusion blood specimens.
3. Carry out the re-grouping of the donor, using a blood specimen from the donor unit being used for the transfusion.
4. Perform a direct Coombs test, using the recipient's cells obtained from pre-transfusion and post-transfusion blood specimens.
5. Repeat the cross-match, using the donor's cells and recipient's sera obtained from pre-transfusion and post-transfusion blood samples.
6. Look for any strongly reacting antibodies in the donor's blood if the patient's blood group is other than O, but received group O blood.
7. Collect the post-transfusion urine and test the same for hemoglobinuria and hematuria.
8. Perform serum bilirubin and plasma hemoglobin determinations from 6 hours post-transfusion blood to know the degree of damage that occurred in the recipient.
9. Perform Gram's staining and plate the blood sample on suitable culture media to find out any bacteriological causes.

Finally, a report is prepared to contain all required test results and submitted to the concerned medical officer without delay.

Hemolytic Disease of the Fetus and Newborn (HDFN)

Hemolytic disease of the fetus and newborn is clinically indicated by jaundice, anemia, and enlargement of the liver and spleen. The disease begins *in utero*. It affects the erythropoiesis of the fetus, causing the appearance of erythroblasts in the circulatory system. This is the reason why this disease was originally called *Erythroblastosis fetalis*.

Blood group incompatibility (i.e., anti-D incompatibility and ABO incompatibility) is the most common cause of hemolytic disease of the fetus and the newborn. Antibodies (IgG type) from the maternal circulation enter the fetal circulation through the placenta. The antibodies so entered attach to blood group antigens available on the red cells, causing sensitization of the red cells. The sensitized red cells are sequestered in the spleen for hemolysis. Furthermore, liberated hemoglobin is broken down into various end products in which bilirubin is an important yellow pigment. Under such circumstances, bone marrow activity is increased to replace the lost red cells. The severity of the disease ranges from mild anemia to stillbirth. The degree of the damage occurring in the fetus and the newborn depends upon the number of red cells destroyed and to what extent the compensation of lost cells is made by increased production of new red cells. As mentioned previously, both causes of hemolytic disease of the fetus and newborn are briefly discussed below:

1. *Anti-D incompatibility:* This is a more common and severe cause than ABO incompatibility. If an Rh-negative mother becomes pregnant with an Rh-positive fetus, Rh-positive fetal red cells enter the mother's body through the placental barrier, inducing the formation of anti-Rho (anti-D). Anti-Rho (anti-D) so formed returns to the fetal circulation through the placenta. Now, anti-Rho (anti-D) will bring about the coating of the fetal Rh-positive red cells (i.e., sensitization of fetal red cells). Finally, hemolysis of sensitized red cells takes place in the spleen, liberating hemoglobin. Thus, severely affected infants can have cord hemoglobin levels as low as 3-4 gms%. Hemoglobin is further degraded to a variety of products, including bilirubin as a major pigment. Peak levels of bilirubin are usually seen by the third day of life in full-term infants. But, it may reach 40-50 mg% in untreated cases of hemolytic disease. Levels in normal full-term babies rarely exceed 13 mg%.

2. *ABO incompatibility:* The disease can occur if the blood groups of a pregnant woman and her child are 'O' and 'A'/'B', respectively. Woman's plasma must have anti-A or anti-B belonging to the IgG class. Fortunately, naturally occurring antibodies namely, anti-A and anti-B belong to the IgM class. Therefore, they fail to cross the placental barrier and thus the baby's red cells are not damaged.

Laboratory diagnosis of the disease includes a direct Coombs test on cord blood or blood collected within the first 24 hours of life. The test result may be only weakly positive or negative[35], although the disease prevails. It can be seen that diagnosis is made after delivery and cannot be predicted by any prenatal testing.

Hemolytic disease of the fetus and newborn (HDFN) is also an example of cytotoxic (Type II) hypersensitivity.

---

[35] Usually, a blood specimen collected 24 hours after birth shows a negative result.

Diagnostic Laboratory tests are:

1. ABO grouping and Rho typing of the infant and the mother
2. Direct Coombs test, using red cells obtained from cord blood
3. Hemoglobin and serum bilirubin determinations
4. Peripheral smear study of a thin stained blood smear
5. ABO incompatibility: Usually, the disease is not serious and hemoglobin values are often nearly normal

Note:

Elution and identification of antibodies of the cord blood are carried out if the Coombs test result is positive. This is done by the acid elution technique. Also, the detection of anti-Rho (anti-D) from the mother's blood specimen is done as a prenatal investigation.

Prevention and treatment

Hemolytic disease of the fetus and newborn can be completely prevented by the administration of RhIG (RhoGAM) within 72 hours post-delivery. The immune globulin should be administered intramuscularly. The dosage of RhIG (RhoGAM) is determined by the number of fetal Rh-positive red cells in the maternal circulation.

Once the screening test (rosette method) result is positive, the next step is to perform a Kleihauer-Betke (KB) stain (or flow cytometry) to assess a fetomaternal hemorrhage-associated risk of the patient in question. The Kleihauer-Betke test helps estimate the volume of fetal Rh-positive red cells in maternal circulation. Usually, this is accomplished by performing a Kleihauer-Betke (KB) stain. The test involves the preparation of a thin smear using the specimen of maternal blood, followed by treatment with an acid/alkali and subsequent staining with erythrosin B-hematoxylin. Microscopically, fetal red cells appear rose-pink as opposed to the pale ghost-like appearance of maternal cells because fetal hemoglobin resists acid/alkali treatment. The percentage of fetal cells is estimated based on a count of 2000 cells in the smear. The volume of fetomaternal hemorrhage is calculated using the following formula:

$$\text{Volume of fetomaternal hemorrhage} = \frac{\text{number of fetal red cells x volume of maternal blood (mL)}}{\text{Number of maternal red cells}}$$

Alternatively, volume (mL) of fetomaternal bleed can simply be calculated by multiplying the percentage of fetal red cells by 50. The multiplication factor, 50, is based on an assumed mother's total circulatory blood volume of 5,000 mL.

Furthermore, an adequate dose of Rh immune globulin (RhIG) is required to be administered for successful neutralization of the effect of fetomaternal hemorrhage (FMH). A single vial of 300 µg (standard) offers protection against 30 mL of whole blood (equivalent to 15 mL of packed red

cells). Additional doses of RhIG are indicated for patients with massive fetomaternal hemorrhages (i.e., exposure to > 30 mL of whole blood). The number of RhIG vials required is calculated based on the volume (mL) of fetal whole blood that passed through the fetomaternal bleed.

This numerical value for the number of the vial(s) required is derived by a simple division of the volume (mL) of fetomaternal bleed by 30 mL. Administration of RhIG to Rh-negative women may be either postpartum (if newborn Rh-positive) or antepartum as a prophylactic measure. Antepartum RhIG candidacy may be associated with one of these causes, namely 26-28 weeks' gestation, amniocentesis, abdominal trauma, ectopic pregnancy, threatened pregnancy loss, or termination of pregnancy. It has been recommended that RhIG is effectively administered to Rh-negative women within three days of delivery or exposure (proven/suspected) to Rh-positive red cells. Treatment of the disease can be done in one of the following three ways:

1. Exchange transfusion
2. Induction of labor
3. Intrauterine transfusions

The most widely used treatment is exchange transfusion carried out in the first few hours of life. The blood for exchange transfusion should be as fresh as possible, not more than three days old. The baby suffering from the hemolytic disease of the fetus and newborn due to anti-D incompatibility must receive Rh-negative blood. It is important to note that the donor's red cells must be cross-matched against the maternal plasma and not that of the baby. A simple rule is followed while selecting the ABO group of blood. Group O blood is always suitable and should be given whenever the ABO blood groups of the baby and the mother differ. If the ABO blood groups of the baby and the mother are the same, there is no reason why the blood of that group should not be used. The type of blood to be selected for various situations is shown in Table 51.2.

Table 51.2: Choice of blood for exchange transfusion

Mother	Baby	Exchange transfusion
Group O	O A B	O
Group A	O B	O
	A AB	A or O
Group B	O A	O
	B AB	B or O
Group AB	A B AB	A *or* O B *or* O A, B, AB, *or* O

The estimated volume of blood for double volume exchange transfusion is determined by the formula below:

$$\text{Weight (Kg)} \times 2 \times 80$$

Then, add approximately 30 mL for the tubing dead space.

Usually, two units (i.e. 900 mL) of blood are transfused in the newborn through the umbilical cord. (Normally the volume of blood in the infant is about 200 mL).
The exchange transfusion therapy serves the following four purposes:

1. To remove bilirubin, preventing its deposition in the tissues e.g., kernicterus (deposition of free bilirubin into the brain tissues)
2. To remove the sensitized red cells and to replace normal red cells
3. To restore normal cardiac function and to improve anemia without increasing the circulatory load
4. To remove the maternal antibody from the baby's circulation for keeping subsequently formed red cells unharmed

Chapter 52

Blood Banking and Automation

Introduction

The author never imagined the existence of a machine capable of doing all operations without the assistance of a human. The era of computers has greatly benefited in designing fully automated machines. Such machines greatly alleviate the possibility of human errors to occur, e.g., switching of specimens, erroneous recording of the test results (i.e., transcription errors), and traceability of variables (e.g., reagents). The author is still very hopeful of more sophisticated automated systems in the days to come, making blood banking more efficient than ever.

1. Column agglutination technology (gel system)

Dr. Yves Lapierre of Lyon, France launched the gel test in 1985, designing a more reproducible and standardized test. First and foremost, the fully automated machine based on gel technology was introduced in North America by Ortho Diagnostic Systems Inc. in 1995. This fully automated machine (ProVue™) is shown in Fig. 52.1.

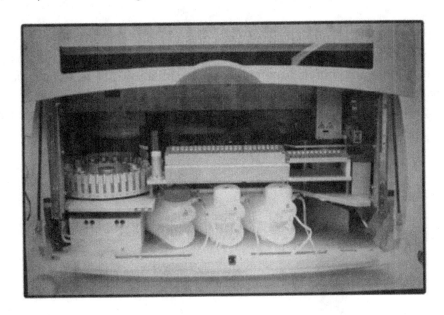

Fig. 52.1: A fully automated machine (ProVue™).
(Reproduced with permission from Ortho Diagnostic Systems Inc.; Raritan, N. J.)

Principle
The principle involved in gel technology is very simple and self-explanatory. Agglutinated red cells form clumps that cannot travel through the porous gel and remain at the top of a microtube, forming a red line of clumped red cells (positive reaction) following centrifugation {see Fig. 52.2 (a)}. On the other hand, the red cells not undergoing agglutination are small enough in size pass through the porous gel. Therefore, the individual red cells can easily travel and settle at the bottom of a microtube, forming a button (negative reaction) following centrifugation {see Fig. 52.2 (b)}.

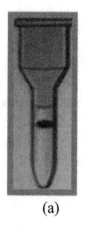 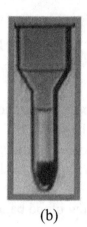

(a)　　　　　　　　　(b)

(a) Positive reaction
(b) Negative reaction

Fig. 52.2: Reactions in gel microtubes.
(Courtesy of Ortho Diagnostic Systems Inc.; Raritan, N. J.)

Gel cards
A gel card used in ID-Micro Typing System™ is a plastic-made card that measures approximately 5x7 centimeters. Each card has six microtubes. Each microtube, in turn, contains pre-dispensed gel (dextran-acrylamide) and diluent, making up approximately 75% of the gel-liquid mixture in each microtube. Since gel particles are porous and approximately 70μ in diameter (10 times larger than red cell diameter), they serve as a filter as well as a reaction medium in some cards as shown in Fig. 52.3.

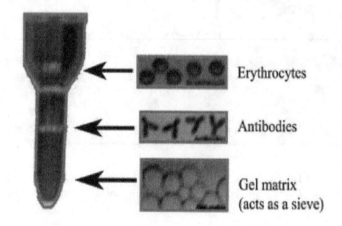

Fig. 52.3: Contents of a gel microtube.
(Courtesy of Micro Typing Systems Inc.; Pompano Beach, FL.)

There are different types of gel cards, depending upon the nature of testing to perform. For example, monoclonal anti-A, monoclonal anti-B (forward grouping sera), and anti-D are pre-dispensed in microtubes of A|B|D cards {see Fig. 52.4 (a)} as opposed to the IgG (rabbit) gel card {see Fig. 52.4 (b)} used for antibody screening.

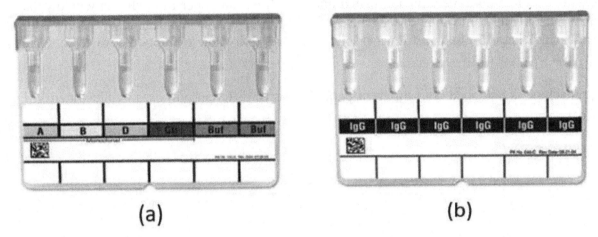

(a) A|B|D monoclonal and reverse grouping gel card
(b) Anti-IgG (rabbit) gel card

Fig. 52.4: Types of gel cards.
(Courtesy of Ortho Diagnostic Systems Inc.; Raritan, N. J.)

The strengths of a specific red cell antigen and its corresponding plasma/serum antibody reaction vary. These reactions are graded as shown in Fig. 52.5.

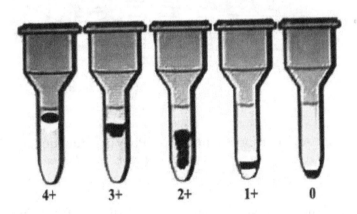

Fig. 52.5: Grading of agglutination reactions.
(Courtesy of Ortho Diagnostic Systems Inc.; Raritan, N. J.)

Reagents
Reverse grouping cells, screening cells, and diluent.

Sample
The patient's red cells are washed and suspended in diluent to make 0.8% suspension as opposed to 2-5% suspension for tube testing. It is strongly recommended that antibody screen and antibody identification procedures should make use of plasma. This eliminates false positives that may be caused by fibrin clots from serum.

Apparatus

ProVue® is a non-portable fully automated machine. It has an upper front sliding window that is used in loading and unloading of reagents, gel cards, diluent, and samples. Also, there is a lower access panel that is useful to refill wash solution bottles (two) and to empty the waste bottle and a tray with used gel cards.

The machine is equipped with different parts that serve different purposes as illustrated in Fig. 52.6.

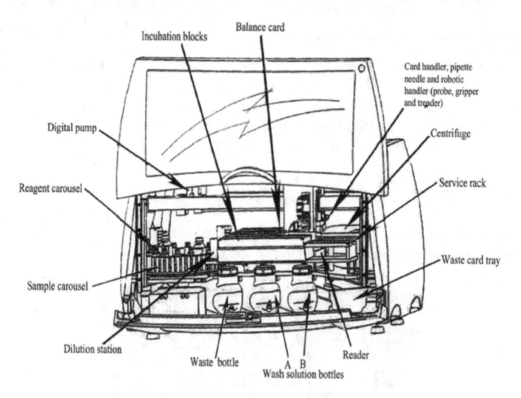

Fig. 52.6: A closer look at the Ortho ProVue™ functional areas.
(Courtesy of Ortho Diagnostic Systems Inc.; Raritan, N. J.)

Working

The key steps involved in the processing of samples for ABO and Rh determinations and antibody screening include:

1. Identification of a specimen by using a bar-code reader
2. Identification of A|B|D and IgG (rabbit) gel cards being used for the sample in question
3. Dispensing of reagent red cells, namely A1 and B red cells, for reverse grouping to the microtubes of A|B|D gel card
4. Dispensing 50µL of reagent red cells for antibody screen to the microtubes of IgG (rabbit) gel card
5. Dispensing 25µL of plasma/serum from the patient's sample to the last two microtubes of A|B|D gel card (reverse grouping) and IgG (rabbit) gel card (antibody screen)
6. Preparation of approximately 0.8% of red cell concentration from the patient's sample being processed

7. Dispensing of pre-diluted patient's red cells (forward grouping) to the microtubes of A|B|D gel card
8. Incubation of IgG (rabbit) gel cards at 37°C for 15 minutes
9. Centrifugation of gel cards at 90 degree angle for pre-set 10 minutes
10. Reading of gel cards on both sides of each microtube immediately (stable for 48-72 hours)

Note: Red cells are added before plasma to the reaction chamber to avoid false negatives.

Uses
1. Determination of ABO (forward and reverse groupings) group
2. Determination of Rho (D) type
3. Detection of irregular antibody/antibodies in plasma/serum (i.e., antibody screen)
4. Compatibility testing
5. Direct antiglobulin testing (DAT)
6. Phenotyping of red cell antigens, e.g., C, E, and e
7. Identification of antibodies, e.g., anti-C, anti-E, and anti-K

Gel technology has several advantages and some disadvantages over the traditional tube methodology.

Advantages
1. Standardization and stability
2. Specificity and sensitivity
3. Improved safety and decreases hazardous waste
4. No cell washing step involved
5. Easy cross-training
6. Improved traceability of samples, reagents, and operating technologist
7. Improved productivity
8. High throughput
9. Enables to detect mixed-field (mf) reactions, e.g., organ transplant patients
10. Availability of automated panels

Disadvantages
1. Longer turnaround time, e.g., a minimum of 20 minutes for ABO-Rh determination
2. Wear and tear (i.e., costly maintenance)
3. False-positive results in the presence of particulate matter, e.g., medications, disease states, infections, Wharton's jelly, and/or cross-contamination
4. Costly investment

Alternatively, a microcolumn prefilled with glass bead microparticles impregnated with a diagnostic reagent (e.g., AHG) may be used (Reis K.J., 1993). The sieving effect is attributed to glass microbeads instead. Like a gel card technique, a glass microbead matrix-based column agglutination method is also specific and sensitive.

2. Solid-phase technology (see Fig. 52.7)

Microwell solid-phase technology is based on the methods of Plapp *et al* and Juji *et al*. Like conventional tube technique, solid-phase red cell adherence (SPRCA) assay involves both washing and centrifugation steps.

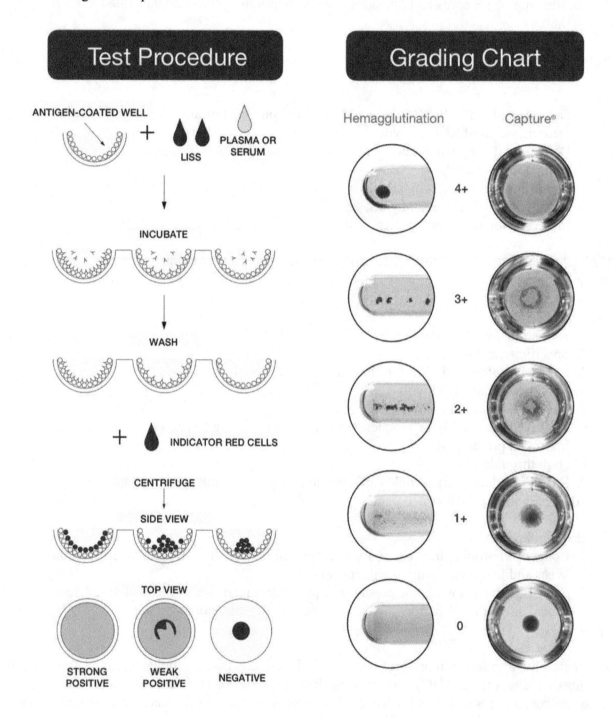

Fig.52.7: Various procedural steps and grading chart of a solid-phase red cell adherence assay.
(Copyrighted material used with the permission of Immucor, Inc.
Copying or reprinting without permission is expressly forbidden.)

484

The system makes use of a microwell plate with pre-coated hemolyzed and dried RBCs (RBC stroma). The patient's plasma/serum and LISS (potentiator) are added to a microtiter well followed by incubation at 37°C, washing, and centrifugation steps. If a red cell-specific antibody is present in the patient's plasma/serum, it reacts with the membrane-bound RBC antigen during incubation. The washing step allows us to remove the unbound antibody molecules and other residues. Finally, antihuman globulin (AHG)-coated red cells (indicator cells) are added and the microwell plate is centrifuged before reading the reaction. A positive reaction is graded (1+ to 4+), depending upon the size of the red-colored circle developed. The size of the circle is proportional to the concentration of plasma/serum antibody in the sample. A fully automated analyzer based on solid-phase technology was launched by Immucor, Inc. (Norcross, GA, USA) in 1999. Currently, an updated version named Galileo ECHO with multiple operations is available.

Results

Positive: Adherence of indicator RBCs with the formation of a small circle (graded as 1+ to 4+)

Negative: A pellet formation at the bottom of the microwell

Advantages

1. Small sample volume
2. Sensitive and accurate
3. Stability of results
4. Compatible with automation
5. Wide range of tests, including platelet IgG antibodies and platelet cross-matching
6. Simple to perform and economical
7. Suitable for hemolyzed, icteric, or lipemic samples

3. Erythrocyte-magnetized technology

New erythrocyte-magnetized technology uses paramagnetic nanoparticles. These nanoparticles are adsorbed on the membrane of erythrocytes. These magnetized RBCs are allowed to react with antibody molecules. Thereafter, both reactive and non-reactive magnetized RBCs are rapidly pulled to the bottom of the microplate well. This pulling effect is exerted by an external magnetic field due to a magnetic plate. Following the shaking step, the technologist can read the result as a positive/negative reaction. Surprisingly, this technology does not need washing and centrifugation steps. A piece of sophisticated equipment, QWALYS 3 (DIAGAST; France), is an example of erythrocyte-magnetized technology. The system is capable of performing a whole spectrum of pre-transfusion tests, ranging from ABO/Rh to antibody identification. Thus, the robustness of the system is exceptionally unique.

Comparison

A comparative study of all the three innovative technologies, including conventional tube technique was undertaken by Bajpai, M. et al. in 2012. Some important findings are summarized below:

Considering column agglutination (gel) and solid phase red cell adherence assay procedures, they exhibit some similarities listed below:

- Can detect IgG antibodies from the sample
- Capable of detecting weaker blood groups
- Amenable to batch testing
- Almost similar sensitivity and susceptibility levels

However, the pitfalls of a solid phase red cell adherence assay include involvement of one washing step and inability to detect IgM antibodies from the sample. Like column agglutination method, the highly specific erythrocyte-magnetized technique does not involve a washing step and amenable to batch testing. However, it cannot detect weaker blood groups and IgM antibodies, and produces false positives with fibrinic/lipemic samples.

Conclusion

All the three innovative technologies supersede the conventional tube technique (CTT), e.g., screening sensitivity for clinically significant antibodies and uniformity of the results. Conventional tube technique suffers from its poor sensitivity, i.e., approximately 43% (LISS-IAT). However, CTT (the gold standard) remains a backup method in rare conditions, e.g., emergency testing of trauma patients.

Review questions

1. What is the total volume of blood in an adult?
2. What is the age limit for prospective blood donors?
3. What is the usual interval between blood donations?
4. What chromosome number possesses the HLA antigens?
5. Which anticoagulant solution is recommended for the collection of blood if it is to be stored for 35 days?
6. What is the storage temperature range for whole blood and red blood cells?
7. What is the recommended concentration of erythrocytes for cross-matching (tube method)?
8. What are the reactants used in the major cross-matching?
9. Which test is carried out to detect antibody bound to erythrocytes?
10. Which antibody is present in the serum of human subjects who belong to the 'A' blood group?
11. What technique is used to identify weak D (D^u antigen)?
12. Which permitted chemical preservative is used in blood grouping sera?
13. Which chemical agent inactivates IgM molecules?
14. Which antigenic substance is absent in the individuals belonging to Bombay blood group (Oh)?
15. Which enzymes are used in the blood bank while working with multiple antibodies?
16. Which technique is recommended to remove antibodies from erythrocytes?
17. What is the cause of the majority of hemolytic transfusion reactions?
18. Which solution should be used for dispersing cells in rouleaux formation?
19. Which blood product is advised in the treatment of hemophilia A?
20. Which antibodies react in cold (4°C)?
21. Which lectin is used to differentiate A_1 from A_2 cells?
22. What percentage of the population inherit at least Se gene, i.e., "secretors"?
23. Which sub-group of the group A exhibits mixed field (mf) agglutination with anti-A, and anti-A,B?
24. What is the temperature range permissible for maintaining red blood cells and whole blood during shipping?
25. Which class of immunoglobulin is generally involved in hemolytic disease of the fetus and newborn (HDFN)?
26. How many vials of RhIG (300 µg standard dose) should be administered to the mother with 65 mL of bleed?
27. Which drugs have been implicated to cause a drug-induced red blood cell sensitization?
28. Which IgG antibodies are called "treacherous" antibodies that may cause delayed hemolytic transfusion reactions (HTRs)?
29. What potentiators can be used to enhance antigen-antibody reactions?
30. What is the most common genotype for the Rh-negative population?
31. Which test is performed in order to confirm the identity of plasma antibody(ies)?
32. What storage temperature is used for platelets?
33. What is the shelf-life of fresh frozen plasma (FFP) after thawing?
34. What is the ABO group of cells used in antibody screens and antibody panels?
35. Which antibodies may show reactivity at any phase?
36. Which antibodies usually react at the AHG phase?

37. What does polyspecific (broad-spectrum) antihuman globulin detect?
38. Which viral infection is the most common in transfusion medicine?
39. What class of antibodies do the most HLA antibodies belong to?
40. Where are lectins, e.g., anti-H lectin, extracted from?

Answers:

1. about 6 liters
2. 17-66 years
3. 8 weeks
4. 6
5. CPDA-1
6. 1°-6°C
7. 2-5%
8. patient's serum and donor's red blood cells
9. direct antiglobulin test
10. anti-B
11. indirect antiglobulin technique
12. sodium azide (0.1%)
13. 2-Mercaptoethanol
14. H-substance
15. ficin, bromelin, and trypsin
16. elution
17. clerical errors
18. physiological or normal saline
19. cryoprecipitate
20. anti-Le^a, anti-Le^b, and anti-P$_1$.
21. *Dolichos biflorus*
22. 80%
23. A$_3$
24. 1°-10°C
25. IgG
26. 3 vials
27. penicillin, cephalosporin, quinine, and methyldopa
28. anti-Jk^a and anti-Jk^b
29. 22% albumin, LISS, and polyethylene glycol (PEG)
30. rr
31. phenotyping of the patient's red blood cells
32. room temperature (20°-24°C) with continuous gentle agitation
33. 24 hours
34. group O cells
35. Lewis
36. Kell, Duffy, and Kidd
37. IgG and C$_3$d
38. hepatitis C
39. IgG
40. plants (usually seeds)

Section VI: Body Fluids

Chapter 53

Routine Urinalysis

Introduction

Several chemical substances are present in urine specimens. It is evident from the chemical composition of normal urine as shown in Table 53.1.

Table 53.1: Chemical substances present in a urine specimen

Constituent	Concentration, g/dL
Water	95
Urea	2
Sodium	0.6
Chloride	0.6
Sulfate	0.18
Potassium	0.15
Phosphate	0.12
Creatinine	0.1
Ammonia	0.05
Uric acid	0.03
Calcium	0.015
Magnesium	0.01

Why is urinalysis required?

Though urinalysis is a simple laboratory test, it discloses many facts about the functioning of various organs as shown in Fig. 53.1.

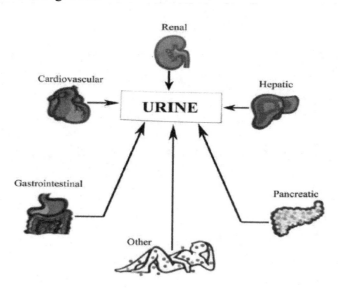

Fig. 53.1: Routine urinalysis provides information about the functioning of various organs.

A. Physical examination

Gross information about urine can be obtained from its physical characteristics. The physical examination of urine includes the following tests:

a. volume
b. color and appearance
c. odor
d. specific gravity

a. Volume

The normal amount of urine secreted in 24 hours by an adult varies widely from 600 to 2,500 mL. The output of urine normally depends on fluid intake, diet, external temperature, and mental and physical state. The formation of urine during activity is more than twice that at sleep.

Increased secretion of urine occurs after increased fluid intake and a protein-rich diet. On the other hand, diminished secretion is due to sweating as a result of exposure to high temperature or exercise. Children form urine 3 to 4 times more than adults per kilogram of body weight.

1. Polyuria (increased secretion of urine)
   - Diabetes mellitus
   - Diabetes insipidus
   - Chronic renal failure
   - Paralysis agitans
   - Tumors of the brain and spinal cord

2. Oliguria (decreased secretion of urine)
   - Dehydration (diarrhea and vomiting)
   - Acute nephritis and nephrosis
   - Cardiac deficiency
   - Acute intestinal obstruction
   - Portal cirrhosis
   - Acute febrile diseases
   - Peritonitis
   - Obstruction of the ureters
   - Poisoning by agents that damage the kidneys

3. Nocturia (secretion of more than 500 mL of urine at night with a specific gravity below 1.018)
   - Chronic glomerulonephritis

4. Anuria (complete cessation of urinary secretion by kidneys)
   - Poisoning with bichloride of mercury

b. Color and appearance

Normally, urine is pale yellow or amber owing to the presence of urochrome (a chief urinary pigment). Moreover, small quantities of uroerythrin, urobilin, and hematoporphyrin are present. Variation in the color of normal urine depends on the quantity and concentration of urine voided.

Color changes of urine due to pathological processes are listed in Table 53.2.

Table 53.2: Color changes of urine due to pathological processes

Color	Cause
Orange-yellow to green-brown	− bilirubin from obstructive jaundice
Clear red to red-brown	− hemoglobinuria in paroxysmal hemoglobinuria, blackwater fever, incompatible blood transfusion, severe burns, exposure to cold, or intra-abdominal hemorrhage
Smoky red to brown	− non hemolyzed red cells from hemorrhage in the urinary tract
Port-wine color	− hemochromatosis, hematoporphyrinuria, or hemolytic jaundice
Brown with black tinge	− melanin from malignant melanoma, or − alkaptonuria
Dark brown	− urobilin in liver infection, malaria, pernicious anemia, or acute infections

Color changes of urine due to drugs and chemicals are listed in Table 53.3.

Table 53.3: Color changes of urine due to drugs and chemicals

Color	Cause
Green-blue	− Methylene blue or thymol
Dark brown to black	− Carbolic acid, guaiacol, creosote, salol, or resorcin poisoning
Deep red	− Pyramidon, prontylin, or rose bengal
Pink (alkaline urine)	− Administration of phenolsulfonphthalein in kidney function test
Orange-red	− Pyridium
Deep yellow	− Santonin, senna, or chrysarobin
Yellow-green	− Acriflavine

Normally, urine is quite transparent. Turbidity may develop by the presence of bacteria, pus cells, and phosphates, and carbonates (alkaline urine). Pink turbidity is caused by the presence of salts of uric acid (acidic urine). The presence of lymph (e.g., filariasis) in the urine develops a milky appearance. In alcohol and phosphorus poisoning, urine is opalescent.

c. Odor
Fresh normal urine has an aromatic odor because it contains volatile fatty acids. On the other hand, old normal urine has an ammoniacal odor as there is bacterial degradation of urea.

Odor changes of urine due to abnormal constituents are listed in Table 53.4.

Table 53.4: Odor changes of urine due to abnormal constituents

Odor	Constituent(s)
Fruity	Acetone (ketosis)
Peppermint	Menthol
Spice-like	Sandalwood oil, tolu, and saffron
Somewhat acrid	Asparagus
Foul	Bacteria and pus cells

d. Specific gravity

The specific gravity of normal urine is directly proportional to the amount of urea and chlorides present. It normally ranges from 1.003 to 1.030. There are three methods to measure the specific gravity of urine:

1. Urinometer
2. Refractometer (*Goldberg refractometer*)
3. Ames reagent strip

Clinical significance

The specific gravity of urine is **high** (above 1.025) in:
- Diabetes mellitus
- Acute glomerulonephritis
- Fever
- Loss of water (sweating, vomiting, or diarrhea)

The specific gravity of urine is **low** (below 1.010) in:
- Diabetes insipidus
- Chronic nephritis
- Endocrine disorder
- Excessive fluid intake
- Low salt intake

B. Chemical examination

Results of chemical tests of urine serve as a valuable guide to the clinician. Therefore, they should carefully be carried out. Routine chemical tests of urine may be listed as under:

a. pH (reaction)
b. Glucose
c. Proteins
   (i) Albumin
   (ii) Bence-jones protein
d. Bile pigments
   (i) Bilirubin
   (ii) Urobilinogen
e. Bile salts
f. Ketones
g. Occult blood
h. Nitrite
i. Leukocyte esterase

a. pH (reaction)
Fluids having a pH of 0-7 are called acidic fluids. On the other hand, fluids with a pH of 7-14 are termed alkaline fluids. Normally, fresh urine is slightly acidic. The urine specimen for pH measurement must be fresh. There are four methods to measure the pH of urine:

1. Litmus papers
2. Indicator papers
3. Reagent strip
4. pH meter

Results:
Normal pH: about 6 (normal pH range: 5-7)
Acid pH: 4.5-5.5 (some types of diabetes, acidosis, and muscular fatigue)
Alkaline pH: 7.8-8 (UTI, renal failure, and a vegetarian diet)

Knowledge of urine pH is also helpful in the detection of certain crystals. For example, Ca-oxalate and uric acid crystals occur in acidic urine while phosphates and carbonate crystals occur in alkaline urine.

b. Glucose
Detectable glucose is not present in normal urine. There are two methods to detect urinary glucose:

1.Enzymatic test (reagent strip)

Principle:

Glucose oxidase converts glucose to gluconic acid and hydrogen peroxide. Hydrogen peroxide so formed, in the presence of peroxidase, reacts with potassium iodide (a chromogen) to form a green to brown color. Thus, this reaction is a double sequential enzymatic reaction:

(i) $$Glucose + 2H_2O + O_2 \xrightarrow{\text{glucose oxidase}} Gluconic\ acid + 2\ H_2O_2$$

(ii) $$3\ H_2O_2 + KI \xrightarrow{\text{peroxidase}} KIO_3 + 3H_2$$

Procedure:

1. Immerse the test area of the strip in fresh urine and remove it immediately.
2. Tap the end of the strip gently against the rim of the container to remove excess urine.
3. After one minute, match the color of the test area with the closest color blocks provided on the bottle label.

Results:

Standard color blocks in mg/dL are: 0 (negative), 100 (trace), 250 (+), 500(+ +), 1000 (+ + +) and over 2000 (+ + + +).

2. Reduction test
Principle:
Glucose reduces copper from a cupric to a cuprous state (Benedict's solution).

Causes of glycosuria (glucose in the urine):

- Diabetes mellitus
- Renal tubular disease
- Cushing's syndrome
- Pregnancy

c. Proteins

(i) Albumin

A trace of albumin is present in the normal urine. Excretion of albumin in the urine may be pathological (e.g., glomerulonephritis, CCF, UTIs, etc.) or physiological (e.g., pregnancy, protein-rich meal, psychological strain, etc.). The presence of albumin in the urine is called albuminuria. There are three methods to detect albumin in the urine:

1. Sulphosalicylic acid (3%) test
2. Heat and acetic acid test
3. Dry reagent strip test (uses bromophenol blue indicator that is sensitive to albumin and less sensitive to globulins and Bence-Jones protein)
4. Nitric acid method

Clinical significance

Physiological
- Pregnancy
- Protein-rich meal
- Fever
- Strenuous exercise

Pathological
- Glomerulonephritis
- UTIs
- Nephrotic syndrome

(ii) Bence-Jones protein (B.J. protein)

Bence-Jones protein is an endogenous protein. It is an abnormal globulin protein with an unusual property of solubility. It is normally present in the bone marrow and WBCs. Moreover, it is almost completely excreted within 12 hours after its formation. There are three methods to detect B J. protein in the urine:

1. Heat and cool method
2. Zone electrophoresis
3. p-Toluene sulfonic acid

1. Heat and cool test:
Principle:
B.J. protein gets precipitated between 40°-60°C and redissolved almost completely at 100°C.

Procedure:
1. Take about 5 mL of clear urine in a clean and dry test tube.
2. If the urine is alkaline to litmus, add 33% acetic acid till it becomes faintly acidic.
3. Place a thermometer and a test tube in the water bath.
4. Heat carefully over a Bunsen flame up to 100°C, observing the temperature at which the precipitate appears.
5. Allow the urine to cool to about 60°C, watching for any cloudiness to reappear.

Clinical significance
B.J. protein is associated with multiple myeloma, lymphoma, and macroglobulinemia.

d. Bile pigments

Certain abnormal types of bile pigments formed under diseased conditions include:
- Bilirubin (a chief bile pigment)
- Urobilinogen
- Urobilin (stercobilin)
- Hemoglobin
- Porphyrins

● Indican

(i) Bilirubin

1. Fouchet test

Bilirubin is concentrated by adsorption on insoluble barium salts. Furthermore, bilirubin is oxidized to biliverdin (green pigment) by $FeCl_3$.

Reagents

10% $BaCl_2$

Barium chloride	10 g
Distilled water	100 mL

Dissolve the chemical in water.

Fouchet's reagent

Trichloroacetic acid	25 g
10% Ferric chloride	10 mL
Distilled water	100 mL

Mix the solutions together.

Procedure

1. Mix 10 mL of urine with 2.5 mL of 10% $BaCl_2$ and filter or centrifuge.
2. Obtain the precipitate and add 2 drops of Fouchet's reagent to the precipitate.

Results:

The appearance of a greenish-blue color indicates the presence of bilirubin.

2. Diazo test

Bilirubin couples with dichloroaniline (diazotized) under strongly acidic medium:

$$\text{Bilirubin} + \text{Diazo salt} \xrightarrow{\text{acidic medium}} \text{Azobilirubin (blue)}$$
(pink to reddish-purple colored compound)

Unlike a gradual development of color in the case of normal urines, pathological urine is characterized by an immediate development and a rapid disappearance of the color.

(ii) Urobilinogen

Urobilinogen is formed from conjugated bilirubin by the action of intestinal bacteria.

1. Modified Ehrlich test

Principle:

$$\text{Urobilinogen} + \text{p-diethylaminobenzaldehyde} \xrightarrow{\text{acidic medium}} \text{pink red color (positive)}$$

Results

Positive: Appearance of deep red color indicates an increased amount of urobilinogen.

Negative: The appearance of a faint pink or brown color indicates a normal amount of urobilinogen.

If its concentration exceeds 2 mg/dL, the cause may be clinical as shown in Table 53.5.

Table 53.5: Clinical applications of bilirubin and urobilinogen

Bile pigment	Normal	Liver disease	Hemolytic disease	Biliary obstruction
Bilirubin	negative	positive	negative	positive
Urobilinogen	positive	elevated	elevated	negative/decreased

e. Bile salts

Bile salts play an important role in digestion because they emulsify fats in the intestine.

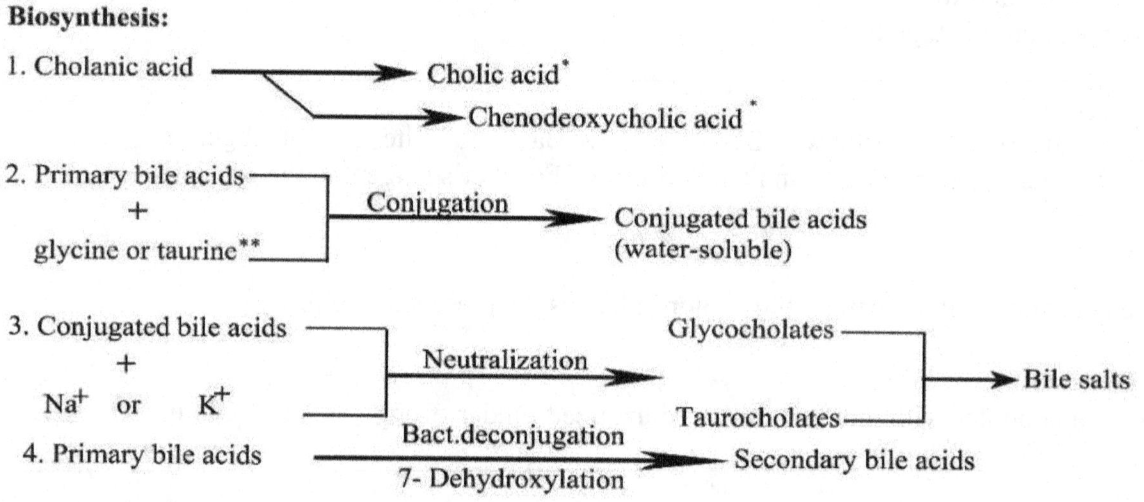

Biosynthesis:

1. Cholanic acid ⟶ Cholic acid[*]
   ⟶ Chenodeoxycholic acid[*]

2. Primary bile acids
   +
   glycine or taurine[**] —— Conjugation ⟶ Conjugated bile acids (water-soluble)

3. Conjugated bile acids
   +
   Na^+ or K^+ —— Neutralization ⟶ Glycocholates ——
   Taurocholates —— ⟶ Bile salts

4. Primary bile acids —— Bact.deconjugation / 7- Dehydroxylation ⟶ Secondary bile acids

[*]Primary bile acids
[**]Taurine is a cystine derivative

There are two methods to detect bile salts in the urine:
1. Hay's test
2. Test based on Pettenkofer's reaction

1. Hay's test

Principle:
The bile salts reduce the surface tension of the urine, making the particles of sulfur sink to the bottom.

Clinical Significance:
Causes of positive bile salts in the urine are obstructive jaundice and liver diseases with the appearance of jaundice.

f. Ketones

The formation of ketone bodies occurs during the catabolism of fatty acids. Acetoacetic acid is formed from acetyl CoA. Thereafter, acetone and β-hydroxybutyric acid is derived from acetoacetic acid as follow:

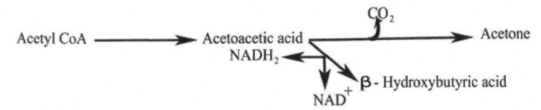

Rothera's test

Principle

An alkaline solution of sodium nitroprusside forms a purple colored complex in the presence of acetone and acetoacetic acid. β-hydroxybutyrate is not detected.

Procedure:

1. Saturate about 3 mL of urine with ammonium sulfate.
2. Add 2 drops of sodium nitroprusside.
3. Add a few drops of ammonia, running along the inner wall of the test tube.

Results:

Positive: The appearance of a purple ring at the junction suggests the presence of ketones.
Negative: No development of a purple ring indicates the absence of ketones.

Other tests that can be used to detect ketone bodies are Gerhardt's test, Lang's test, Linderman's test, Han's test, and Tablet test.

Clinical Significance:

- Diabetes mellitus
- Starvation
- Prolonged vomiting and diarrhea
- Dietary imbalance

g. Occult blood

The presence of red cells in the urine is called 'hematuria'. If hemolysis of red cells (e.g., black-water fever) occurs, free hemoglobin is found in the urine called 'hemoglobinuria'.

Stool Guaiac test (see chapter 54)

Causes of hematuria:

- Acute nephritis
- Renal calculi
- Renal carcinoma
- Polycystic kidneys
- Nephrotic syndrome
- Bacterial endocarditis

Causes of hemoglobinuria:

- Severe burns
- Hemolytic anemias
- Transfusion reactions
- Allergic reactions
- Multiple myeloma
- Poisonous mushrooms

h. Nitrite

The nitrite test[36] is used for the early detection of significant and asymptomatic bacteriuria:

$$\text{Nitrate} \xrightarrow{\text{Bact. reduction}} \text{Nitrite}$$
$$(E.\ coli,\ Klebsiella,\ Enterobacter,\ Proteus,\ \text{and}\ Citrobacter\ \text{spp.})$$

1. N-Multistix (dry reagent strip)

Principle:

$$\text{Nitrite + p-Arsanilic acid} \xrightarrow{\text{Acid pH}} \text{diazonium compound}$$
$$+$$
$$1, 2, 3, 4\text{- tetrahydro-benzo [h] quinolin-3-ol}$$
$$\downarrow \text{(after 40 seconds)}$$
$$\text{Pink color}$$

i. Leukocyte esterase

Leukocyte esterase test is an indirect screening test to rule out urinary tract infections (UTIs). Normally, urine specimens contain 0-5 leukocytes per high power field. A clean-catch urine specimen is needed for this test. A ready-made reagent strip is immersed in the urine and taken out. The color change on the pad suggests positive/negative results (follow manufacturer's directions). The interfering substances include trichomonas infection and vaginal secretions (e.g., blood or heavy mucus discharge) that lead to falsely positive results. False-negative results can be caused by the presence of high content of vitamin C and protein.

---

[36] First morning urine is preferable as a specimen.

3. Microscopic examination: (see Fig. 53.2)

About 5-10 mL of urine is centrifuged to obtain sediment or deposit. The supernatant fluid is poured off, and the deposit is mixed by tapping the bottom of the tube. The deposit is transferred to a slide, covered with a cover glass, and examined microscopically using the 10x and 40x objectives, with a reduced condenser aperture.

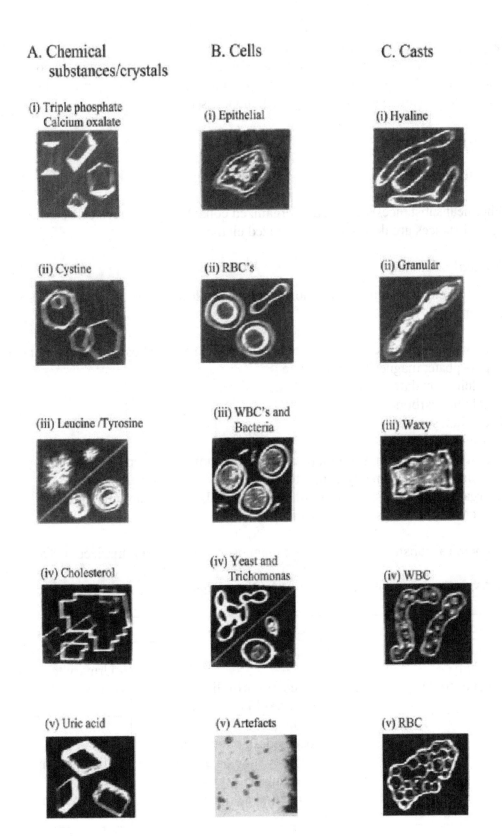

A. Chemical substances/crystals

(i) Triple phosphate Calcium oxalate

(ii) Cystine

(iii) Leucine /Tyrosine

(iv) Cholesterol

(v) Uric acid

B. Cells

(i) Epithelial

(ii) RBC's

(iii) WBC's and Bacteria

(iv) Yeast and Trichomonas

(v) Artefacts

C. Casts

(i) Hyaline

(ii) Granular

(iii) Waxy

(iv) WBC

(v) RBC

Fig. 53.2: Chemical substances, cells, and casts found in the urinary deposit.

505

Urinary deposits are detected in the first morning specimen collected in a clean and dry container. Furthermore, it is advisable to examine the urine within an hour or so after collection. Alternatively, it is stored at 2°-8°C no longer than 24 hours to examine for urinary deposits. Urinary deposits can be grouped into four main classes:

a. chemical substances
b. cells
c. casts

The chemical substances are called unorganized constituents whereas cells, casts, organisms, and foreign substances are described as organized elements.

a. Chemical substances

They may be either crystalline or amorphous. The following chemical substances can be found in urine sediment:

1. phosphates: magnesium ammonium phosphate (triple phosphate), calcium hydrogen phosphate, magnesium phosphate
2. calcium oxalate
3. calcium carbonate
4. calcium sulfate
5. uric acid
6. urates: ammonium, sodium, potassium, calcium, and magnesium
7. amino acids: cystine, tyrosine, leucine
8. organic substances: Cholesterol, hippuric acid, indigo, xanthine, bilirubin, and occasionally drugs or their metabolites

Those chemical substances which are of diagnostic value are summarized in Table 53.6.

Table 53.6: Chemical substances and their clinical significance

Chemical substance	Characteristics	Clinical significance
Magnesium ammonium phosphate (triple phosphate)	− seen in alkaline urine − colorless − prism-shaped or coffin lid type or the feathery, fernlike variety	- Urinary tract infection (UTI)
Calcium oxalate	− seen in acidic urine − usually, octahedral, or envelope-shaped, but they may be ellipsoidal (side view dumb-bell shaped) − soluble in mineral acids, but not in acetic acid.	− renal calculi − idiopathic hypercalciuria − primary hyperparathyroidism

Table 53.6 (cont.): Chemical substances and their clinical significance

Chemical substance	Characteristics	Clinical significance
Uric acid	– seen in acidic urine – color may be red-brown, yellow, or colorless	– although increased in 16% of patients with gout and patients with malignant
	– may assume various forms e.g., rhombic plates, rosettes, or barrel – soluble in sodium hydroxide, but not in HCl or acetic acid	-lymphoma or leukemia, their presence does not usually indicate pathology or increased uric acid concentrations
Cystine	– colorless – thin, hexagonal-shaped structures – soluble in alkalis and mineral acids, but not in the water, acetic acid, ethanol, and ether. – formation of stones occur at an acidic pH when the concentration of cystine exceeds 300 mg	– genetic defect – cystinuria and homocystinuria
Leucine and tyrosine	– leucine is yellow, oily, appearing spheres with radial and circular striations. – tyrosine is yellow, tufts of fine needles arranged as sheaves or rosettes – both are insoluble in acetone and ether, but soluble in acids.	– severe liver disease (e.g., acute yellow atrophy)
Cholesterol	– appear as irregularly or regularly notched, transparent plates. – soluble in ether, ethanol, and chloroform, but not in the water, acids, and alkalis.	– some diseases of the kidneys and renal tract

b. Cells

Various types of cells found in urine sediments are summarized in Table 53.7.

Table 53.7: Cells found in urine sediments

Type(s) of cell	Characteristics	Clinical significance
Epithelial: *(i) squamous*	– originate in the bladder, urethra, or vagina – large and flat with abundant cytoplasm – prominent small oval-shaped nucleus – cell edge is often folded	– seen in urine sediments of normal persons
(ii) renal tubular	– slightly larger than a leukocyte (<15μm) – contains a large round nucleus	– rarely seen in normal urine, but found in some renal diseases
(iii) transitional	– originate from the bladder, prostate, ureters, and pelvis – two to three times the size of a leukocyte – have a round nucleus (sometimes two nuclei) – tend to be pear or spindle-shaped	– frequently seen after prostate massage and ureteric catheterization
Pus	– originate from any part of the renal system. – appear as round granular spheres – larger than red blood cells (about 12μ in diameter) – 'Glitter' cells are polymorphonuclear leukocytes showing Brownian movement in their cytoplasmic granules	– presence of >1 pus cell per high power field in males or >5 pus cells per high power field in females or children indicates infection, cystitis, or pyelonephritis
Red blood cells	– may originate from any part of the renal system – appear round or biconcave in shape – yellow colored – lack nucleus – the shape varies, depending upon the concentration of the dissolved solutes in the urine – lysis in acetic acid	– The presence of large numbers of R.B.Cs indicates infection, trauma, tumors, renal calculi **Note:** Blood from menstrual contamination should not be considered abnormal.

Table 53.7 (cont.): Cells found in urine sediments

Type of cell	Characteristics	Clinical significance
Yeast cells	– colorless – vary in size – ovoid – asexual reproduction by budding – are mistaken for red blood cells – lysis does not occur by treatment with 2% acetic acid	– *Candida albicans* causes candidiasis and is often found in diabetes, pregnancy, obesity, and other debilitating conditions
Trichomonas vaginalis	– appears as leukocytes – flagellate protozoan	– causes urethritis in males and vaginitis in females
Bacteria	– Gram-ve small rods, occurring singly, in pairs, or clusters – Gram +ve cocci (e.g., *Streptococcus faecalis*), occurring in chains	– cause urinary tract infections
Spermatozoa	– Long and slender structures, consisting of the head, middle-piece and tail	– seen normally in the urine of males after emission of semen – after prostatic massage

c. Casts

Casts seen in urine are listed in Table 53.8.

Table 53.8: Casts seen in urine specimens

Type of cast	Characteristics	Clinical significance
Hyaline	– have a pale, transparent, homogeneous structure – are cylindrical – vary considerably in length and breadth – composed of a protein gel in the renal tubule – dissolve very rapidly in alkaline urine and acetic acid	– presence of more hyaline casts per high power suggests pathological proteinuria
Granular	– contain closely packed granules of varying degrees of coarseness – may contain a certain amount of fat	– presence in fairly high numbers suggest degeneration of the tubular epithelium

Table 53.8 (cont.): Casts seen in urine specimens

Type of cast	Characteristics	Clinical significance
Waxy (Colloid)	– composed of a highly refractile substance which often has a yellowish tinge and a dull opaque luster – are shorter and wider than other casts – insoluble in acetic acid	– severe chronic renal disease and renal amyloidosis
WBC	– leukocytes are incorporated within the cast matrix	– presence suggests pyelonephritis and glomerular diseases
RBC	– contain erythrocytes in a bag like structure within the cast matrix	– renal hematuria – acute glomerulonephritis – copus, bacterial endocarditis, septicemias

Also, artifacts in urine can be confusing to the inexperienced examiner. Common artifacts include cotton fibers, powder, and oil droplets.

Chapter 54

Examination of Stool

Introduction

Laboratory personnel hesitate to approach the feces because of their obnoxious nature. But, the examination of stool is of great diagnostic value. For example, microscopic examination reveals the type of parasite involved in the infestation.

The stool is to be carefully collected in a well-rinsed bedpan lined with a plastic sheet. Thereafter, the specimen of stool is transferred to a suitable container (e.g., leak-proof cardboard, plastic, or glass), using a spatula or tongue depressor. In the case of some tests (e.g., occult blood), a carefully selected portion of the stool is sent in a waxed carton. Furthermore, care is to be taken to avoid contamination of stool with urine, since urine harms protozoa.

It is highly desirable to examine fresh specimens of stool. Feces are examined from four aspects:

- A. Physical examination
- B. Chemical examination
- C. Microscopic examination
- D. Microbiological examination

A. Physical Examination

The stool is inspected for the following preliminary tests:

a. Quantity

Two-thirds of the weight of the average stool is due to its water content. Moreover, bacteria contribute about one-third of the total weight of stool. The stool is soft and bulky from a person consuming a diet rich in vegetables. On the other hand, it is dry and less bulky if the diet consists largely of meat. Normally, 100-200 g of stool is excreted per day.

b. Consistency

- firm and formed (normal)
- hard and dry (diuretics, aging, and other causes)
- soft and formed
- soft and unformed
- semi-solid
- mushy, foul-smelling, and gray (steatorrhea)
- firm and spherical masses (constipation)
- liquid and watery (diarrhea)
- watery; like rice-water (cholera)
- oily stool (malabsorption)

c. Color

- light to dark brown due to stercobilin (normal)
- yellow-brown or yellow-green (children)
- clay-colored (obstructive jaundice)
- black-tarry (upper GIT)

d. Odor

Due to the formation of indole and skatole from tryptophan by bacteria, stool specimens normally smell unpleasant. It mainly depends upon the type of food people eat and the microbial flora of the colon.

Abnormal characteristics

- flakes of mucus
- streaks of pus
- blood-stained mucus (dysentery)
- blood in the stool (*Cl. difficile* colitis)
- mucous membranes
- worms or segments of worms, e.g., *A. lumbricoides*, *E. vermicularis* (infestation)

B. Chemical examination

Fecal occult blood test (FOBT)

The fecal occult blood test is routinely performed to detect occult (hidden) blood in the stool specimen. This screening test aids to detect digestive tract-related bleeding disorders e.g., peptic ulcer, colon cancer, gastritis, Crohn's disease, hemorrhoids, and colon polyps. Guaiac, a plant substance, is used in disposable test cards. Guaiac (colorless) turns blue (i.e., oxidized) in the presence of hydrogen peroxide if stool contains red cells. Patients are instructed not to consume some foods (e.g., red meat, radish, horseradish, turnip, uncooked broccoli, and cantaloupe) to avoid false-positive results. Also, some medicines (e.g., vitamin C and aspirin) may interfere with the test.

Unlike guaiac-based tests (gFOBT, cFOBT), immunological occult blood tests (iFOBT) are more sensitive and specific. Thus, the false-positive results of guaiac-based testing are avoided. This explains why immunological fecal occult blood test (iFOBT) rendered guaiac fecal occult blood test (gFOBT) obsolete.

C. Microscopic examination: (see Fig. 54.1)

Usually, saline and iodine preparations are examined for the identification and differentiation of stool parasites. One has to look for ova, cysts, and larvae of worms and protozoa. In addition to this, pus cells, red blood cells, yeast cells, and free-living forms of amoebae (i.e., flagellates or ciliates) are also to be reported.

1. Saline preparation

Since physiological saline is isotonic with living organisms, organisms remain alive in this preparation. Crystal clear saline must be used for this purpose.

The pea-sized stool is mixed with saline and is covered with a coverslip. This preparation is examined under low power and high power objectives, keeping the condenser racked down and with a reduced condenser aperture. In the case of slimy stools, preparation can be made without saline. Here, excess mucus is pressed out on a slide under a coverslip and cleaned with the help of blotting paper.

2. Iodine preparation

This preparation is made in the same way as saline preparation. It allows one to examine the nuclear structure of cysts, thus differentiating them from host white blood cells. Iodine stains the chromatin granules and karyosome of nuclei, brown. But, the chromatoid bars remain unstained. The differences between amoebic and bacillary dysentery are listed in Table 54.1.

Intestinal parasites: (see Fig. 54.1)

1. *Entamoeba histolytica*: Fully developed four-nucleated cyst, containing chromatid bodies (saline preparation)

2. *Entamoeba histolytica:* Four-nucleated cyst (iodine preparation)

3. *Entamoeba histolytica:* Active form, containing included red blood cells (saline preparation)

4. *Iodamoeba buetschlii:* Cyst (saline preparation). Note the unstained glycogen vacuole

5. *Entamoeba coli:* Fully developed eight-nucleated cyst (saline preparation)

6. *Entamoeba coli:* Eight-nucleated (stained by Lugol's iodine solution)

7. *Entamoeba coli:* Active form (saline preparation)

8. *Iodamoeba buetschlii:* Cyst (stained by Lugol's iodine solution)

9. *Giardia lamblia:* Cyst form (stained by Heidenhain's hematoxylin)

10. *Giardia lamblia:* Active form (stained by Heidenhain's hematoxylin)

11. *Trichomonas hominis:* Stained by Giemsa's method

12. *Isospora belli (I. hominis):* Undeveloped oocyst as passed in human feces

13. *Balantidium coli:* Active form (stained by Heidenhain's hematoxylin)

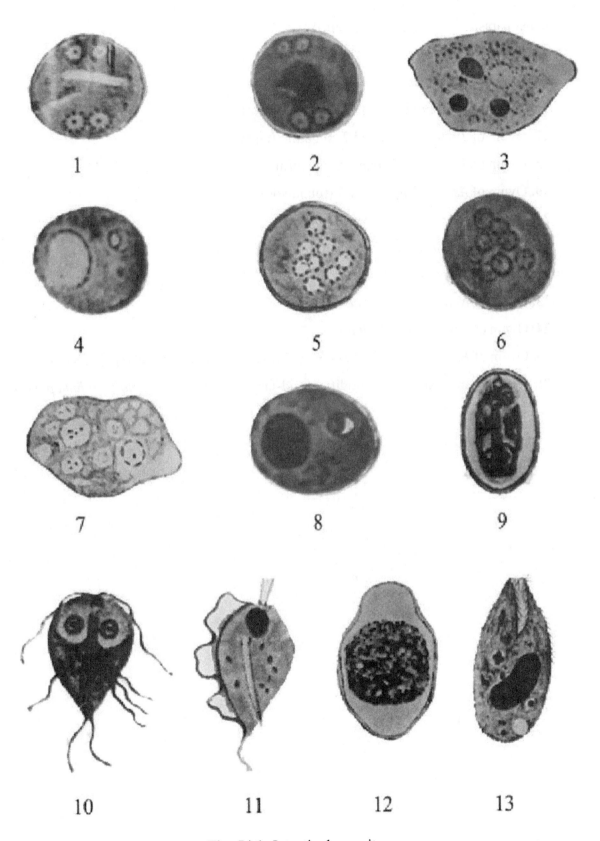

Fig. 54.1: Intestinal parasites.

Intestinal parasites: {see Fig. 54.1 (cont.)}

14. *Strongyloides stercoralis*: The rhabditiform larva

15. Ovum of *Ancylostoma duodenale* (hookworm)

16. Ovum of *Enterobius vermicularis* (threadworm)

17. Ovum of *Taenia solium* and *T. saginata* (tapeworm)

18. Ovum of *Trichuris trichiura* (whipworm)

19. Ovum of *Ascaris lumbricoides* (roundworm)

20. Ovum of *Schistosoma haematobium*

21. Ovum of *Schistosoma japonicum*

22. Ovum of *Schistosoma mansoni*

23. Ovum of *Necator americanus*

24. Ovum of *Diphyllobothrium latum*

25. Ovum of *Paragonimus westermani* and Charcot-Leyden crystals (polarized light)

26. Red oocysts (stained by a modified acid-fast technique) of *Cryptosporidium parvum*

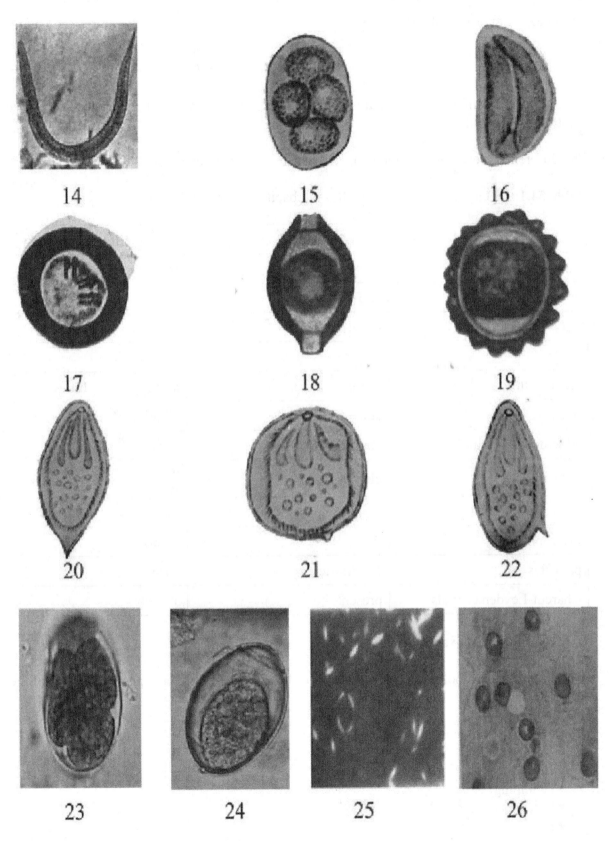

Fig. 54.1 (cont.)**:** Intestinal parasites.

Preparation of normal saline

Sodium chloride	0.90 g
Distilled water	to 100 mL

Note: If saline is infected with organisms (e.g., algae, small flagellates), it is discarded and a fresh solution is prepared.

The differences between amoebic and bacillary dysentery are listed in Table 54.1.

Table 54.1: Differences between amoebic and bacillary dysentery

Test	Amoebic dysentery	Bacillary dysentery
number of stools/day	6 - 8	more than 10
amount	copious	small
odor	offensive	odorless
color	dark red	bright red
fecal matter	present	absent or very little
reaction	acid	alkaline
adherence to container	absent	present
red cells	clumps	discrete or rouleaux formation
pus cells	scanty	plenty
macrophages	few	plenty
parasites	*E. histolytica*	absent
Charcot-Leyden crystals	present	absent

D. Microbiological examination

A microbiological stool test (stool culture) is ordered by the health care provider in one of the following conditions:

- Presence of mucus or blood in the stool
- Nausea
- Vomiting
- Cramping
- Diarrhea (if lasts > 3 days)
- Fever

To collect an acceptable stool specimen for a culture test, the patient needs to strictly follow the instructions during the collection. The most common intestinal pathogenic bacteria include:

- *E. coli* 0157:H7
- *Salmonella* spp.
- *Shigella* spp.
- *Yersinia enterocolitica*
- *Vibrio* spp.
- *Campylobacter* spp.
- *Clostridium difficile*

A request for *Helicobacter pylori* is processed only in case of a special complaint from the patient.

Since stool samples largely contain coliforms, it is difficult to isolate the causative agent of the disease for identification. Therefore, various selective media and enrichment techniques are employed as a part of the stool processing protocol. For more details, the reader should refer to chapter 37.

Chapter 55

Semen Analysis

Introduction

Examination of semen (seminal fluid) is carried out in the following situations:

1. Infertility problems
2. Forensic studies (e.g., the examination of vaginal secretions or clothing stains for the presence of semen in alleged or suspected rape cases)
3. To disprove a denial of paternity on the grounds of sterility
4. Semen donors for semen bank
5. Investigation for the effectiveness of vasectomy (Usually, semen is examined after 3 months of operation without sexual abstinence)

Collection

It is recommended that the semen specimen should be collected following three days of sexual abstinence. Semen is usually collected by masturbation in the laboratory. Alternatively, it is collected by coitus interruptus at the patient's residence. If the condom is to be used in the collection of semen, it must first be washed with soap and water, rinsed, and finally dried. Thus, the effect of any spermicidal agents is avoided. Semen specimens can be collected in a wide-mouth clean glass jar or plastic or polyethylene containers.

After its collection, it must be sent to the laboratory, preferably within 30 minutes. It is advisable to examine it soon after its liquefaction. Examination of seminal fluid is channeled in three ways:

A. Physical examination
B. Chemical examination
C. Microscopic examination

A. Physical examination

Tests routinely performed under physical examination are summarized in Table 55.1.

Table 55.1: Physical examination of semen

Test	Normal value
color	greyish-white
odor	fishy
appearance	thick and viscous
volume	2-4 mL
reaction (pH)	alkaline (pH 7.2-8.0)
liquefaction time	within 30 minutes

B. Chemical examination
Seliwanoff's test for fructose

Principle: Hot HCl converts fructose to hydroxymethylfurfural which, in turn, combines with resorcinol to form a red-colored compound.

Reagent

Resorcinol	50 mg
Conc. HCl	33 mL
Distilled water to	100 mL

Note: Dissolve resorcinol in conc. HCl, add distilled water to make the final volume of 100 mL.

Procedure

1. Take 5 mL of the reagent in a clean and dry test tube.
2. Add 0.5 mL of semen.
3. Keep in a boiling water bath for 2 minutes.
4. Record the results.

Results: The development of the red color indicates the positivity of the test.

C. Microscopic examination

a. Motility

This is a valuable test, grading the semen specimen as very good, good, and poor. Normally, 80 percent of the spermatozoa are actively motile and 20 percent are sluggish or completely non-motile.

Procedure

1. Place a drop of liquefied semen on a clean and dry glass slide and cover it with a coverslip.
2. Apply petroleum jelly at the edge of the coverslip to prevent dehydration.
3. Examine under low-power and high-power.
4. Record the proportion of motile to non-motile forms as an average value by examining various fields.
5. Save the slide by keeping it in a damp chamber at room temperature and examine after 3 hours, 6 hours, 12 hours, and 24 hours (There is a little or no reduction of motility at the end of 3 hours. On the other hand, the total loss of motility occurs at the end of 12 hours in normal semen specimens).
6. Record the number of hours of motility of spermatozoa.

Note: Report if there are any pus cells, red blood cells, epithelial cells, or crystals.

b. Viability

Sperm viability (vitality) assessment is based on a dye exclusion method. The dye fails to enter the viable sperms because their plasma membrane is intact (unbroken). Dead spermatozoa have a damaged membrane, allowing the dye to color them.

The assay is performed immediately after liquefaction. Equal amounts of both semen and a vital stain (trypan blue) are mixed on a slide. Then, a coverslip is placed and left for at least 5 minutes for the reaction to occur. Differentiation is made between the stained (dead) and unstained (living) while counting 100 sperms (motile and non-motile).

Eosin-nigrosin can also be used as a vital stain. This method allows for easier identification of the viable sperms against the dark background due to nigrosin. Heads of dead sperms stain red/dark pink as opposed to white/light pink heads of the living ones.

The viability assessment test of sperms is valuable, particularly in the case of a low percentage of progressively motile counts, i.e., 30-40%.

c. Total count

Counting spermatozoa by the use of a counting chamber is a relatively inaccurate method. This is easy to understand because of the viscous nature of semen. Therefore, it is advisable to take an average value of the number of counts made (at least two times) from the specimen.

Procedure

1. Mix the completely liquified semen specimen by gentle shaking.
2. Fill a small graduated test tube or a cylinder with semen up to the 1 mL mark accurately.
3. Add the semen diluting fluid up to the mark of 20 mL to make 1 in 20 dilutions.
4. Mix the contents of the container well.
5. Charge the improved Neubauer counting chamber, using a Pasteur pipette.
6. Allow the spermatozoa to settle by leaving the chamber undisturbed for 3-4 minutes.
7. Count the spermatozoa in four large corner squares (4 sq mm) as in total leukocyte count.
8. Calculate the number of spermatozoa per mL of undiluted semen as under:

$$\text{Spermatozoa/mL} = \frac{N \times 10 \times 20 \times 1000}{4}$$

$$= N \times 50,000 \text{ (Normal count: 40-300 million/mL)}$$

d. Abnormal forms

Abnormalities of the morphology of spermatozoa are studied in the stained smear.

Procedure

1. Prepare a thin smear of liquefied semen on a glass slide.
2. Allow the smear to air-dry.
3. Fix the smear by passing it quickly over the Bunsen flame and allow it to cool.
4. Cover the smear with a 0.25% aqueous solution of basic fuchsin for 5 minutes.
5. Wash it with tap water and dry it in the air after blotting.
6. Examine under the oil-immersion lens.
7. Count all spermatozoa in the microscopic field (see Fig. 55.1).
8. Count abnormal forms seen in the microscopic field (see Fig. 55.2).
9. Calculate the percentage of abnormal forms seen.

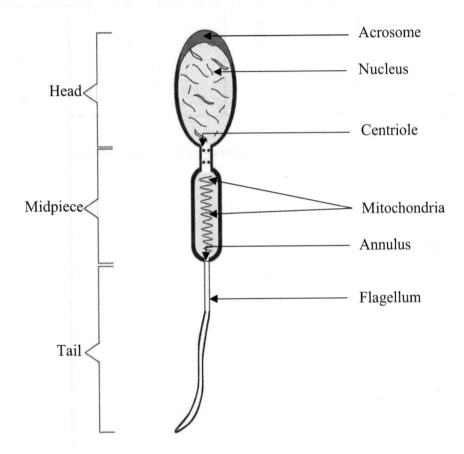

Fig. 55.1: Normal spermatozoan.

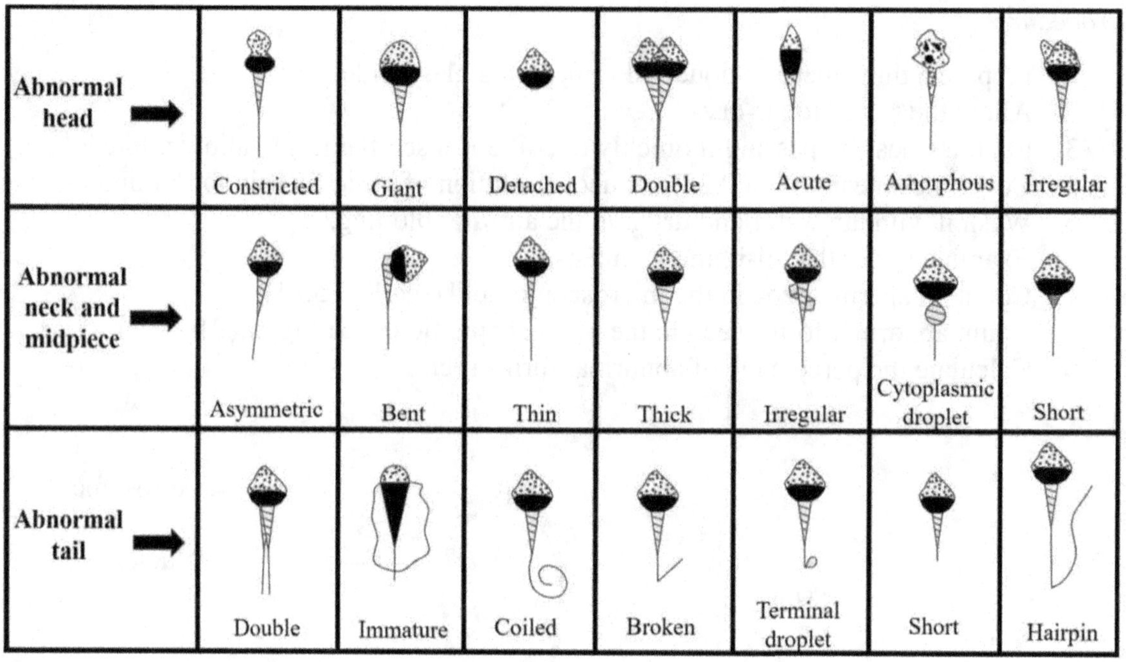

Abnormal head →	Constricted	Giant	Detached	Double	Acute	Amorphous	Irregular
Abnormal neck and midpiece →	Asymmetric	Bent	Thin	Thick	Irregular	Cytoplasmic droplet	Short
Abnormal tail →	Double	Immature	Coiled	Broken	Terminal droplet	Short	Hairpin

Fig. 55.2: Abnormal forms of spermatozoan.

Questions

1. Intracorpuscular defect-related hemolysis occurs in:

    A. Thalassemia
    B. Hereditary spherocytosis
    C. Sickle cell disease
    D. Paroxysmal nocturnal hemoglobinuria (PNH)
    E. All of the above

2. Which of the following characteristics are associated with the plasma cell?

    A. Eccentric nucleus
    B. Deep blue cytoplasm
    C. Presence of vacuoles in the cytoplasm
    D. Perinuclear halo
    E. All of the above

3. A low level of leukocyte alkaline phosphatase may be detected in:

    A. Leukemoid reactions
    B. *Polycythemia vera*
    C. Chronic lymphocytic leukemia
    D. Chronic myelogenous leukemia
    E. None of the above

4. What age group is commonly victimized by acute lymphocytic leukemia?

    A. 3- 6 years
    B. 13-16 years
    C. 23-26 years
    D. 1- 2 years
    E. 63 years and older

5. Differentiation between T and B lymphocytes can best be done by:

    A. Leukocyte alkaline phosphatase (LAP)
    B. Monoclonal antibodies to surface antigens
    C. Supravital stains
    D. New methylene blue
    E. None of the above

6. Toxic granulation is an indication of:

    A. Relative lymphocytosis
    B. Severe septicemia

C. Reactive lymphocytosis

D. Myelofibrosis

E. None of the above

7. Elevated prothrombin time (PT) is seen in:

A. Congenital factor VII deficiency

B. Obstructive liver disease

C. Hemorrhagic disease of the newborn

D. Venous thrombosis treated with warfarin

E. All of the above

8. Hypersegmentation is an outstanding laboratory finding in:

A. Iron deficiency anemia

B. Pernicious anemia

C. Aplastic anemia

D. Acute loss anemia

E. None of the above

9. Which of the following hemoglobins is composed of four beta chains?

A. Hemoglobin A

B. Hemoglobin F

C. Hemoglobin H

D. Hemoglobin Barts

E. None of the above

10. Which of the following hemoglobins is composed of two alpha and two beta chains?

A. Hemoglobin F

B. Hemoglobin A_2

C. Hemoglobin A

D. Hemoglobin D

E. None of the above

11. Sickling is seen in patients with:

A. Hemoglobin D

B. Hemoglobin S

C. Hemoglobin C

D. Hemoglobin F

E. None of the above

12. Differentiation between sickle cell disease and sickle cell trait can be made by:

A. ELISA

B. Electrophoresis

C. Examination of the peripheral blood smear

D. Schilling test

E. None of the above

13. Which of the following main factors can be associated with anemia?

A. Bone-marrow (e.g., leukemia or lymphomas)

B. Nutrition (e.g., iron, vitamin B12, and folate)

C. Kidneys

D. Alcoholism

E. All of the above

14. Which of the following characteristics are commonly associated with hereditary spherocytosis?

A. Red cell membrane disorder

B. RBCs are small and almost spherical

C. Excessive fragility in hypotonic saline solutions

D. Can be cured by the removal of the spleen

E. All of the above

15. Which of the following disorders are associated with an elevated leukocyte percentage?

A. Hemolytic disorders (intrinsic and extrinsic)

B. Recovery from a nutritional anemia

C. Recovery of erythropoiesis following bone-marrow suppression

D. Acute reticulocytosis following acute blood loss

E. All of the above

16. All of the following causes are etiologic causes of thrombocytopenia *except*:

A. Idiopathic thrombocytopenic purpura (ITP)

B. Megaloblastic anemia

C. Post-splenectomy

D. Acute myeloproliferative disorders

E. Splenic sequestration

17. All of the following causes are etiologic causes of thrombocytosis *except*:

A. *Polycythemia vera*

B. Iron deficiency

C. Post-splenectomy

D. Chronic myeloproliferative disorders

E. Disseminated intravascular coagulation (DIC)

18. Which of the following coagulation factor deficiencies cause an elevated prothrombin time?

A. Factor V
B. Fibrinogen
C. Factor X
D. Factor VII
E. All of the above

19. Which of the following coagulation factors is *NOT* vitamin-k dependent?

A. Factor VIII
B. Factor X
C. XI
D. Thrombin
E. Factor VII

20. Which chemical compound in the urine is associated with bacteriuria?

A. Cholesterol
B. Nitrite
C. Triple phosphate
D. Tyrosine
E. Bilirubin

21. Which of the following diseases are associated with normocytic-normochromic RBCs?

A. Sickle cell disease
B. Sickle cell trait
C. Hemoglobin C trait (AC) and hemoglobin C disease (CC)
D. Hereditary spherocytosis and acute blood loss
E. All of the above

22. Which of the following disorders are linked with microcytic-hypochromic RBCs?

A. Sideroblastic disorder
B. Chronic blood loss
C. Beta thalassemia minor and beta-thalassemia major (cooley's anemia)
D. Iron deficiency anemia
E. All Of the above

23. Which of the following urinary crystals can be described as hexagonal, monomorphic, transparent, ammonia soluble, and insoluble in water?

A. Calcium oxalate
B. Phosphate
C. Cystine

D. Uric acid

E. None of the above

24. Which of the following urinary crystals can be detected in acidic urine?

    A. Ca-oxalate

    B. Tyrosine

    C. Cholesterol

    D. Leucine and cysteine

    E. All of the above

25. Which of the following diseases is associated with decreased excretion of 17 - hydroxycorticoids and 17-ketosteroids?

    A. Multiple myeloma

    B. Addison's disease

    C. Cystinuria

    D. Hepatitis B

    E. Acute pancreatitis

26. Which of the following disorders can be held accountable for elevated ESR?

    A. Agglutination of RBCs

    B. Multiple myeloma

    C. Pregnancy

    D. Anemia

    E. All of the above

27. Which of the following disorders can be linked with the presence of nucleated RBCs in the peripheral smear?

    A. Myelogenous leukemia

    B. *Erythroblastosis fetalis*

    C. Normal newborn

    D. Severe anemia

    E. All of the above

28. What is the developmental stage of a white blood cell where there is a disappearance of nuclei and a differentiation of granules occur?

    A. Myeloblast

    B. Promyelocyte

    C. Myelocyte

    D. Metamyelocyte

    E. Band neutrophil

29. Which of the following is the breakdown product of heme?

A. Albumin
B. Globulin
C. Bilirubin
D. Urobilin
E. None of the above

30. Which of the following pairs of LDH isoenzymes play an important role in cardiac disease?

A. LDH_1 and LDH_2
B. LDH_4 and LDH_5
C. LDH_2 and LDH_3
D. LDH_2 and LDH_5
E. None of the above

31. Which of the following formulae is a correct formula for the standard deviation (SD)?

A. $-\log [H^+]$

B. $\quad s = \sqrt{\dfrac{\sum (x - \bar{x})^2}{n - 1}}$

C. $pK' + \log \dfrac{salt}{acid}$

D. $2 - \log 10\%T$

E. None of the above

32. Which of the following equations is a correct equation for the coefficient of variation (CV)?

A. $\%CV = \dfrac{SD}{X}$

B. $C = \dfrac{UV}{P}$

C. $mEq/L = \dfrac{mg/L}{eq.wt.}$

D. $M = \dfrac{\% \times 10}{mol.wt.}$

E. None of the above

530

33. **Which of the following sugars is a monosaccharide?**

   A. Sucrose
   B. Lactose
   C. Glycogen
   D. Glucose
   E. None of the above

34. **Which of the following sugars is a polysaccharide?**

   A. Glucose
   B. Sucrose
   C. Fructose
   D. Glycogen
   E. None of the above

35. **Which of the following methods for the determination of glucose is used as a reference method?**

   A. *o*-Toluidine
   B. Glucose dehydrogenase
   C. Glucose oxidase
   D. Hexokinase
   E. None of the above

36. **Which of the following terms is used to describe the conversion of hexoses into pyruvic acid?**

   A. Glycogenolysis
   B. Glycolysis
   C. Gluconeogenesis
   D. Glycogenesis
   E. None of the above

37. **Which of the following characteristics can be associated with Type I diabetes mellitus?**

   A. Autoimmune destruction of B cells and absolute deficiency of insulin
   B. Early-onset (under 20 years of age)
   C. Susceptible to Diabetic ketoacidosis (DKA)
   D. Occurs less frequently than Type II (IDDM)
   E. All of the above

38. **Which of the following hormones are linked with the increase of blood glucose levels?**

   A. Cortisol
   B. Glucagon

C. Epinephrine
D. Growth hormone
E. All of the above

39. **Which of the following tests is recommended to reveal the blood glucose level in the past 2- to 3-month period?**

   A. Glucose tolerance test (GTT)
   B. Lactose tolerance test
   C. Glycosylated hemoglobin (A1c)
   D. D-Xylose absorption test
   E. Ketone bodies test

40. **Which of the following descriptions are associated with ketone bodies?**

   A. Formation of ketone bodies from fatty acids
   B. Includes acetone, acetoacetic acid, and β-hydroxybutyric acid
   C. Detection by sodium nitroprusside
   D. Formation under starvation
   E. All of the above

41. **Which of the following disorders are linked with the rise of blood urea nitrogen (BUN)/urea levels?**

   A. Kidney disease
   B. Dehydration
   C. High dietary protein intake
   D. Obstruction of urine flow
   E. All of the above

42. **Which of the following methods is used in the determination of urea?**

   A. Diacetylmonoxime (DAM)
   B. Uricase
   C. *o*-Toluidine
   D. Jaffe reaction
   E. Folin-Wu method

43. **Which of the following cations is a major extracellular cation?**

   A. Sodium
   B. Potassium
   C. Magnesium
   D. Bicarbonate
   E. Chloride

44. **Which of the following cations is a major intracellular cation?**

   A. Potassium
   B. Sodium
   C. Chloride
   D. Magnesium
   E. None of the above

45. **Which of the following diseases is linked with an elevated level of uric acid?**

   A. Alkaptonuria
   B. Phenylketonuria
   C. Gout
   D. Maple syrup disease
   E. Liver disease

46. **Which of the following methods is a reference method in the determination of proteins?**

   A. Biuret
   B. Kjeldahl
   C. Refractometry
   D. Electrophoresis
   E. All of the above

47. **Which of the following descriptions are associated with albumin?**

   A. Synthesis in the liver
   B. 60% of total serum protein
   C. Maintains plasma osmotic pressure
   D. Transportation of substances
   E. All of the above

48. **Which of the following facts can be linked with serum protein electrophoresis?**

   A. At buffer pH of 8.6, the order of migration of the serum proteins is albumin, alpha$_1$-globulin, alpha$_2$-globulin, beta-globulin, and gamma-globulin
   B. After the electrophoretic run, agarose gel (commonly used as a support medium) is stained by Coomassie Blue or Ponceau S to visualize the protein bands
   C. Absence of fibrinogen
   D. Most proteins possess a negative electrical charge at an alkaline pH of 8.6, enabling them to migrate toward the anode
   E. All of the above

49. **Which of the following factors influence the enzyme activity?**

   A. Temperature and pH
   B. Presence or absence of activator or inhibitor

533

C. Nature and concentration of enzyme and substrate
D. Presence or absence of a coenzyme
E. All of the above

50. **Which of the following disorders are associated with elevated levels of alkaline phosphatase?**
A. Paget's disease
B. Gout
C. Biliary obstruction
D. Both A and C
E. None of the above

51. **Which of the following disorders is associated with a rise in aldolase levels?**

A. Muscle necrosis
B. Biliary obstruction
C. Bone disease
D. Alcoholic cirrhosis
E. Carcinoma

52. **Which of the following isoenzymes of creatine kinase (CK) is elevated in myocardial infarction (MI)?**

A. CK (MB)
B. CK (BB)
C. CK (MM)
D. Both B and C
E. LD$_4$

53. **Which of the following statements is *true* while assaying the enzyme activity?**

A. Zero-order kinetics
B. First order kinetics
C. Reaction rate is independent of the concentration of an enzyme
D. Reaction rate is not dependent on the concentration of a substrate
E. Both A and D

54. **Which of the following screening tests is a suitable test method for heavy metals e.g., lead?**

A. Trinder reaction
B. Reinsch test
C. Gas chromatography
D. Absorbance spectrophotometry
E. None of the above

55. **Which of the following vitamins are fat-soluble *except?***

   A. Vitamin A
   B. Vitamin B
   C. Vitamin D
   D. Vitamin E
   E. Vitamin K

56. **Which of the following facts apply to the deficiency of cyanocobalamin (vitamin B$_{12}$) *except?***

   A. Megaloblastic anemia
   B. Pernicious anemia
   C. Neuropathy
   D. Macrocytic-normochromic RBCs
   E. Microcytic-hypochromic RBCs

57. **Which of the following trace elements can be measured by atomic absorption spectrophotometry (AAS)?**

   A. Arsenic
   B. Zinc
   C. Mercury
   D. Copper
   E. All of the above

58. **Which of the following conditions affect the serum drug levels?**

   A. Age
   B. Underlying disease(s), e.g., renal, hepatic
   C. Genetics
   D. Smoking
   E. All of the above

59. **Which of the following diseases is associated with hyperthyroidism?**

   A. Adrenal carcinoma
   B. Addison's disease
   C. Graves' disease
   D. Cushing's syndrome
   E. None of the above

60. **Which of the following diseases can be linked with the reduced secretion of antidiuretic hormone (ADH)?**

   A. Diabetes mellitus
   B. Diabetes insipidus

C. Graves' disease
D. Addison's disease
E. Testicular tumors

61. **Which of the following disorders is associated with vitamin C deficiency?**

A. Beriberi
B. Scurvy
C. Hepatitis B
D. Pellagra
E. Cushing's syndrome

62. **Which of the following chemical compounds can be quantitated by radioimmunoassay (RIA) technique?**

A. Drugs
B. Ethanol
C. Vitamins
D. Both A and C
E. Carbon monoxide

63. **Which of the following drugs has a toxic effect on the liver?**

A. Digoxin
B. Barbiturate
C. Acetaminophen
D. Opiates
E. All of the above

64. **Which of the following hormones affect the plasma calcium levels?**

A. Parathyroid hormone (PTH)
B. Aldosterone
C. Cortisol
D. Progesterone
E. All of the above

65. **Abnormal accumulation of bilirubin in brain tissues is referred to as:**

A. Hepatitis
B. Kernicterus
C. Obstructive jaundice
D. Post-hepatic jaundice
E. None of the above

66. **Which of the following diseases is associated with the deposition of lipid in the liver, bone marrow, and spleen?**

   A. gout
   B. Addison's disease
   C. Gaucher's disease
   D. Tay-Sachs disease
   E. Obstructive jaundice

67. **Excessive concentration of dissolved carbon dioxide ($cdCO_2$) in the arterial blood leads to:**

   A. Metabolic acidosis
   B. Respiratory acidosis
   C. Metabolic alkalosis
   D. Respiratory alkalosis
   E. None of the above

68. **Coronary artery disease (CAD) assessment involves the measurement of:**

   A. low-density lipoprotein cholesterol (LDL-Cholesterol)
   B. High-density lipoprotein cholesterol (HDL-cholesterol)
   C. Fatty acids
   D. Chylomicron
   E. Alpha-lipoprotein

69. **Which of the following substances is combined with antigen to enhance the formation of antibodies?**

   A. Complement
   B. Haptens
   C. Adjuvant
   D. Normal saline
   E. None of the above

70. **Which of the following classes of immunoglobulins is a dimer found in tears?**

   A. IgD
   B. IgE
   C. IgA
   D. IgM
   E. IgG

71. **Which of the following classes of immunoglobulins is a pentamer and an excellent complement activator?**

A. IgA
B. IgG
C. IgE
D. IgM
E. IgD

72. **A stronger and faster secondary antibody response that produces a higher titer of IgG over IgM is called:**

A. Anamnestic reaction
B. Allergic reaction
C. Primary response
D. Inflammatory response
E. None of the above

73. **Which of the following antigen-antibody reactions use sheep RBCs, hemolysin, and complement as an indicator system?**

A. Agglutination
B. Precipitation
C. Complement-Fixation test
D. ELISA
E. Neutralization

74. **Failure of the immune system to recognize as "self" versus "non-self" is termed as:**

A. Prozone phenomenon
B. Autoimmunity
C. Active immunity
D. Passive Immunity
E. Zoning reaction

75. **Which of the following cells are transformed into plasma cells capable of producing antibodies?**

A. T cells
B. B cells
C. Giant platelets
D. Natural killer cells
E. T helper cells

76. **Which of the following cells is the main source of interleukin 2 (IL-2)?**

   A. Basophils
   B. B cells
   C. T cells
   D. Plasma cells
   E. None of the above

77. **Which of the following factors can be valid in the case of a *false negative* antiglobulin test?**

   A. Omission of anti-human globulin (AHG) reagent
   B. Inadequate cell washing
   C. Use of inactive AHG reagent
   D. Inadequate centrifugation
   E. All of the above

78. **Which of the following procedural steps are crucial while doing compatibility testing?**

   A. Checking of the recipient's history
   B. Determination of ABO, Rh as well as the detection of abnormal antibody (ies), if any, present in the recipient's serum
   C. Performing the ABO and Rh testing on a prospective donor unit before the compatibility testing
   D. Major cross-matching: immediate spin cross-match or full cross-match as the case may be
   E. All of the above

79. **Which of the following clotting factors are normally present in fresh frozen plasma?**

   A. Factor X
   B. Factor V
   C. Factor VIII
   D. Factor IX
   E. All of the following

80. **Which of the following red cell antibodies are commonly associated with hemolytic disease of the newborn (HDN)?**

   A. Anti-Kell
   B. Anti-D
   C. Anti-A
   D. Anti-s
   E. All of the following

81. **Which of the following red cell antibodies commonly cause hemolytic transfusion reactions?**

   A. Anti-E
   B. Anti-A
   C. Anti-Fy^a
   D. Anti-Kell
   E. All of the above

82. **Which of the following descriptions are *true* about Anti-A$_1$?**

   A. Reacts at room temperature (RT)
   B. Can be seen in 26% of A$_2$B individuals
   C. Extracted from *Dolichos biflo*rus (anti-A$_1$ lectin)
   D. Can be seen in 1-2% of A$_2$ individuals
   E. All of the above

83. **Which of the following descriptions are *true* about the Bombay phenotype (Oh)?**

   A. Serum contains a strong anti-H
   B. Individuals lack not only A and B substances but also H substance
   C. Persons have hh genotype
   D. Red cells of the Bombay group give a negative reaction with anti-H lectin (*Ulex europaeus*)
   E. All of the above

84. **Which of the following antibodies are classified as cold antibodies?**

   A. Anti-N
   B. Anti-M
   C. Anti-P
   D. Anti-Le^a
   E. All of the above

85. **Which of the following diseases are blood transfusion-related diseases?**

   A. Malaria
   B. Viral hepatitis (both hepatitis B and hepatitis C)
   C. Acquired immune deficiency syndrome (AIDS)
   D. Cytomegalovirus (CMV) infection
   E. All of the above

86. **Which of the following techniques can be valuable in resolving antibody identification problems?**

   A. Use of enzymes (ficin and papain) and lectins (anti-A$_1$ and anti-H)
   B. Elution

C. Neutralization
D. Adsorption
E. All of the above

87. **Which of the following descriptions are true about the Duffy blood group system** *except*?

A. Linked with transfusion reaction and hemolytic disease of the newborn
B. Activity enhanced by enzyme treatment
C. Resistance to *Plasmodium vivax* associated with Fy (a⁻b⁻)
D. Well developed at birth
E. Present on chromosome #1

88. **Which of the following descriptions are true about anti-M** *except*?

A. Usually IgM antibody
B. Reacts best at room temperature (RT) or 4°C
C. Exhibits dosage effect
D. Clinically significant
E. Causes irregularities in back typing

89. **Which of the following descriptions are true about Dᵘ** *except*?

A. Common in blacks
B. Detectable only in antiglobulin test (AGT)
C. Dᵘ positive donor blood can be transfused to D positive recipients
D. Dᵘ positive donor blood can be transfused to D negative pregnant women
E. All D negative donors need Dᵘ testing

90. **All of the following causes can be valid in ABO discrepancies** *except*:

A. Absence of unexpected antibodies
B. Chimerism
C. Rouleaux
D. Immunodeficiency
E. Acquired B antigen

91. **Which of the following biochemical changes in red cells ("storage lesion") is** *incorrect* **during blood storage?**

A. Accumulation of lactic acid (decreased pH)
B. Decrease in ATP levels
C. Decreased plasma Na⁺ levels
D. Decreased 2,3-diphosphoglycerate (2,3-DPG) levels
E. Decreased plasma hemoglobin levels

92. Which of the following preservatives/additive solutions/anticoagulants is *not* used in the storage of blood?

A. Heparin
B. Adsol (AS-1)
C. Acid-citrate-dextrose (ACD)
D. Ethylene diamine tetraacetate (EDTA)
E. Citrate-phosphate -dextrose-adenine (CPDA-1 and CPDA-2)

93. Which of the methodologies can be used in the preparation of leukocyte-poor red blood cells?

A. Use of microaggregate filters
B. Washing by saline solution
C. Glycerolization/freezing/deglycerolization of red blood cells
D. Inverted centrifugation
E. All of the above

94. Given the following blood bank results of a trauma patient:

Forward group				Reverse group			
antisera →				reagent red cells →			
A	B	A_1B	A_1 lectin	A_1	A_2	B	O
3+	0	3+	0	1+	0	4+	0

Which of the following blood groups does the patient have?

A. Patient's blood group "A_2" with anti-A_1
B. Patient's blood group "A" with leukemia

C. Patient's blood group "A_x" with anti-A_1
D. Patient's blood group "A" with multiple myeloma
E. None of the above

95. Which of the following descriptions is *not true* for "single donor" platelets?

A. Storage at room temperature (RT) on the agitator
B. Increases platelet count by 30-60,000/μL per unit
C. Shelf life of 5 days (closed system)
D. Reduced risk of hepatitis
E. Aspirin enhances platelet aggregation

96. **Which of the following descriptions is *incorrect* in delayed hemolytic transfusion reaction?**

   A. No fever
   B. Extravascular hemolysis
   C. Anamnestic reaction
   D. Positive DAT
   E. Mostly caused by anti-Fy^a, anti-Jk^a, anti-Jk^b, anti-E, and anti-C

97. **Which of the following is *incorrect* for cryoprecipitate?**

   A. Storage at -18°C or lower for 1 year
   B. Contains Factor VIII-C and Factor VIII-von Willebrand factor
   C. Prepared from fresh frozen plasma (FFP)
   D. Useful in the treatment of classic hemophilia, hypofibrinogenemia, and Factor XIII deficiency
   E. Does not contain fibrinogen and fibronectin

98. **Which of the following test techniques can be used in the detection of HBsAg?**

   A. Gel electrophoresis
   B. High-performance liquid chromatography (HPLC)
   C. Radioimmunoassay
   D. Gas-liquid chromatography (GLC)
   E. All of the above

99. **Given the following laboratory findings on a pregnant mother:**

   • Mother is Rh negative.
   • The infant is Rh positive.
   • Fetal-maternal hemorrhage is 1.4% (based on Kleihauer-Betke acid elution stain)

   How many vials of RhIg (300 ug/mL each vial) as a postpartum dose need to be administered within 72 hours to the mother for successful prophylaxis?

   A. 4
   B. 3
   C. 2
   D. > 4
   E. < 2

100. **Which of the following tests is a diagnostic test for paroxysmal cold hemoglobinuria?**

   A. Kleihauer-Betke acid elution stain
   B. Radioimmunoassay
   C. Donath-Landsteiner test
   D. Acid elution

E. Autoadsorption

101. **Which of the following culture media is highly selective in the isolation of *Salmonella* species from stool specimens?**

A. MacConkey agar
B. Brilliant green agar
C. Bismuth sulfite agar
D. Eosin methylene blue agar
E. Both B and C

102. **Which one of the following genera is associated with a high lipid content in the cell wall and acid-fastness?**

A. *Bordetella*
B. *Mycobacterium*
C. *Haemophilus*
D. *Staphylococcus*
E. *Klebsiella*

103. **Which of the following descriptions is (are) *true* in the case of *Mycobacterium leprae*?**

A. Cause of Hansen's disease
B. Has never been cultured on artificial cell-free media
C. Chronic disease of the skin and mucous membrane
D. Laboratory diagnosis involves the acid-fast stain of biopsy specimens
E. All of the above

104. **Which of the following descriptions is (are) *correct* in the case of *Helicobacter pylori*?**

A. Etiologic agent of peptic ulcer in human beings
B. Urease positive
C. Gastric tissue biopsy is the specimen of choice
D. Formerly *Campylobacter pylori*
E. All of the above

105. **Which of the following features are associated with *Campylobacter jejuni*?**

A. Cause of bacterial enteritis
B. Grows at 42°C but not at 35°C
C. Shows "darting" motility
D. S-shape or "gull-winged" gram-negative rods
E. All of the above

106. **Which of the following statements are *true* about *Escherichia coli except*?**

A. Cause of "traveler's diarrhea"

B. Indole = positive

C. Citrate = negative

D. Green metallic sheen on EMB agar

E. Voges Proskauer = positive

107. **Which one of the following bacteria is characterized by a yellow zone surrounding the colony on mannitol salt agar (MSA) medium?**

    A. *Serratia marcescens*

    B. *Staphylococcus aureus*

    C. *Staphylococcus epidermidis*

    D. *Streptococcus pneumoniae*

    E. *Streptococcus pyogenes*

108. **What basic nutrients, in general, are essential in designing a growth medium?**

    A. Carbon and nitrogen

    B. H_2O

    C. Phosphorus

    D. Minerals

    E. All of these

109. **Which one of the following listed granulocytes increases in case of bacterial infections?**

    A. Eosinophils

    B. Basophils

    C. Neutrophils

    D. Both A and B

    E. None of these

110. **Which of the following granulocytes increase during protozoan infestations?**

    A. Eosinophils

    B. Basophils

    C. Neutrophils

    D. Both B and C

    E. None of the above

111. **Which of the following viruses produce multinucleated giant cells in tissue culture?**

    A. Mumps

    B. Measles

    C. Parainfluenza

    D. Respiratory syncytial virus (RSV)

    E. All of the above

112. **Which one of the following viral agents causes the outbreaks of acute gastroenteritis during late winter in young children?**

A. Rotavirus
B. Adenovirus
C. Rhinovirus
D. Retrovirus
E. Enterovirus

113. **Which of the following techniques are valuable in the detection of viruses?**

A. Enzyme-linked immunosorbent assay (ELISA)
B. Immunofluorescence
C. Cytopathic effect (CPE)
D. Electron microscopy (EM)
E. All of these

114. **Which of the following viruses is "double-stranded" and "enveloped" *except*?**

A. Cytomegalovirus (CMV)
B. Epstein-Barr virus (EBV)
C. Varicella-zoster (VZ)
D. Herpes simplex virus (HSV) 1
E. Rabies virus

115. **Which of the following characteristics of rickettsiae are in support of bacteria?**

A. Have most of the bacterial enzymes
B. Have a typical bacterial cell wall
C. Have structural features of bacteria
D. All of the above
E. None of the above

116. **Which one of the following bacterial agents is implicated with human plague?**

A. *Bacillus anthracis*
B. *Listeria monocytogenes*
C. *Corynebacterium diphtheriae*
D. *Yersinia pestis*
E. *Yersinia enterocolitica*

117. **Which one of the following modes of transmission occurs in rickettsial diseases?**

A. Food and water
B. Aerial
C. Arthropod vector
D. Sexual
E. Fecal-oral route

118. Which one of the following diseases is caused by *Francisella tularensis*?

A. "Rabbit fever"
B. Scarlet fever
C. Typhoid fever
D. Q fever
E. Relapsing fever

119. Which one of the following techniques is commonly used in the confirmation of human immunodeficiency virus (HIV) infection?

A. Enzyme-linked immunosorbent assay (ELISA)
B. Western blot
C. Hemagglutination
D. Isotope labeling
E. Southern blot

120. Which one of the following selective enrichment broths is feasible during the isolation of enteric pathogens?

A. Selenite broth
B. Thioglycollate broth
C. Nutrient broth
D. Lauryl sulfate broth
E. Peptone broth

121. Which one of the following tests is a valuable test for the quick presumptive identification of *Candida albicans*?

A. Germ tube formation
B. H2S formation
C. Alkali formation
D. KOH wet mount
E. None of these

122. Which one of the following bacterial agents produces the CAMP factor?

A. *Staphylococcus aureus*
B. *Staphylococcus epidermidis*
C. *Streptococcus agalactiae*
D. *Streptococcus lactis*
E. *Streptococcus pneumoniae*

123. Which of the following etiological agents implicated in whooping cough?

A. *Bordetella pertussis*

B. *Haemophilus ducreyi*

C. *Citrobacter freundii*

D. *Brucella abortus*

E. *Neisseria gonorrhoeae*

124. **Which of the following fungal pathogenic agents exhibit "dimorphism"?**

   A. *Histoplasma capsulatum*
   B. *Sporothrix schenckii*
   C. *Blastomyces dermatitidis*
   D. *Paracoccidioides brasiliensis*
   E. All of the above

125. **Which of the following fungal agents can cause systemic mycoses?**

   A. *Nocardia brasiliensis*
   B. *Coccidioides immitis*
   C. *Nocardia asteroides*
   D. *Actinomyces israeli*
   E. All of the above

126. to 130. **Match the bacterial agents listed in column "A" with correct answers in column "B".**

Column "A"	Column "B"
126. *Staphylococcus aureus* _____	**A.** Mimics acute appendicitis
127. *Yersinia enterocolitica* _____	**B.** Toxic shock syndrome
128. *Pseudomonas aeruginosa* _____	**C.** Double zone of beta hemolysis
129. *Streptococcus pyogenes* (Group A) _____	**D.** Growth at 42°C
130. *Clostridium perfringens* _____	**E.** Sensitive to 0.04 U bacitracin

131. **Which of the following laboratory tests can be used as confirmatory tests for TB?**

   A. Cytochrome oxidase test
   B. Polymerase chain reaction (PCR)
   C. Culture
   D. Both B and C
   E. Fluorescent stain

132. **Which of the following specimen(s) is (are) acceptable for AFB culture?**

   A. Morning sputum
   B. Cerebrospinal fluid (CSF)
   C. Blood
   D. Stool
   E. All of these

133. Which of the following predisposing factors accounted for the development of tuberculosis (TB) in individuals infected with TB?

A. Malaria
B. Diabetes mellitus
C. Human immunodeficiency (HIV) infection
D. Hansen's disease
E. Hepatitis B infection

134. Which of the following infection(s) is (are) caused by Group *A Streptococcus*?

A. Scarlet fever
B. Erysipelas
C. Impetigo
D. Bacterial pharyngitis
E. All of these

135. Which of the following fermentable sugars are present in triple sugar iron (TSI) slant?

A. Lactose
B. Sucrose
C. Glucose
D. All of these
E. None of these

136. Which one of the following anticoagulants is used in blood cultures?

A. Heparin
B. Ethylene diamine tetraacetate (EDTA)
C. Sodium polyanethol sulfonate (SPS)
D. Sodium citrate
E. Potassium oxalate

137. Which one of the following bacterial infections is *not* a zoonotic infection?

A. Lyme disease
B. Anthrax
C. Brucellosis
D. Tularemia
E. Filariasis

138. Which of the following bacteria are cytochrome oxidase positive *except*?

A. *Acinetobacter*
B. *Neisseria gonorrhoeae*

C. *Neisseria meningitidis*
D. *Moraxella catarrhalis*
E. *Kingella denitrificans*

139. **Which one of the following reagents is used for the catalase test?**

    A. Potassium hydroxide (KOH)
    B. 3% hydrogen peroxide (H_2O_2)
    C. Methylene blue
    D. Rabbit plasma
    E. Sheep erythrocytes

140. **Which one of the following pigments is associated with *Pseudomonas aeruginosa*?**

    A. Bilirubin
    B. Pyocyanin
    C. Urobilin
    D. Hemin
    E. Hemoglobin

141. **Which of the following factors affect the accuracy assay results?**

    A. Storage of the specimen
    B. Choice of the assay method
    C. Instrumentation
    D. Controls and standards
    E. All of the above

142. **Which one of the following causes the "random" error?**

    A. Inappropriately reconstituted reagents
    B. Malfunctioning of the instrument
    C. Clerical error
    D. Incorrectly prepared controls
    E. All of these

143. **Which one of the following terms is correct for a substance capable of resisting the shifts in the pH?**

    A. Acid
    B. Alkali
    C. Buffer
    D. Indicator
    E. Electrolyte

144. What term is appropriate to refer to "the difference between a current value and the one preceding that value"?

   A. Coefficient of variation
   B. Standard deviation
   C. Clerical error
   D. Delta Check
   E. None of the above

145. How often do micropipettes need to be verified for their reliable performance?

   A. Monthly
   B. Biweekly
   C. Quarterly
   D. Yearly
   E. When the laboratory is fully-staffed

146. Which one of the following tools is useful in checking the speed of a laboratory centrifuge?

   A. A ruler
   B. A camera
   C. Tachometer
   D. Forceps
   E. None of these

147. to 150.: Mark "True" statements as A and "False" statements as B:

147. A tachometer is used to check the speed of a clinical laboratory centrifuge _____.

148. In a *Levey-Jennings chart*, plotted points around the mean within +2SD are indicative of the proper performance of an analytical method _____.

149. Comparison of the standard deviations (i.e. precision) of two different analytical methods is called Paired t-Test _____.

150. All clinical laboratory scientists must have easy access to safety data sheets (SDS) _____.

Answers:

1. E	31. B	61. B	91. E	121. A
2. E	32. A	62. D	92. D	122. C
3. D	33. D	63. C	93. E	123. A
4. A	34. D	64. A	94. A	124. E
5. B	35. D	65. B	95. E	125. E
6. B	36. B	66. C	96. A	126. B
7. E	37. E	67. B	97. E	127. A
8. B	38. E	68. B	98. C	128. D
9. C	39. C	69. C	99. B	129. E
10. C	40. E	70. C	100. C	130. C
11. B	41. E	71. D	101. E	131. D
12. B	42. A	72. A	102. B	132. E
13. E	43. A	73. C	103. E	133. C
14. E	44. A	74. B	104. E	134. E
15. E	45. C	75. B	105. E	135. D
16. C	46. B	76. C	106. E	136. C
17. E	47. E	77. E	107. B	137. E
18. E	48. E	78. E	108. E	138. A
19. A	49. E	79. E	109. C	139. B
20. B	50. D	80. E	110. A	140. B
21. E	51. A	81. E	111. E	141. B
22. E	52. A	82. E	112. A	142. C
23. C	53. E	83. E	113. E	143. C
24. E	54. B	84. E	114. E	144. D
25. B	55. B	85. E	115. D	145. C
26. E	56. E	86. E	116. D	146. C
27. E	57. E	87. B	117. C	147. A
28. C	58. E	88. D	118. A	148. A
29. C	59. C	89. D	119. B	149. B
30. A	60. B	90. A	120. A	150. A

Appendix I (a)

Sorensen's phosphate buffers:

Solution A for Sorensen's buffer

Potassium dihydrogen phosphate (anhydrous) (KH_2PO_4)	9.0727g
Distilled or boiled clean water	to 1L

Solution B for Sorensen's buffer

Disodium hydrogen phosphate (hydrated) ($Na_2HPO_4.2H_2O$)	11.867g
Distilled or boiled clean water	to 1L

Note: The above two solutions must be clear and should give no test for chloride or sulfates.

Sorensen A solution, mL	Sorensen B solution, mL	pH
0.25	9.75	5.288
0.5	9.5	5.589
1.0	9.0	5.906
2.0	8.0	6.239
3.0	7.0	6.468
4.0	6.0	6.643
5.0	5.0	6.813
6.0	4.0	6.979
7.0	3.0	7.168
8.0	2.0	7.381
9.0	1.0	7.731
9.5	0.5	8.043

Glycine-HCl (Sorensen) buffer

Volume (mL) of glycine - sodium chloride mixture, 100 mmol/L of each, to be diluted to 1 liter with 100 mmol/L hydrochloric acid.

pH	ml.	pH	ml.
1.2	150	2.6	702
1.4	287	2.8	756
1.6	382	3.0	808
1.8	457	3.2	856
2.0	523	3.4	903
2.2	583	3.6	945
2.4	645		

Appendix I (b)

Indicators

Indicator	pH range	Color change
Phenol red (acid range)	0.0-2.0	Pink to yellow
Bromocresol green	3.8-5.4	yellow to blue
Methyl red	4.2-6.3	red to yellow
Litmus	5.0-8.0	red to blue
Bromothymol blue	6.0-7.6	yellow to blue
Neutral red	6.8-8.0	yellow to red
Phenol red	6.8-8.4	yellow to red
Phenolphthalein	8.3-10.0	colorless to purple-red

Appendix II

Metric values

1 milliliter	(mL)	= 1 cubic centimetre (cc)
1 liter	(1)	= 1000 mL = 1.76 pints
1 pint	(P)	= 568 mL
1 gallon	(gal)	= 4.55 liters
1 fluid ounce	(fL oz)	= 24.4 mL
1 deciliter	(dL)	= 100 mL
1 microgramme	(mg)	= 1/1000 m. gram
1 milligram	(mg)	= 1/1000 gram
1 kilogram	(kg)	= 1000 g = 2.2 lb
1 ounce	(oz)	= 28.35 g
1 pound	(lb)	= 454 g
1 micrometer (micron)	(μm)	= 1×10^{-6} m
1 millimetre	(mm)	= 0.039 inches
1 inch	(in)	= 25.4 mm

Temperature conversions

To change Centigrade temperatures into Fahrenheit: Multiply by 9/5 and add on 32.
To change Fahrenheit temperatures into Centigrade: Subtract 32 and multiply by 5/9.

Appendix III

International atomic weights of commonly used elements
(based on carbon-12)

	Symbol	Atomic number	Atomic weight
Aluminum	AI	13	26.982
Antimony	Sb	51	121.75
Arsenic	As	33	74.912
Barium	Ba	56	137.34
Beryllium	Be	4	9.0122
Bismuth	Bi	83	208.98
Boron	B	5	10.811
Bromine	Br	35	79.909
Cadmium	Cd	48	112.40
Calcium	Ca	20	40.08
Carbon	C	6	12.011
Chlorine	Cl	17	35.453
Chromium	Cr	24	51.996
Cobalt	Co	27	58.933
Copper	Cu	29	63.54
Fluorine	F	9	18.998
Gold	G	79	196.97
Hydrogen	H	1	1.0080
Iodine	I	53	126.90
Iron	Fe	26	55.847
Lead	Pb	82	207.19
Lithium	Li	3	6.939
Magnesium	Mg	12	24.312
Manganese	Mn	25	54.938
Mercury	Hg	80	200.59
Molybdenum	Mo	42	95.94
Nickel	Ni	28	58.71
Nitrogen	N	7	14.007
Oxygen	O	8	15.999
Phosphorus	P	15	30.974
Potassium	K	19	39.102
Selenium	Se	34	78.96
Silicon	Si	14	28.086

(cont.) International atomic weights of commonly used elements (based on carbon-12)

	Symbol	Atomic number	Atomic weight
Silver	Ag	47	107.87
Sodium	Na	11	22.990
Strontium	Sr	38	87.62
Sulfur	S	16	32.064
Thallium	T1	81	204.37
Tin	Sn	50	118.69
Tungsten	W	74	183.85
Zinc	Zn	30	65.37

Appendix IV

Serology

TEST	NORMAL VALUE
Antibovine milk antibodies	Negative
Antideoxyribonuclease (ADNAase)	<1:20
Antinuclear antibodies (ANA)	<1:10
Antistreptococcal hyaluronidase (ASH)	< 1:256
Antistreptolysin O (ASLO)	<160 Todd units
Brucella agglutinins	<1:80
Coccidioidomycosis antibodies	Negative
Cold agglutinins	<1:32
Complement, C3	100-170 mg/dL C-
Reactive protein (CRP)	0
Fluorescent treponemal antibodies (FTA)	Non Reactive
Hepatitis-associated antigen (HAA or HBAg)	Negative
Heterophile antibodies	<1:56
Histoplasma agglutinins	<1:8
Latex fixation	Negative
Leptospira agglutinins	Negative
Ox cell hemolysin	<1:480
Rheumatoid factor	
sensitized sheep cell	<1:160
latex fixation	<1:80
bentonite particles	<1:32
Streptococcal MG agglutinins	<1:20
Thyroid antibodies	
antithyroglobulin	<1:32
antithyroid microsomal	<1:56
Toxoplasma antibodies	<1:4
Trichina agglutinins	0
Tularemia agglutinins	<1:80
Typhoid agglutinins	
O	<1:80
H	<1:80
VDRL	Nonreactive
Weil-Felix (*Proteus* OX-2, OX-K and OX-19 agglutinins)	Fourfold rise in titre between acute and convalescent sera

Appendix V

Licensure examinations and credential evaluation services

Since it is a requirement of a valid license for clinical laboratory scientists (CLSs) as well as medical laboratory technicians (MLTs) to practice in the US, some certifying agencies administer examinations:

(1) American Society for Clinical Pathology (ASCP): Board of Registry

> Address: 33 West Monroe Street; Suite 1600
> Chicago, IL 60603
> Phone: 1-800-267-2727
> Fax: (312) 541-4845
> Website: www.ascp.org

(2) American Medical Technologists (AMT)

> Address: 10700 W Higgins Rd.; STE 150
> Rosemont, IL 60018
> Phone: (847) 823-5169
> Fax: (847) 823-0458
> Email: mail@americanmedtech.org

(3) New York State License

> Address: NYS Education Department
> Office of the Professions
> PO Box 22063
> Albany, NY 12201

(4) California State License

> California Department of Health Services
> Laboratory Field Services Personnel Licensing Section
> 850 Marina Bay Pkwy Bldg P, 1st floor
> Richmond, CA 94804
> Phone: (510) 620-3834
> Fax: (510) 620-3697

Note: California does not recognize any certification or any other state license. Must pass California state examination. All foreign graduates MUST SUBMIT educational evaluation obtained from:

(1) International Education Research Foundation, Inc.

Post Office Box 3665
Culver City, CA 90231-3665

For Courier Service only (no walk-in service available):
International Education Research Foundation, Inc.
6133 Bristol Parkway, Suite 300
Culver City, CA 90230
Phone: (310) 258-9451
Fax: (310) 342-7086
Mon-Fri: 8:00 AM – 4:00 PM (Pacific Standard Time)
e-mail: info@ierf.org

(2) Scholaro Inc.

29 E Madison St., Suite 1005
Chicago, IL 60602
Phone: (312) 801-3319
Mon-Fri: 9:30 AM – 5:00 PM (central time)

(3) World Education Services (WES)

Postal Address:
WES Reference No. -----------------------
World Education Services
Attention: Documentation Center
P.O. Box 5087
Bowling Station
New York, N.Y. 10274 – 5087
USA
Courier Address:
WES Reference No. --------------------
World Education Services
Attention: Documentation Center
64 Beaver St. #146
New York, N.Y. 10004
USA
Phone: (212) 966-6311
Fax: (212) 739-6100
Mon-Fri: 9:00 AM - 6:00 PM (Eastern Time)

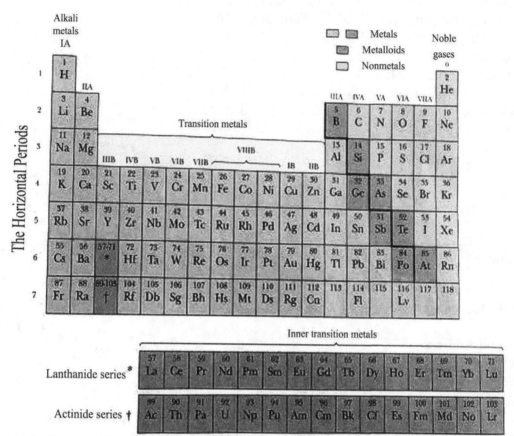

Evidence for the discovery of elements 113 through 118 has been reported. See www.webelements.com for the latest information and newest elements. The names and symbols for elements 114 and 116 have been suggested but are not official.

Periodic table of the elements.
(Reproduced with permission by Wiley Global)

Parts of the human body

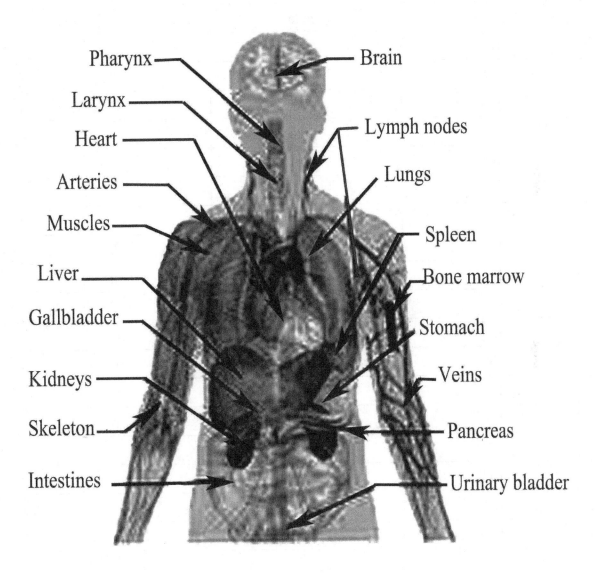

Pharynx — Brain

Larynx — Lymph nodes

Heart — Lungs

Arteries — Spleen

Muscles — Bone marrow

Liver — Stomach

Gallbladder — Veins

Kidneys — Pancreas

Skeleton — Urinary bladder

Intestines —

Appendix VIII

Metric prefixes of SI Units

Factor	Prefix	Symbol
10^{24}	yotta	Y
10^{21}	zetta	Z
10^{18}	exa	E
10^{15}	peta	P
10^{12}	tera	T
10^{9}	giga	G
10^{6}	mega	M
10^{3}	kilo	k
10^{2}	hecto	h
10^{1}	deka	da
10^{-1}	deci	d
10^{-2}	centi	c
10^{-3}	milli	m
10^{-6}	micro	μ
10^{-9}	nano	n
10^{-12}	pico	p
10^{-15}	femto	f
10^{-18}	atto	a
10^{-21}	zepto	z
10^{-24}	yocto	y

Laboratory mathematics: Hematology

(A) Hematological indices: are a set of values that can assist, together with other test values, in investigating an anemic patient. These are the calculated values useful in the classification of various types of anemia.

(i) mean corpuscular volume (MCV)

Formula:

$$MCV\ (fL) = \frac{Hematocrit(\%) \times 10}{RBC\ count\ (x\ 10^{12}/L)}$$

Example: Calculate the MCV for a given subject with a 27.5% of hematocrit (packed cell volume) and RBC count of 3.01 x 10^{12}/L.

Solution:
Substituting these values in the above formula,

$$MCV(fL) = \frac{-b \pm \sqrt{b^2 - 4ac}}{3.01\ x\ 10^{12}/L}$$

$$= 91.3\ fL$$

Reference values: 80-97 fL

Clinical significance: Red blood cells are of normal size (normocytic). If MCV is high (>97fL), cells are macrocytic. On the other hand, cells are microcytic where MCV is low (<80fL).

Note: Some hematology analyzers directly measure MCV.

(ii) mean corpuscular hemoglobin (MCH)

Formula:

$$MCH(pg) = \frac{Hemoglobin\ (g/L)}{RBC\ count\ x\ 10^{12}/L}$$

Example: Calculate the MCH for a given subject with hemoglobin of 101 g/L and RBC count of 2.34 x 10^{12}/L.
Solution: Substituting these values in the above formula,

$$MCH(pg) = \frac{101 g/L}{2.34 \times 10^{12}/L}$$

$$= 43 \text{ pg}$$

Reference values: 27-31 pg

Clinical significance: The MCHC is a better indicator of color than the MCH because the MCH tends to follow the volume of the red blood cell.

(iii) mean corpuscular hemoglobin concentration (MCHC)

Formula:

$$MCHC \text{ (g/L)} = \frac{\text{hemoglobin (g/dL)} \times 100}{\text{hematocrit (\%)}}$$

Example: Calculate the MCHC for the given subject with hemoglobin concentration of 7 g/dL and hematocrit of 20%.

Solution: Substituting these values in the above formula,

$$MCHC \text{ (g/L)} = \frac{70 \text{ g/L}}{0.20 \text{ L/L}}$$

$$= 350 \text{ g/L}$$

Reference values: 320-360 g/L

Clinical significance: Red blood cells are of normal color (normochromic). If MCHC values are low (<320 g/L), cells are hypochromic. On the other hand, elevated MCHC is rare but can occur when there is spherocytosis.

(B) Corrected WBC count: Most automated hematological analyzers do not differentiate between the WBCs and nucleated RBCs. In other words, automated WBC count = WBC + nRBCs. If the number of nucleated RBCs exceeds 5, it is necessary to correct the WBC count. Therefore, the number of nRBCs per 100 WBCs is recorded while performing a differential count of WBCs.

Formula:

$$cWBC = \frac{WBC \times 100}{nRBCs + 100}$$

Example: Calculate the corrected WBC for a given subject with an automated WBC count of 8,400/μL and 40 nRBCs/100 WBCs.

Solution: Substituting these values in the above formula,

$$= \frac{8,400 \times 100}{40 + 100}$$

$$= \frac{8,400 \times 100}{140}$$

$$= 6,000/μL$$

Clinical significance: Nucleated RBCs can be found in the case of myelogenic leukemia, severe anemia, *erythroblastosis fetalis* and normal newborn.

(C) LAP test: The LAP test is a simple and valuable test in differentiating between bacterial and nonbacterial stimuli. A blood smear is prepared from a drop of capillary blood or heparin anticoagulated blood (EDTA is inhibitory). Then, a smear is stained and examined while making a consecutive count of 100 segmented neutrophils and bands as well as scoring each as follows:

0 = no reddish-brown granules in the cytoplasm of neutrophil
1+ = barely visible, occasional reddish-brown granules
2+ = diffuse staining with moderate reddish-brown granules
3+ = numerous reddish-brown granules
4+ = very numerous coarse reddish-brown granules

Example: Calculate the LAP score for a subject having the following numbers of LAP activity in neutrophils:

Degree of activity	⟶	0	1+	2+	3+	4+
Number of neutrophils	⟶	37	23	20	14	6
LAP score	⟶	0	23	40	42	24

Solution: There are two steps: (1) multiplication of the number of neutrophils by the corresponding activity grade (2) addition of all numbers to obtain a final score.

Therefore, total score = 0+23+40+42+24
                       = 129
Normal values: 30-100

Clinical significance:
- Increase in polycythemia vera and leukemoid reactions
- Decrease in chronic myelogenous leukemia (CML) and paroxysmal nocturnal hemoglobinuria (PNH)

(D) Absolute counts of a specific leukocyte: are determined by multiplying the total number of leukocyte count with the relative percentage of that particular cell type.

Formula: Absolute count of a specific leukocyte = Total WBC count x 1000 x relative percentage of that specific leukocyte.

Example: Calculate the absolute lymphocyte count for a given subject with a total WBC count of 5×10^9/L and 50% of lymphocytes (expressed as a decimal) on the differential count.

Solution: Substituting these values in the above formula,

So, absolute lymphocyte count = 5×10^9/L x 0.25
$$= 2.5 \times 10^9/L$$

Normal values:
Total WBC count = $1.0\text{-}4.0 \times 10^9$/L
Relative percentage of lymphocyte = 20-44%

Clinical significance: Absolute count must be used in the process of evaluation of the differential leukocyte count. In this case, the absolute count (2.5×10^9/L) lies within the reference range ($1.0\text{-}4.0 \times 10^9$/L)) but the relative percentage of lymphocytes is elevated (50%). Therefore, this is called relative lymphocytosis.

(E) Total Iron Binding Capacity (TIBC): is a test that measures indirectly the level of the transferrin (protein) in the blood. The serum is preferred to plasma (lithium heparin) as a specimen of choice. Plasma (EDTA) falsely decreases the results.

Formula:

$$\text{Transferrin saturation (\%)} = \frac{\text{serum iron x 100\%}}{\text{TIBC}}$$

Example: Calculate the transferrin saturation (%) for the subject with the serum iron = 100 µg/dL and TIBC = 300 µg/dL.

Solution:
Plugging these values in the above equation,

$$\text{Transferrin saturation (\%)} = \frac{100\mu g/dL \times 100\%}{300\mu g/dL}$$

$$= 33\%$$

Normal values:
Serum iron: 60-170 µg/dL
TIBC: 250-450µg/dL
Transferrin saturation: 25-35 %

Clinical significance: Normally, transferrin is one-third saturated with iron, leaving about two-third in reserve. In iron deficiency anemia, usage of all of the stored iron causes more production of transferrin in order to enhance the iron transfer. This leads to the higher TIBC values concurrent with a decrease in transferrin saturation (%). TIBC is often decreased in hemochromatosis and sideroblastic anemia.

Note: The sum of the serum iron and UIBC represents the TIBC.

Appendix IX (b)

Laboratory mathematics: Clinical chemistry

(A) Beer's Law

Formula: Absorbance (A) = 2 – log %T
Example: Convert 30% T to absorbance (A)
Solution: Absorbance (A) = 2 –log%T

$$A = 2 – 1.477$$
$$A = 0.523$$

(B) Spectrophotometric determination of the concentration of an unknown solute in a given sample:

Formula:

$$Ctest = \frac{Atest}{Astd.} \times Cstd.$$

Where,

Ctest = conc. of test (unknown)
Cstd. = conc. of standard
Atest = absorbance of the test (unknown)
Astd. = absorbance of the standard

Example: Calculate the conc. of glucose in a sample for the given subject with the following data:

$$Astd. = 0.300, Atest = 0.250, \text{ and } Cstd. = 80 \text{ mg/dL}$$

Solution:
Substituting these values in the above formula,

We get,

$$Ctest \left(\frac{mg}{dL}\right) = \frac{0.250}{0.300} x \, 80$$

$$= 66.7 mg/dL$$

(C) Creatinine Clearance: is a valuable kidney function test.

Formula:

$$\text{Creatinine clearance (mL/min)} = \frac{U}{P} \times V$$

Where,

U = urine creatinine (mg/dL)
P = plasma creatinine (mg/dL)
V = volume of urine (mL/min)

Since creatinine clearance is affected by the body surface area as well as the size of the kidney of a subject being tested, correction is required as under:

$$\text{Corrected creatinine clearance (mL/min)} = \frac{U}{P} \times V \times \frac{1.73 \text{ meter}^2}{A}$$

Where,
>   1.73 meter² = standard adult body surface area
>   A = patient's body surface area

Example: Calculate the creatinine clearance for an average size subject whose laboratory findings are as follows:

>   urine volume for 24 hours = 1500 mL
>   plasma creatinine = 1.1 mg/dL
>   urine creatinine = 114 mg/dL

Solution:
Substituting these laboratory values in the above formula,

$$\text{Creatinine clearance (mL/min)} = \frac{114\ \text{mg/dL}}{1.1\ \text{mg/dL}} \times \frac{1500\ \text{mL/24 hr}}{1440\ \text{min/24 hr}}$$

$$= 103.6 \times 1.04$$
$$= 104.6\ \text{mL/min}$$

Normal values:
Male (uncorrected): 90-139 mL/min
Female (uncorrected): 80-125 mL/min

Clinical significance: Assessment of the glomerular filtration rate (GFR). It should be noted that creatinine clearance often overestimates by 10-20 % of the true GFR.

(D) Anion gap: Beyond its application in the detection of some disorders, it is also useful in the assessment of the performance of the instrument as a quality control tool in electrolyte measurements.

Formula: $(\text{mmol/L}) = (Na^+ + K^+) - (Cl^- + CO_2)$...............(i)

or

$$= (Na^+ - (Cl^- + CO_2)) ....(ii)$$

Example: Calculate the anion gap for the given subject using the following data:

$Na^+ = 140$ mmol/L ; $K^+ = 4.4$ mmol/L; $Cl^- = 100$ mmol/L; $CO_2 = 24$ mmol/L

Solution:
Plugging the analytical results in the above equation,

Anion gap (mmol/L) = (140 4.4) – (106 + 24)
>   = 14 mmol/L

Reference values: 10-20 mmol/L for equation (i) and 8-16 mmol/L for equation (ii)

Clinical significance: Increased values can be seen in metabolic ketoacidosis, renal failure, salicylate poisoning high albumin levels and a decrease in cations. Oppositely, decreased values can be associated with the presence of abnormal proteins, a decrease in anions and low albumin levels.

(E) Henderson–Hasselbalch equation: is an important equation that shows the relationship between pH, the concentration of dissolved carbon dioxide ($cdCO_2$) and the concentration of bicarbonate ions ($cHCO_3^-$).

Formula:

$$pH = pK' + \log \frac{cHCO}{cdCO}$$

Where,

pH = negative log of H_+ activity
pK' = dissociation constant (6.1)
$cHCO_3^-$ = concentration of bicarbonate ($cHCO_3^-$)
$cdCO_2$ = concentration of dissolved carbon dioxide ($cdCO_2 = pCO_2 \times 0.03^*$)

Example: Calculate the arterial blood pH for the subject having total CO_2 = 30 mmol/L; pCO_2(artery) = 44 mm Hg.

Solution:

(i) Conversion of pCO_2 to dissolved CO_2: by multiplying the pCO_2 by the solubility constant for CO_2 gas (0.03) as under:

So, $cdCO_2$ = 44 mm Hg x 0.03 mmol/L
            = 1.32 mmol/L

(ii) Find the concentration of bicarbonate: by subtracting the concentration of dissolved CO_2 from the total CO_2 as follows:

$cHCO_3^-$ = 30 mmol/L – 1.32 mmol/L
             = 28.68

(iii) Finally, substituting the values in the above equation,

$$pH = 6.1 + \log \frac{26.68}{1.32}$$
$$= 6.1 + \log 21.72$$
$$= 6.1 + 1.3$$
$$= 7.43$$

Reference values: The normal ratio of the concentrations of bicarbonate ions ($cHCO3^-$) to dissolved carbon dioxide ($cdCO2$) is 20:1.

Clinical significance: The Henderson-Hasselbalch equation is a very valuable equation in the assessment of acid-base balance.

(F) Osmolality and osmolal gap: There are two forms of osmolality: (i) measured in the laboratory and (ii) calculated. Osmolal gap is, then, derived by subtracting the calculated osmolality from the measured one.

(i) measured osmolality:

Example: Find mOsm/Kg in an aqueous solution that depresses the freezing point of the solution to -0.80°C

Solution:

$$= \frac{1}{0.00186\,°C} \times \frac{?}{0.80}$$

0.00186 x (?) = 0.80
Measured osmolality (?) = 430.1 mOsm/Kg

(ii) Calculated osmolality:

Formula:

$$\text{(mOsm/kg)} = 1.86\,(Na^+;\ mmol/L) + \frac{(\text{glucose; mg/dL}^{37})}{18} + \frac{(\text{BUN; mg/dL}^{37})}{2.8} + 9$$

Example: Calculate the serum osmolality if Na^+ = 141 mmol/L; glucose = 100 mg/dL; BUN
$$= 20\ mg/dL.$$

Solution:
Substituting these values in the above formula,

$$\text{(mOsm/kg)} = 1.86(141) + \frac{100}{18} + \frac{20}{2.8}$$

$$= 262.2 + 5.6 + 7.1 + 9$$
$$= 284$$

Reference range $= 0 \pm 6$

(G) Enzyme activity: The *international unit* (U)[38] is that quantity of enzyme capable of catalyzing the reaction of one micromole (μmole) of substrate per minute under specified conditions.

Formula:

$$U/L = \frac{\Delta Abs./min \times Vt\ (mL) \times 106\mu mol/mol}{\text{Absorptivity} \times \text{light path (cm)} \times Vs\ (mL)\text{constant}}$$

---

[37] Needs to convert to mmol/L.
[38] Nowadays, *katal* (SI Unit) expresses the enzyme activity in moles per second.

Where,

Δ Abs./min. = Change in absorbance per minute
Vt(mL) = Total volume of test (substrate + sample)
absorptivity constant = Molar absorptivity for NADH at 340 nm (6.22 x 103 L/mol·cm)
Vs (mL) = Volume of serum specimen
Light path (cm) = 1

Example: Calculate the enzyme activity in U/L of a given serum sample with the following data:

Change in ΔAbs. per one minute	= 0.250
The volume of a serum specimen	= 0.02mL (20µL)
The volume of reagent	= 2.8 mL
Light path	= 1 cm.

Solution:
Plugging these values in the above equation,

$$= \frac{0.250 \times 2.82 \text{ mL} \times 106 \text{ /µmol/mol}}{6.22 \times 10^3 \text{ L/mol} \cdot \text{cm} \times 1 \text{ cm} \times 0.02 \text{ mL}}$$

$$= \frac{0.705 \times 106 \text{µmol/mol}}{0.124 \times 10^3 \text{ L/mol} \cdot \text{cm}}$$

$= 5.66 \times 10^3$ µmol/mol
$= 5660$ U/L

Reference values = see Table 16.1
Clinical significance: Some enzymes (e.g., LDH) are measured because they help in the clinical diagnosis.

(H) Conversion of concentrations: In many instances, it is required to prepare the desired concentration from a given concentration of a solution in any chemistry laboratory. The units used for the volume as well as the concentration on both sides must be the same. Therefore, the volume or the concentration (or both) of a given solution are changed before plugging these values in the formula, if needed.

Formula:
$$V_1 \times C_1 = V_2 \times C_2$$

Where,

V_1 = volume of the first solution
C_1 = concentration of the first solution
V_2 = volume of the second solution and
C_2 = concentration of the second solution

Example: Find the volume in liters of a given 3% NaCl solution needed to prepare 4 liters of a 0.95% NaCl solution.

Solution:
Substituting the values in the above formula,

$$V_1\,(?) \times 3 \;=\; 4 \times 0.95$$

$$V_1\,(?) = \frac{4 \times 0.95}{3}$$

$$V_1\,(?) = \frac{3.8}{3}$$

$$= 1.2\ \text{L}$$

(I) Temperature conversions: Sometimes, it becomes essential to change the temperature from Degrees Fahrenheit (°F) to Degrees Celsius (°C) and vice versa.

Formulae:

(i) °F = (°C x 9/5) + 32 and
(ii) °C = (°F - 32) x 5/9

Example: Convert (i) 50°C to °F and 92°F to °C:

Solution:
Substituting these values in the above formulae (i) and (ii) respectively,

(i) °F = (50 x 9/5) + 32
    = 90 +32
    = 122°F

(ii) °C = (92 - 32) x 5/9
    = 60 x 5/9
    = 33.3°C

(J) Conversions among the concentration expressions of normality (N), molarity (M), percent (%), mmol/L and mEq/L.

Formula:
(i) N = M x valence

Example: change 5 M H_2SO_4 to normality (N)

Solution: normality (N) = 5 x 2 (valence)
$$= 10 \text{ N } H_2SO_4$$

(ii) $\dfrac{N}{valence}$

Example: change 4 N H_2SO_4 to molarity (M)

Solution:

$$\text{molarity(M)} = \frac{4}{2}$$

$$= 2 \text{ M } H_2SO_4$$

(iii) $M = \dfrac{\% \times 10}{2\,mol.\,wt.}$

Example: change 20% NaCl to molarity (M)

Solution:

(iv) $\text{molarity(M)} = \dfrac{20 \times 10}{58.5^*}$ (* mol. wt. of NaCl)

$$= \frac{200}{58.5}$$

$$= 3.4 \text{ M NaCl}$$

Example: convert 8 mg/dL. of magnesium (Mg^{2+}) to millimoles per liter (mmol/L.)

Solution:

$$= \frac{8 \text{ mg/dL} \times 10^*}{24}$$ (* conversion factor from dL to L)

$$= \frac{80}{5823.5}$$

$$= 3.3 \text{ mmol/L}$$

(v) $\text{mEq/L} = \dfrac{\text{mg/dL x } 10^*}{\text{eq. wt.}}$ (* conversion factor from dL to L)

Example: change 15 mg/dL of NaCl to mEq/L

Solution:

$$\text{mEq/L} = \frac{15 \text{ x } 10}{58.5}$$

$$= \frac{150}{58.5}$$

$$= 2.6 \text{ mEq/L}$$

GLOSSARY

A

Abdomen: The part of the human body that includes the stomach, intestines, etc.

ABO blood group system: a set of glycoproteins found on the surface of red blood cells. The presence or absence of specific carbohydrates determines the blood types.

Abscess: pus-filled cavity formed in a damaged tissue.

Absorption: A process in which uptaking of molecules takes place throughout the volume of the absorbent.

Acellular: not made up of cells.

Acidophile: an organism that grows best at a pH between 4 -5.

Acquired immunodeficiency syndrome (AIDS): a disease caused by HIV and is characterized by opportunistic infections and rare cancers.

Active immunity: stimulation of one's own adaptive immune responses.

Active site: location within an enzyme where substrate(s) binds.

Adaptive immunity: a third-line defence mechanism and is characterized by specificity and memory.

Adjuvant: is a chemical agent that enhances the antibody response to that antigen.

Adsorption: A process in which uptaking of molecules takes place only at the surface of the adsorbent.

Aerobe: an organism that depends on atmospheric oxygen to grow.

Aerosol: a cloud of fine droplets containing live pathogenic organisms.

Agar: a polysaccharide extracted from marine algae and is used as a solidifying agent in growth media.

Agglutination: binding of different pathogenic cells by Fab regions of the same antibody to aggregate and enhance elimination from body.

Agglutinin: an antibody produced against the agglutinogen (antigen).

Agglutinogen: an antigen capable of stimulating the formation of agglutinin (antibody).

Albumin: protein present in the highest concentration in human plasma and is used as a potentiator solution in serologic reactions, enhancing antigen-antibody interactions.

Algae: photosynthetic plant-like eukaryotes that inhabit places such as marine and freshwater.

Alkaliphile: an organism that grows optimally at a pH between 8-11.

Allele: a gene that occupies the same locus as an alternative form on chromosomes.

Allergen: an antigen capable of inducing type I hypersensitivity reaction.

Allergy: an IgE-mediated exaggerated immune response to a foreign substance (allergen). Also called hypersensitivity).

Ames test: a method that uses auxotrophic bacteria to detect mutations resulting from exposure to potentially mutagenic chemical compounds.

Amino acid: an organic acid that serves as a building block of proteins.

Amphitrichous: the presence of flagella at both poles of a microbe.

Anabolism: a set of energy-requiring chemical reactions that result in the formation of large molecules from simpler ones.

Anaerobe: an organism that grows in the absence of atmospheric oxygen.

Anamnestic response: a rapid rise in antibody titer following secondary exposure to an antigen.

Anemia: a condition where oxygen-delivery to the tissues is low; may occur due to (i) increased destruction of red cells, (ii) excessive blood loss, or (iii) decreased production of red cells.

Angstrom: unit that is used for the measurement of very small distances, e.g., wavelengths of light

Anion: an ion that carries a negative electrical charge.

Anisocytosis: variation in red cell size.

Antecubital: at the bend of the elbow; usual site for blood collection.

Antenatal: occurring before birth.

Anti-A_1 lectin: a reagent produced from the seeds of the plant *Dolichos biflorus*; reacts with A_1 antigen red cells but not with A subgroup red cells e.g., A_2, A_3, etc.

Antibiotic: a chemical substance produced by microorganisms and/or synthesized in the laboratory; capable of inhibiting the growth or killing other microbes.

Antibody: a Y-shaped protein molecule made by certain white blood cells which is produced by the body's immune system in response to a foreign substance (antigen).

Anticoagulant: an agent that prevents blood clotting.

Anticodon: a set of three base sequences of transfer RNA that is complementary to the codon (a set of three base sequences) of messenger RNA.

Antigen: a foreign substance such as a pathogen that stimulates the body's immune system to produce antibodies.

Antihistamine: a drug that counteracts the effects of histamine and is used in the treatment of allergy.

Antiseptic agent: a chemical agent used safely on external parts of the body to destroy microbes.

Antiseptic: an antimicrobial chemical that can be used safely on living tissues.

Apheresis: a method in which whole blood is collected from the donor; the desired component is separated and retained, and the remainder of the blood returned to the donor e.g., plateletpheresis and plasmapheresis.

Apoenzyme: an enzyme without its cofactor or coenzyme.

Apoptosis: the genetically programmed destruction of cells.

Archaea: prokaryotic unicellular organisms that live in harsh environmental conditions.

Asthma: a type of chronic allergy in the respiratory system caused by inhaled or ingested allergens.

Atom: the smallest unit of an element.

Atrichous: an organism that lacks flagella.

Attenuation: a method of weakening the virulence of an organism through a serial transfer in a non-native host.

Atypical antibodies: an antibody other than anti-A, anti-B, or anti-A,B.

Autoclave: an instrument designed for sterilization using moist heat under pressure.

Autoimmune disease: loss of tolerance to self, resulting in immune-mediated destruction of self-cells and tissues.

Autosome: any chromosome other than the sex (X and Y) chromosomes.

Autotroph: organisms that do not need organic nutrients for growth.

B

B lymphocyte: a type of leukocyte that gives rise to antibody-synthesizing plasma cells.

Bacillus: a bacterial cell that is rod-shaped.

Bacteremia: the presence of bacteria in the blood.

Bacteria (singular-bacterium): are single-celled prokaryotic organisms with spherical, rod, spiral, or filamentous shapes.

Bactericidal agent: an agent that kills bacteria permanently; irreversible effect.

Bacteriophage: a virus that attacks bacteria; also called *phage*.

Bacteriostatic agent: an agent that inhibits the growth and multiplication of bacteria for the time being-reversible effect.

Bacteriuria: the presence of bacteria in the urine.

Benign: harmless.

Bilirubin: the orange-yellow pigment in bile; produced from hemoglobin (red blood cell pigment) by reticuloendothelial cells (bone marrow, spleen, and elsewhere); two forms of bilirubin (i) Direct bilirubin (conjugated) is water-soluble, and (ii) Indirect bilirubin (unconjugated) is water-insoluble.

Binary fission: the asexual process of cell division in bacteria, making two daughter cells.

Binocular: a light microscope equipped with two eyepieces.

Biochemistry: the discipline of organic chemistry that deals with the chemical reactions of biological systems.

Bioinformatics: the integration of software programs to automate analytical techniques.

Bioluminescence: the generation of light by some species of bacteria, insects, fish, and animals through the conversion of chemical energy into photo form.

Biota: harmless or beneficial resident microbial flora found internally and/or externally in humans.

Biphasic: reactivity taking place in two phases.

Bombay (Oh) group: individuals who possess normal A or B genes but unable to express them because they lack the gene needed to produce H antigen (precursor for A and B); these individuals often have a potent anti-H in their serum, which reacts with all cells other than the Bombay type.

Bradykinin: a polypeptide produced during anaphylaxis and causes vasodilation.

Broad-spectrum antimicrobial: a drug that targets many different types of microbes.

Bronchitis: an inflammation of the bronchi.

Bubo: the swelling of inflamed lymph node(s) due to the accumulation of pus.

Budding: a process is seen in yeasts and a handful of bacteria in which a small structure develops on the surface of a parental cell.

Buffy coat: light stratum of a blood clot (mostly white blood cells) between the plasma and the red blood cells obtained at the end of the centrifugation of a blood specimen.

Burst size: the number of virus particles produced at the end of a lytic cycle.

C

Cancer: any malignant neoplasm that invades the neighboring tissues and can spread to other locations.

Capnophile: an organism that requires carbon dioxide for growth.

Capsid: a protein coat of a virus particle.

Capsule: a polysaccharide or protein made structure surrounding the cell walls of certain microorganisms (e.g., *Streptococcus pneumoniae)*.

Carbohydrate: an energy-rich organic compound containing carbon, hydrogen, and oxygen in the proportion of 1:2:1 (CH_2O).

Carbuncle: a deep pus-filled lesion due to an infection.

Carcinogen: a cancer-causing substance.

Catabolism: a set of energy-liberating chemical reactions aimed at the breakdown of complex compounds into simpler ones.

Catalyst: any substance that accelerates the rate of a chemical reaction without being altered or used up.

Cation: an ion that carries a positive electrical charge.

Cell coincidence: is an inherent error (in impedance-based techniques) in which two or more cells passing through an orifice at one time generate a single voltage pulse, recording as one cell (also called *coincidence doublets*).

Cell: The basic unit of all living things.

Cellular immunity: adaptive immunity involving T cells and the destruction of pathogens and infected cells.

Central dogma: a scientific principle explaining the flow of genetic information from DNA to RNA to protein

Central nervous system (CNS): portion of the nervous system made up of the brain and spinal cord.

Chemostat: a device that maintains the steady-state growth (stationary phase) through a controlled continuous inflow of nutrients and outflow of waste products.

Chemotherapeutic agent: a chemical substance that is used in the treatment of disease(s).

Chitin: A primary component of the cell walls of fungi and composed of a polymer of *N*-acetylglucosamine.

Chlorophyll: a green photosynthetic pigment usually found in organelles called chloroplasts.

Chloroplast: a chlorophyll-containing organelle found in photosynthetic eukaryotes.

Cholera: a gastrointestinal illness caused by *Vibrio cholerae* characterized by severe diarrhea.

Chromosome: a long continuous piece of DNA that carries genetic information.

Chronic disease: any disease that progresses and persists over a long time.

Cilium (plural, cilia): a tiny hair-like structure on the surface of some micro-organisms or cells which beats rhythmically to either propel trapped material out of the body (e.g., lungs) or make a free-living microbe to move.

Coenocytic: hyphae without cross-walls (septa).

Cofactor: an inorganic ion that helps stabilize enzyme conformation and function.

Competitive inhibitor: a molecule that binds to an enzyme's active site, preventing substrate binding.

Complement system: a set of serum proteins that act in a definite sequence when activated.

Complement-fixation test: a test for antibodies against a specific pathogen using complement-mediated hemolysis.

Congenital: existing at birth.

Constitutive enzyme: an enzyme that is produced irrespective of the presence or absence of its substrate in the medium.

Convalescent stage: the period after active infection has subsided.

Coombs test: a test developed by R. Coombs and is useful to detect IgG classes of antibodies.

Cryoprecipitate: a concentrated product prepared from a single unit of donor blood; mainly contains coagulation Factor VIII; also contains Factor XIII, fibrinogen, and von Willebrand factor.

Cyanosis: bluish skin discoloration due to hypoxia.

Cyst: a thick-walled resistant and dormant stage of protozoa.

Cytomegalovirus: one of the group of species-specific herpesviruses.

Cytopathic effect (CPE): the visible destructive changes; usually seen with virus-infected tissue culture cells.

Cytotoxic T cells: effector cells of cellular immunity that target and eliminate cells infected with intracellular pathogens through induction of apoptosis.

Cytotoxicity: harmful effects to the host cell.

D

Dark-field microscopy: a form of microscopic technique in which micro-organisms appear bright against a dark background; valuable method in the examination of spirochetes in their living state.

Defined medium: a culture medium that contains known specific kinds and concentrations of chemical ingredients.

Dermatophytes: fungi that infect the skin, hair, and nails

Deuteromycotina: a class of fungi in which a true sexual cycle has not yet been known; also called the Fungi imperfecti.

Dimorphism: a phenomenon in which the tissue form (in the host) and the free-living form (cultures in the laboratory) differ markedly.

Diphtheria: a serious infection of the larynx and is caused by the toxigenic bacterium *Corynebacterium diphtheriae.*

DNA: deoxyribonucleic acid

Drug resistance: ability of a microbe to persist and grow in the presence of an antimicrobial drug.

E

Electrolyte: a substance that is in a solution capable of conducting an electric current.

Electrophoresis: a separation technique in which the charged particles move through a medium (paper, agar gel) in the presence of an electrical field; useful in the separation and analysis of proteins.

Elution: a process whereby antibody is removed from the red blood cells; the antibody may be freed by physical (heating, shaking) or chemical (acid, ether) method; the harvested antibody-containing fluid is called an eluate.

Embolism: obstruction of a blood vessel by a blood clot or foreign substances.

Enteric: bacteria of the family *Enterobacteriaceae*, which live in the human intestinal tract.

Enteritis: an inflammation of the lining of the intestine.

Enzyme: a thermolabile organic catalyst liberated by a living cell and can function independently of the cell; can be recovered in an unaltered form at the end of an enzymatic reaction.

Enzyme-linked immunosorbent assay (ELISA): a highly specific immunologic test; involves the linking of soluble antibodies or antigens to an insoluble solid surface to retain the reactivity of the antibody or antigen.

Epidemic disease: an illness with a higher-than-expected incidence in a given period within a given population.

Epidemiology: the study of where and when infectious diseases occur in a population and how they are transmitted and maintained in nature.

Epidermis: the outermost layer of human skin.

Epitope: the antigenic determinant; is directly involved in the interaction with the antibody.

Eukaryote: a cell having a well-defined nucleus surrounded by a nuclear envelope.

Exogenous: outside of an organ or part.

Extravascular: outside of the blood vessel.

F

Facultative: an organism that can grow and reproduce in the presence as well as the absence of oxygen.

Febrile reaction: a transfusion reaction characterized by fever.

Fermentation: the catabolic process that involves an organic compound as the final electron acceptor.

Fibrin: a whitish protein clot formed by the action of thrombin on fibrinogen.

Fibrinogen: a protein produced in the liver.

Ficin: a proteolytic enzyme obtained from the fig.

Flagellum (plural, flagella): a long thin appendage present on the surface of some cells, e.g., bacteria, enabling them to move.

Fluorescence: is the emission of light by a substance that has absorbed light or other electromagnetic radiation.

Formalin: 40% solution of formaldehyde.

Fungus (plural, fungi): an eukaryotic organism occurring as a long, branching filament (mold) or a single cell (yeast).

G

Gamete: a sex cell with a single set of chromosomes (haploid).

Gametocyte: either the female or male form of the malarial parasite and related parasites (sex cell).

Gamma hemolysis: no enzymatic breakdown of hemoglobin; red blood cells in a blood agar medium remain intact (absence of a clear zone surrounding the bacterial colony).

Gelatinase: the extracellular enzyme (exoenzyme) that breaks down gelatin (protein).

Gene: a unit of inheritance within a chromosome.

Generation time: the time it takes for a bacterial population to double.

Genetic engineering: the technology of manipulating, transferring, and exchanging the segments of genetic material in and among organisms.

Genital: about the reproductive organs.

Graft-versus-host (GVH) disease: a disorder in which the grafted tissue invades the host tissue.

Granulomatous: tumorous.

H

Hapten: the specificity-determining portion of an antigen.

Helminth: a parasitic worm.

Helper T cells: class of T cells that is the central orchestrator of the cellular and humoral defenses of adaptive immunity.

Hematuria: the presence of blood in the urine.

Hemorrhage: bleeding.

Hepatitis: an inflammation of the liver.

Hepatomegaly: enlargement of the liver.

Herd immunity: a reduction in disease prevalence brought about when few individuals in a population are susceptible to an infectious agent.

Hermaphrodite: the presence of both male and female sex organs in the same organism.

Heterotroph: an organism that needs organic substances for nutrition and survival.

Histogram: a one-dimensional graphic representation of cell number (Y-axis) versus one measured cell characteristic (X-axis), e.g., cell size.

Holoenzyme: an enzyme with a bound cofactor or coenzyme.

Host cell: a cell that is infected by a virus or another type of micro-organism.

Humoral immunity: adaptive immunity mediated by antibodies produced by B cells.

Hyaline: hyphae and conidia lightly pigmented when observed under the microscope; includes shades of green and blue.

Hydatid (cyst): the larval stage of the sheep tapeworm (*Echinococcus granulosus*) consisting of a cystic structure filled with fluid.

Hydrodynamic focusing: is a process in which laminar flow is induced through the injection of a slow-moving sample dilution into a stream of fast-moving sheath fluid to prevent mixing (also called *focused flow*).

Hypha (plural, hyphae): the structural vegetative unit of a mycelium; can be non-septate (without cross-walls) or septate (with cross-walls).

Hypoxia: deficiency of oxygen.

I

Icosahedral: a geometric figure with twenty faces and twelve corners.

Idiopathic: about conditions without clear pathogenesis; spontaneous origin.

Immunogen: a substance capable of stimulating the formation of an antibody (immunoglobulin).

Immunoglobulin: an antibody molecule.

Immunology: the study of the immune system.

In utero: within the uterus.

In vitro: outside the living body e.g., a laboratory setting.

In vivo: inside the living body.

Induration: hardness

Inflammation: A reaction of tissue to irritation, injury, or infection. It is a beneficial process as it destroys or contains the pathogen within a small area, enabling the healing process to begin.

Intercalary: developing within the hyphal strand.

Ischemia: temporary and local deficiency of blood supply; caused by obstruction of the circulation to a cell, tissue, or organ.

Isoagglutinins: the ABO antibodies (anti-A, anti-B, anti-A,B).

Isotype: the subclasses of an immunoglobulin molecule.

J

Jaundice (icterus): a condition in which bile pigments (bilirubin) enter the circulation, giving a yellowish tint to the skin, whites of the eyes, mucous membranes, and body fluids.

K

Kaposi's sarcoma: malignant neoplastic (cancerous) growths of small blood vessels.

Kernicterus: accumulation of indirect bilirubin in brain tissue.

Kinin: a group of polypeptides that have considerable biologic activity.

L

Labile: susceptible to deterioration.

Larva: a developmental stage of an insect or a worm.

Lectin: proteins found in plants (usually seeds).

L-forms: It is a phase in which bacterial cells are devoid of cell wall components.

Ligase: an enzyme capable of influencing the formation of a chemical bond between two molecules.

Lumen: cavity.

Lymphatic system: Lymph nodes linked by a network of small tubes spread throughout the body that transport the lymph fluid.

Lymphocyte: a type of white blood cell that arises in lymphoid tissues; important cells in specific immunity; not phagocytic.

Lysis: chemical destruction.

M

Macrophage: end-stage development for monocytes; can ingest various substances for subsequent digestion or storage; located at various sites in the body (e.g., liver, lung, spleen); exist as free mobile cells or fixed cells.

Major crossmatch: a compatibility test that involves the recipient's serum and donor red blood cells.

Malaise: fatigue.

Medium: a preparation that contains nutrients to support the growth of microorganisms; can be a liquid or a solid.

Meiosis: a process that involves cell division of germ cells whereby two successive divisions of the nucleus occur, producing cells with half the number of chromosomes present in somatic cells.

Memory cell: A cell which is produced as part of a normal immune response. These cells remember a specific antigen and are responsible for the rapid immune response (i.e., production of antibodies) on exposure to subsequent infections by that particular antigen.

Metastasis: movement of body cells (e.g., cancer cells) or microbes from one part of the body to another, changing the location of a disease or of its manifestations without direct involvement; spread by the lymph or blood circulation.

Microorganism (microbe): a small living thing. The group includes bacteria, archaea, protozoa, algae, fungi, and viruses.

Mitosis: a process that involves cell division, resulting in daughter nuclei with the same number of chromosomes as the parent cell; occurs in all cells except sex cells.

Mold: filamentous fungus.

Monoclonal: antibody produced by a single ancestral antibody-forming parent cell.

Mordant: an agent that increases the affinity of the stain towards the cell structure e.g., iodine in the Gram stain.

Multiple myeloma: a neoplastic proliferation of plasma cells; characterized by highly elevated immunoglobulin levels of monoclonal origin.

Mycelium (plural, mycelia): a branched network of fungal hyphae.

Myelofibrosis: replacement of bone marrow by fibrous tissue.

N

Necrosis: death and decay of the tissue.

Nematode: a roundworm.

Neonate: a newborn infant ≤ 4 months of age.

Neuraminidase: an enzyme that cleaves sialic acid from the red cell membrane.

Nitrate reduction: formation of nitrite (NO_2) or ammonia (NH_3) from nitrate (NO_3).

Nitrification: conversion of ammonia (NH_3) to nitrate (NO_3).

Normal body flora: Microbes that have adapted to living on the body, are usually present, and rarely cause harm.

Nosocomial: an infection acquired in a hospital or other health care setting.

Nucleus (plural, nuclei): The nucleus is the control center of the cell containing chromosomes.

O

Obligate aerobes: organisms that use only oxygen as their final electron acceptor; also called strict aerobes.

Obligate anaerobes: organisms that fail to grow in the presence of oxygen; also called strict anaerobes.

Oliguria: decreased amount of urine formation.

Operon: a group of genes that function to turn on or turn off the biosynthesis of a protein.

Opsonin: a substance in serum that facilitates phagocytosis by the reticuloendothelial system (R.E.S); the phenomenon is called opsonization.

Organelle: a membrane-enclosed structure (inside of cells) that has a specialized function.

Osmosis: the movement of fluid from one compartment to another, where both compartments are separated by a semipermeable membrane.

Oxyhemoglobin: the combination of hemoglobin with Oxygen.

P

Panagglutination: an antibody that agglutinates all red blood cells, including patient's own cells.

Passive immunity: adaptive immune defenses received from another individual or animal.

Pathogen: an organism that causes a disease.

Pathogenic: capable of causing disease.

Penia: few.

Phagocyte: A white blood cell that can surround, engulf (phagocytosis), and destroy invading micro-organisms including viruses and bacteria. There are two separate groups: macrophages and neutrophils.

Phagocytosis: a type of endocytosis in which large particles are engulfed by membrane invagination, after which the particles are enclosed in a pocket, which is pinched off from the membrane to form a vacuole.

Phagolysosome: a compartment in a phagocytic cell that results when the phagosome is fused with the lysosome, leading to the destruction of the pathogens inside.

Phialide: tube or vase-shaped conidiogenous cell.

Plaque: a clear area in the confluent growth of a cell or bacterial culture due to the lytic action of a bacteriophage or virus.

Poikilocytosis: variation in red cell shape.

Proglottid: One of the segments of a tapeworm; a mature proglottid contains both male and female sex organs and a gravid proglottid contains eggs.

Prokaryote: a cell without a membrane-bound nucleus and membrane-bound organelles.

Protein: a folded long-chain molecule consisting of amino acids. Proteins are required for the structure, function, and regulation of an organism's cell/cells, tissues, and organs.

Protozoan (plural, protozoa): an eukaryotic, single-celled organism that usually lacks chlorophyll.

Pseudopodium (plural, pseudopodia): a temporary extension of the cytoplasm of an amoeboid cell. It is used in both motility and feeding processes.

R

Recombinant: a cell with a complement of genes that did not belong to either parent cell.

Replication: a duplication.

Restriction: a point along a strand of DNA where enzymes can cleave the strand.

Rhino: referring to the nose.

Rhizoid: rootlike hypha.

S

Saprobe: an organism that lives on decaying organic matter.

Satellitism: It is *in vitro* phenomenon where one bacterial species produces a key metabolite that facilitates the growth of another bacterial species near colonies of the first species.

Scatterplot: Two-dimensional graphic representations of two or more cell characteristics plotted against each other (also called *scattergram* or *cytogram*).

Scolex: the head of a tapeworm.

Septicemia: the presence of pathogens or their toxic products.

Septum (plural, septa): A cross-wall that separates cytoplasm and nuclei in a hypha.

Sessile: arising on the sides of a hypha.

Splenomegaly: enlargement of the spleen.

Sporangium (plural, sporangia): A round bag-like structure filled with endogenous asexual spores called sporangiospores.

Spore: A reproductive structure that is formed by either meiosis or mitosis.

Sterigma (plural, sterigmata): A small slender structure on which a basidiospore is produced.

Stolon: a hyphal runner that connects a group of sporangiophores.

Strain: a group of organisms that belong to the same species.

Substrate: a substance acted upon by an enzyme.

T

Taxonomy: classification of organisms by kingdoms, divisions, subdivisions, classes, orders, families, genera, and species.

Template: a strand of DNA or RNA that provides the sequence of nucleotides for a new strand of DNA or RNA being synthesized.

Thresholds: are electronically set size limits that include wanted particles (above the threshold), excluding the ones falling below the threshold (also called *discriminators*).

Tinea: ringworm.

Toxin: any substance that is poisonous to other organisms.

V

Vaccine: a suspension of an infectious agent or its component that is administered as a form of passive immunization to develop resistance against the disease caused by that organism.

Venipuncture: puncture of a vein.

Viral envelope: a spiky coat that covers the viral protein coat or capsid.

Viruses: the smallest infectious agents that contain only one kind of nucleic acid (DNA or RNA); incapable of reproduction without a living host cell and metabolism.

von Willebrand's disease: a congenital bleeding disorder.

Y

Yeast: a form of fungus characterized by cells without hyphae.

Z

Zoonosis: a contagious disease primarily of animals and can be transmitted to humans through direct or indirect contact with infected animals.

Zygospore: a large, thick-walled spore that develops from the fusion of the tips of approximating hyphae followed by meiosis.

Zygote: the cell formed when a male cell and a female cell fuse together.

Bibliography

A

Alcamo, I.E., and Elson, L. M., The microbiology coloring book, 1996, HarperCollins College Publishers, New York, U.S.A.

Alexander JT. EI-Ali AM, Newman JL et al. (2013), *Transfusion,* Red blood cells stored for increasing periods produce progressive impairments in nitric oxide-mediated vasodilation.

Alter, A. A.; Bryan, D. E. and others (Editors), *Medical Technology Examination Review' Vol. 2,* 1978 (fourth edition), Medical Examination Publishing Co., Inc., N.Y.

American chemical society, Reagent chemicals, 2006 (10th edition), American chemical society specifications, Washington, D.C.

An experienced Professor, *Clinical Pathology,* 1978-79 (fifth revised edition), New Literature Publishing Company, Bombay, India.

An experienced Teacher, *Aids to Experimental* Physiology for Medical students, 1972, India.

Anna Salleh (2 March 2009) "Researchers knock down gastro bug myths" ABC Science online Archived.

Atlas, R.M. and Parks, L.C., Microorganisms in our world, 1995,Mosby-Year Books, Inc., Missouri, U.S.A.

Aulbach, A.D., Amuzie, C.J. Biomarkers in Nonclinical Drug Development. A Comprehensive Guide to Toxicology in Nonclinical Drug Development (Second edition, 2017).

Ayyanar, K.; Pichandi, S.; Janakiraman P. Evaluation of Glucose Oxidase and Hexokinase Methods. International Journal of Biotechnology and Biochemistry. ISSN 0973-2691 Volume 14, Number 1 (2018) pp. 51-58.

B

Bauer, J.D., et.al., *Clinical Laboratory Methods,* 1982 (ninth edition), C.V. Mosby Co., St. Louis.

Bernard, K. A., Funke, G. (2012) "*Genus I. Corynebacterium*". In Goodfellow, M.; Kampfer, P.; Busse, H.J.; Trujillo, M.E., Suzuki, K.; Ludwig, W.; Whitman, W.B. (eds.).

Bergey's Manual of Systematic Bacteriology (2nd ed.). Springer. P. 245.

Bhagat, *Viva in Pathology,* 1986 (second edition), Scientific book Corporation, Patna, India.

Bharucha, Chitra; Meyer, Hermina; Bharucha, Hoshang; Moody, Anthony and Carman, R.H. (Editors), *Hand-book of Medical Laboratory Technology,* 1970 (first edition), Department of Clinical Pathology and Blood Bank of the Christian Medical College and Hospital, Vellore, India. -Bhave, *V.N., A Handbook of First Aid,* 1943 (first edition), New Kitabkhana, Poona-2, India.

Black, J.G., *MICROBIOLOGY Principles and Explorations,*2002(5th edition), John Wiley & Sons, Inc. New York, NY.

Blacklock, D.B.; Southwell, T. and Davey, T.H.,.4 *Guide to Human* Parasitology,1953 (fifth edition), H.K. Lewis & Co. Ltd., London. -Blood Bank of the Christian Medical College and Hospital, Vellore, India. -Bramfitt, W. (Editor), *New Perspectives in Clinical Microbiology,* 1978, Kluwer Medical Martinus, Nijhoff Medical Division, London.

Boase S, Foreman A, Cleland E, Tan L, Melton-Kreft R, Pant H, Hu FZ, Ehrlich GD, Wormald PJ (2013). The microbiome of chronic rhinosinusitis: culture, molecular diagnostics, and biofilm detection. *BMC Infect. Dis.* PubMed. Google Scholar.

Bradford, M.M.(1976). A rapid and sensitive method for the quantitation of microgram quantities of protein utilizing the principle of protein-dye binding. Anal. Biochem 72: 248-254.

Brown, B.A., *Hematology: Principles and procedures,* 1984 (fourth edition), Lea and Fabiger, Philadelphia.

Brooks, Geo. F. et al., "Jawetz, Melnick, & Adelberg's Medical microbiology", The McGraw-Hill Companies, Inc., 24th edition, 2007.

Bruggemann H. (2012) *Propionibacterium acnes* host cell tropism contributes to vimentin-mediated invasion and induction of inflammation. *Cell. Microbiol.* PubMed. Google Scholar.

Burch, B. Interpreting Hematology Scatter-Plots. One Cancer Center's Keys to Seeing the BIG Picture. New York University Clinical Cancer Center. Webinar, Dec. 2011.

Burtis, C.A. and Ashwood, E.R. (Editors), *Tietz Fundamentals of Clinical Chemistry*, 1996 (4th edition), W.B. Saunders Company, Philadelphia.

C

Calderone, R. and Fonzi, W. *"Virulence factors of Candida albicans". Trends in Microbiology.* 2001 Jul;9 (7): 327-35.

Cassagne *et al.*; Identification of filamentous fungal isolates by MALDI – TOF mass spectrometry: clinical evaluation of an extended reference spectra library. *Medical Mycology*, Volume 52, Issue 8, Nov. 2014, pages 826-834.

Chaudhry, K., *Biochemical Techniques,* 1989 (first edition), Jaypee Brothers, New Delhi, India.

Cheesbrough, Monica and McArthur, John, *A Laboratory Manual for Rural Tropical Hospitals,* 1976 (first edition), Churchill Livingstone, London.

Ching, E. Solid Phase Red Cell Adherence Assay: a tubeless method for pretransfusion testing and other applications in transfusion science. Transfusion Apheresis Science. 2012, Jun; 46(3):287-91.

Ciulla, A.P., Buescher, G.K. and Youse, J.H., *Medical Technology Examination Review, and Study Guide,* 1988, Appleton and Lange, California.

Clifton, C.E., *Introduction to the Bacteria,* 1958 (second edition), McGraw-Hill Book Company, Inc., London.

Clinical Chemistry, Vol. 31, No. 9,1985 (Symposium issue).

Collee, J.G., *Applied Medical Microbiology,* 1981 (second edition), Blackwell Scientific Publications, London.

Cooke, E., Mary and Gibson, George, L., *Essential Clinical Microbiology,* 1983, John Wiley & Sons, New York, Toronto.

Criswell, K. Interpretation of Hematology Veterinary Scattergrams in Normal, Webinar, Feb.23, 2018.

D

Dacie, Sir J.V.; Lewis, S.M., *Practical Hematology,* 1984 (sixth edition), Churchill Livingstone, N.Y.

Davidsohn, Israel and Henry, J.B., *Todd-Sanford Clinical Diagnosis by Laboratory Methods,* 1977 (15th edition), The Macmillan Company of India Limited, India.

Deepak Kumar, Dibyajyoti Banerjee. Methods of albumin estimation in clinical biochemistry: Past, present, and future. Clinica Chimica Acta. Vol. 469, June 2017, pages 150-160.

Deepak, A. Rao; Le, Tao; Bhusan, Vikas (2007). *First Aid for the USMLE Step 1* 2008. McGraw-Hill Medical.

Di Salvo, A. *"Mycology"*. http:// pathmicro.med.sc.edu/mycology-3 htm.

Dingle, TC, Butler-Wu SM. Maldi-tof mass spectrometry for microorganism identification. Clin. Lab. Med. 2013 Sep; 33(3): 589-609.

District tuberculosis program, *Laboratory Technician's Manual,* 1977, The National Tuberculosis Institute, Banglore, India.

Doucet, L.D.; Packard, A.E., *Medical Technology Examination Review,* 1984 (second edition), J.B. Lippincott Company, Philadelphia, U.S.A.

Dubowski, Kurt M. An o-toluidine method for body fluid glucose determination" Clinical Chemistry. 1962).

Duerden, B.I., Reid, T.M.S.; Jewsbury, J.M. and Turk, D.C., *A New short Text-book of Microbial and Parasitic Infection,* 1987, Hodder & Stoughton Ltd., Kent.

E

Eastam, R.D., *A Laboratory Guide to Clinical Diagnosis,* 1983 (fifth edition), K.M. Varghese Company, Bombay, India.

Evashin Pillay et al. Evaluation of automated malaria diagnosis using the Sysmex XN-30 analyzer in a clinical setting. Malaria Journal; Jan 22, 2019. Springer Nature, Singapore.

F

Foodborne illnesses and Germs. Centers for Disease Control and Prevention (CDC). Retrieved 18 Feb.,2018.

Funke G., Monnet D., deBernardis C., von Graevenitz A., Freney J. (1998). Evaluation of the VITEK 2 system for rapid identification of medically relevant gram-negative rods. J. Clin. Microbiol. 36: 1948-1952.

G

Ganesh, M. et al. (2016). Detection of *Clostridium tetani* in human clinical samples using tetX specific primers targeting the neurotoxin. J. Infect. Public Health. National Institutes of Health. US National Library of Medicine.

Gartner, Leslie P.; Hiatt, James L., " Color Atlas of Histology", Lippincott Williams & Wilkins, Fourth edition, 2006.

German Campuzano-Zuluaga, Thomas Hanscheid, Martin P Grobusch. Automated haematology analysis to diagnose malaria. Malar. J. 2010 Nov 30; 9:346.

Ghoshal, K. and Bhattacharyya, M., *ScientificWorldJournal*, 2014 Mar. 3.

Goljan, E. F., Pathology review, 1998, W.B. Saunders Company, Philadelphia, Penn. U.S.A.

Goodale, R.H., *Clinical Interpretation of Laboratory Tests,* 1950, E. A. Davis Company, Philadelphia.

Gray, C.H. and Howorth, *Clinical Chemical Pathology,* 1980 (ninth edition), Edward Arnold Ltd., London.

Guh, AY; Kutty, PK (Oct. 2018). "*Clostridium difficile* Infection" Annals of Internal Medicine. 169 (7).

Gupta, M.; Chauhan, K.; Singhvi, T.; Kumari, M.; Grover, R. Useful information provided by graphic displays of automated cell counters in hematological malignancies. Journal of Clinical Laboratory Analysis. Volume: 32; Issue: 5. First Published Jan. 21, 2018.

H

Handoo, A. and Dadu, T. Flow Cytometry in Pediatric Malignancies. Indian Pediatrics, 2018; 55: 55-62.

Harpreet Virk, Neelam Varma, Shano Naseem, Ishwar Bihana, Dmitry Sukhachev. Sep. 2018 "Utility of cell population data (VCS parameters) as a rapid screening tool for Acute Myeloid Leukemia in resource-constrained laboratories. Journal of Clinical Laboratory Analysis.

Hartenstein, V. "Blood cells and blood cell development in the animal kingdom". *Annu Rev Cell Dev Biol.* 2006, 22: 677-712.

Henry *Clinical Diagnosis and Management by Laboratory Methods,* 1984 (seventeenth edition), W.B. Saunders, Philadelphia.

Hillman, Robert S. and Finch, Clement A., *Red cell Manual,* 1985 (fifth edition), F.A. Davis Company, Philadelphia.

Hoff brand, A. V. (Editor), *Recent Advances in Hematology,* 1982 (first edition), Churchill Livingstone, London and New York.

Hoffman, Barbara (2012). *Williams gynecology* (2nd edition), McGraw-Hill Medical, New York.

Hood, W., *A-Z of Clinical Chemistry* (a guide for trainee), 1980 (first edition), MTP Press Limited, International Medical Publishers.

I

Ilya Berim, Sanjay Sethi, in (2012) Clinical Respiratory Medicine (4th edition).

Inaba, T.; Nomura, N.; Takahashi, M.; Ishizuka, K.; and others. Characteristic Scattergram of White Blood Cells Obtained Using the Pentra MS CRP Hematology Analyzer in a patient with Neutral Lipid Storage Disease. Laboratory hematology. December 2013.

J

Jana Chalupova, Martin Raus, Michaela Sedlarova, Marek Sebela. Identification of fungal microorganisms by MALDI-TOF mass spectrometry. Biotechnology advances. 2013.

Javiya, V.A., Ghatak, S.B., Patel, K.R., and Patel, J.A., *Indian Journal of Pharmacology*, 2008 Oct., 40(5):230-234.

Jawetz, Ernest; Melnick, J.L. and Adelberg, E.A., *Review of Medical Microbiology,* 1978, Lange Medical Publications, California, U.S.A.

Jean Francois Lesesve, Loic Garcon, Thomas Lecompte. "Finding knizocytes in a peripheral blood smear" Feb. 2011: American Journal of hematology.

Jennifer, M., Sandrine, A., Beatrice, C., Priscilla, C., Pierre-Jean, Cotte-Pattat., Heather, T., Parampal, D., Virginie, M., Victoria, G., Joanne, T., Vanessa, B., Jean-Philippe, L., David, O'Callaghan, Valerie M., Anne, K. (2018) A MALDI-TOF-MS database with broad genus coverage for species-level identification of Brucella. journal. Pntd.

Judy Gopal and Hui-Fen Wu. "A briefcase study demonstrating the applicability of MALDI mass spectrometry for detecting bacteria in dental samples". (2015); Issue 19. Royal Society of Chemistry, UK.

K

Kaswan, K.K.; Varikar, A.V.; Feroz, A.; Patel, H.V.; Gumber, M.; Trivedi H.L.; Saudi, J. (2011). *Nocardia* infection in a renal transplant recipient.

Klainer, A.S., Le Frock, J.L., Allender, P., and Moore, Jr., D.W., Use of the Gram stain in clinical infectious diseases, 1975 (Second edition), Schering Corporation, Kenilworth, N.J.,U.S.A.

Kulkarni, K.P. (Editor), *Medifacts,* Vol.5, Alkem Laboratories, Bombay, India.

Kurokawa I, Nishijima S, Kawabata S, (1999). Antimicrobial susceptibility of Propionibacterium acnes isolated from acne vulgaris. *Eur. J. dermatol.* PubMed. Google Scholar.

Kwiterovich, Peter O. Lipoprotein Analytical Laboratory. University School of Medicine. Laboratory Procedure Manual. 2003-2004. Baltimore, MD. USA.

L

L. Thompson, I. Turko, and F. Murad. Mol. Immunol. 2006, 43, 1485.

Labbe, R.G.; Juneja, V.K. 2017). *"Clostridium perfringens"*, *Foodborne Diseases,* Elsevier.

Levinson, W. Review of Medical Microbiology and Immunology. 2010: McGraw-Hill.

Lewis SM. Reference ranges and normal values. In: SM Lewis, BJ Bain, I Bates, eds. *Dacie and Lewis Practical Haematology*, 11th edn. Philadelphia, PA: Churchill Livingstone; 2011:11-22.

Li H and Lykotrafitis, *Phys Rev E Stat Nonlin Soft Matter Phys*: Vesiculation of healthy and defective red blood cells. 2015 Jul;92(1).

Li-Hua Li, Ewelina P. Dutkiewicz, Ying-Chen Huang, Hsin-Bai Zhou, Cheng-Chih Hsu. Analytical methods for cholesterol quantification. Journal of Food and Drug Analysis. 2019. Vol. 27, Issue 2, pages 375-386.

Liqiang Zhang, Fengyu Su, Sean Buizer, Hungguang Lu, Weimin Gao, Yanqing Tian, and Deirdre Meldrum. A dual sensor for real-time monitoring of glucose and oxygen. Biomaterials. Dec.2013; 34(38).

Lynnsay M. Dickson, Eckhart J. Buchmann, Charl Janse Van Rensburg, and Shane A. The impact of differences in plasma glucose between glucose oxidase and hexokinase methods on estimated gestational diabetes mellitus prevalence. Scientific Reports 9, Article number: 7238 (2019).

M

Mader, Sylvia S. and Windelspecht, "Inquiry into life", McGraw-Hill Education, Sixteenth edition, 2020.

M.H. yang, L.H. Lo, Y.H. Chen, J. Shiea, P.C. Wu, Y.C. Tyan, and Y.J. Jong, Rapid Commun. Mass Spectrom. 2009, 23, 3220.

Maria Siller-Ruiz et al. Fast methods of fungal and bacterial identification by MALDI-TOF mass spectrometry, chromogenic media. Enfermedades Infecciosas Y Microbiología Clínica (English Edition). 2017 Vol. 35. Issue 5, pages 303-313.

Marshall Don. Graham (2003) "The Coulter Principle: Foundation of an industry" Journal of Laboratory Automation: 8 (6): 72-81.

Mary Louise Turgeon. (2004), Clinical Hematology: Theory and Procedures, Vol. 936. Chapter 6. Lippincott Williams & Wilkins.

Mather, A.; Roland, D. The Automated Thiosemicarbazide Diacetyl Monoxime Method for Plasma Urea. May 1969. The American Association of Clinical Chemists, Inc.

Maurizio S., Brunella P. Identification of Molds by Matrix-Assisted Laser Desorption Ionization –Time of Flight Mass Spectrometry. 2016. Colleen Suzanne Kraft (editor) Journal of Clinical Microbiology.

McCartney and *Mackie, Medical Microbiology, Vol. l: Microbial infections,* 1978 (13th edition), Churchill Livingstone, London.

Michael A. Reeve, Denise Bachmann. A method for filamentous fungal growth and sample preparation aimed at more consistent MALDI-TOF MS spectra despite variations in growth rates and/or incubation time. Biology Methods and Protocols, Volume 4, Issue 1, 2019.

Michael Mcmillin J. Blood Glucose. Clinical Methods: The History, Physical, and Laboratory Examinations. (3rd edition).

Miguel A, Orero M, Simon R, et al. Automated neutrophil morphology and its utility in the assessment of neutrophil dysplasia. Lab Hematol. 2007; 13: 98-102.

Miller, William V. (Editor-in-chief), *Technical Methods and Procedures,* 1974 (first edition), American Association of Blood Banks, Washington, D.C.

Mohandas N. et al.," Malaria and human red blood cells". Med Microbiol and Immunol. Nov. 2012, 201(4):593-8.

Moini, Jahangir, "Anatomy and Physiology", Jones & Bartlett Learning, Second edition, 2016.

Mukherjee, Kanai L. (Chief Editor*), Medical Laboratory Technology', Vol. I, II, and 111,* 1988 (first edition), Tata McGraw-Hill Publishing Company Limited, New Delhi, India.

Murray P.R., Barron, E.J., Pfaller M.A., Tenover F.C., Yolken R.H. (editors). *Manual of clinical microbiology* (1999). American Society for Microbiology, Washington, D.C. (7th edition)

Murray, et al. (2009). *Medical Microbiology* (6th edition). Mosby Elsevier.

Muttaiyah S.; Best EJ; Freeman JT Taylor Sl; Morris J; Roberts S.. *Corynebacterium diphtheriae endocarditis:* a case series and review of the treatment approach. Int. J. Infect. Dis. 2011.

Myhre, Byron A. (Editor), *Blood component Therapy, -A Physician's Handbook,* 1975, American Association j) f Blood Banks.

N

Nagao K, Mori T, Sawada C, Sasakawa C, Kanezaki Y. (2007) Detection of the tetanus toxin gene by polymerase chain reaction: a case study. Jpn J Infect Dis. PubMed, Google Scholar.

Naik, S.P. and Karmarkar, M.G., A *Handbook of Practical Microbiology,* 1983 (first edition), Vora Medical Publications, Bombay, India.

Neuschlova, M. et al. (2017) *"Identification of Mycobacterium species by MALDI-TOF-MS".* Department of Microbiology and Immunology , Jessenius Faculty of Medicine in Martin, Comenius University in Bratislava, Mala Hora 4B, 036 01, Martin, Slovakia.

O

Olender, Alina (2013). "The cause of Actinomyces canaliculitis" Annals of Agricultural and EnvironmentalMedicine.

Ortho Diagnostics Inc., *Hemolytic Disease of the Newborn,* 1968, Ortho Diagnostics, Raritan, N.J. 08869, U.S.A.

P

Pant, M.C., *Biochemistry,* 1966 (first edition), Technical Publishers of India.

Patel R. A Moldy Application of MALDI: MALDI-ToF Mass Spectrometry for Fungal Identification. Journal of Fungi. Jan. 2019.

Patel, A.H., *A Text-book of Microbiology,* 1982 (first edition), Patel Publication, Nadiad, India.

Pelczar, M.J.; Chan, E.C.S. and Krieg, N.R., *Microbiology,* 1986 (fifth edition), McGraw Hill Book Company, New York.

Poller, L. (Editor), *Recent Advances in Blood Coagulation,* 1981 (first edition), Churchill Livingstone, London, and New York.

Praharaj, I.; Sujatha, S.; Ashwini, M.A.; Parija, S.C. (8 August 2013). Co-infection with *Nocardia asteroides* Complex and *Strongyloides stercoralis* in a patient with Autoimmune Hemolytic Anemia.

R

Robertson William S. Optimizing Determination of PlasmaAlbumin by the Bromocresol Green Dye-Binding Method. CLIN. CHEM. (1981) 144-146.

Roy, AB (1976). "Sulfatases lysosomes and disease" *The Australian Journal of Experimental Biology and Medical science*. 54 PMID.

Ryan, Kenneth J.; Ray, C. George (2004). *Sherris Medical Microbiology: An Introduction to Infectious Diseases* (4th edition). New York: McGraw-Hill.

S

Saleh, Ayache, Monica Panelli, Francesco M. Marincola, and David F. Stroncek. "Effects of storage time and exogenous protease inhibitors on plasma protein levels". Am J Clin Pathol. 2006,126: 174-184.

Sehgal, S.; Sharma, S.; Sethi, N.; Kushwaba, S.; Chauhan, R. (2013). Abnormal WBC Scattergram: A clue to the diagnosis of malaria. Hematology, 18:2, 101-105.

Severino Jefferson Ribeiro da Silva et al.; Clinical and Laboratory Diagnosis of SARS-CoV-2, the Virus Causing COVID-19., American Chemical Society Infectious Diseases, August 4, 2020, 6, 9, 2319-2336.

Shanaz Khodaiji, Newer CBC Parameters of Clinical Significance. Springer eBook. Jan. 1, 2019. Springer Nature, Singapore.

Simmons, N.A. (Editor), *An Introduction to Microbiology for nurses,* 1980 (third edition), William Heinemann Medical Books Ltd., London.

Singh, Niva; Khardori, Romesh and Agarwal, Savita, *Science Reporter,* May 1991, Publications and Information Directorate, New Delhi, India. -Sodeman, W., *Pathologic Physiology-Mechanisms of Disease,* sixth edition.

Singh, Saumya, Patil, D.Y., (Dec. 2013). Biochemical Reactions. Published in: Education, Technology, Business.

Sood, Ramnik, *Medical Laboratory Technology,* 1985, Jaypee Brothers, New Delhi, India.

Sood, Ramnik, *Multiple Choice Questions in Pathology',* 1984, Jaypee Brothers, New Delhi, India.

Spencer, K.; PriceC.P. Kinetic immunoturbidimetry: the estimation of albumin. Clinica Chimica Acta. Vol. 95, Issue 2, 16 July 1979, pages 263-276.

Stevens, Alan; Lowe, James S.; and Young, Barbara, " WHEATER'S Basic Histopathology", Churchill Livingstone, Fourth edition, 2002.

Stokes, E. Joan, and Ridgway, G.L., *Clinical Microbiology,* 1987 (sixth edition), Edward Arnold (publishers) Ltd., London.

Stroup, Marjory, and Treacy, Margaret, *Blood group Antigens and Antibodies,* 1982, Ortho Diagnostic Systems, N.J. U.S.A.

Swash, M. and Mason, *SHutchison's Clinical Methods,* 1984 (18th edition), Bailliere Tindall, Eastbourne.

Swetha, V.V., Rao, U.S., Prakash, P.H., and Subbarayudu, S., *International Journal of Current Microbiology and Applied Sciences*, Vol. 3 Number 3 (2014) pp. 120-125.

T

Thompson, R.A. (Editor), *Techniques in Clinical Immunology,* 1981 (second edition), Blackwell Scientific Publications, London.

Thomson, Jean M., *Blood Coagulation and Hemostasis* (a practical guide), 1985, (third edition), Churchill Livingstone, London, and New York.

Tilkian, Conover and Tilkian, *Clinical Implications of laboratory tests,* 1979 (second edition), The C.V. Mosby Company, London.

Transfusion Medicine Technical Manual, 2003 (2nd edition), WHO.

Tsutomy Momose, Osuke Ohkura, and Jun Tomita. Determination of urea in Blood and Urine with Diacetyl Monoxime-Glucuronolactone Reagent. July 1964. Clinical chemistry. Vol. ii, No. 2.

V

Vaishnav, V.P., *Text-book of Clinical Pathology,* 1986 (second edition), Medical publishers, Baroda.

Vaishnavi, C; Bhasin, D; Kochhar, R; Singh, K (2000). "Clostridium difficile toxin and fecal lactoferrin assays in adult patients" Microbes and Infection /Institut Pasteur.

Valerie Bush and Roberta G. Reed. Bromcresol Purple Dye-Binding Methods Underestimate Albumin That Is Carrying Covalently Bound Bilirubin. CLIN. CHEM. (1987) 821-823.

Vander, Sherman, Luciano, *Human Physiology-The mechanisms of body function,* 1981 (third edition), Tata McGraw-Hill Publishing Company Ltd., New Delhi, India.

Vani, R., Soumya, R., Manasa, K., and Carl, H., *Oxid Antioxid Med Sci*, Storage lesions in blood components,2015, Vol 4, Issue 3.

Varley, Harold; Gowenlock, A.H. and Bell Maurice, *Practical Clinical Biochemistry Vol. I,* 1980 (fifth edition), William Heinemann Medical Books Ltd., London.

Veloo, A.C.M. et al. (2014). *Clinical Microbiology and Infection.* The influence of incubation time, sample preparation, and exposure to oxygen on the quality of the MALDI-TOF-MS spectrum of anaerobic bacteria.Netherlands.

Vidyarthi, R.D., *A Text-book of Zoology,* 1986 (16th edition), S.Chand and Company (Pvt.) Ltd., New Delhi, India.

W

Wani, D.B., *Transfusion Bulletin* Vol.4, No.2,1991.

Wayne, PA; (2007); Clinical and Laboratory Standards Institute. Performance Standards for Antimicrobial Susceptibility Testing; 17th Informational Supplement.

Weir, D.W., *Immunology,* 1983 (fifth edition), Churchill Livingstone, Edinburgh.

William's Haematology (7th edition), 2005. Published by McGraw-Hill Professional.

Williams, W.J., et al., *Hematology',* 1983 (third edition), McGraw-Hill, New York.

Wistreich, G., Microbiology perspectives, 1999, Prentice-Hall, Inc., New Jersey, U.S.A.

Y

Y. Abiko, M. Saitoh, Curr. Pharm. Des. 2007, 13, 3065.

Yunsheng Zhao, Xiaoyan Yang, Wei Lu, Hong Liao, Fei Liao. Uricase-based methods for determination of uric acid in serum. Microchim Acta (2009) 164: 1-6.

Index

C

C3d, 482, 501
C4, 482
Calcitonin, 208, 218
Calomel electrode, 28
CAMP test, 325, 332
Campylobacter jejuni, 291, 349, 556
Candida albicans, 242, 285, 302, 378, 382, 386–87, 391–92, 521, 559
Candida glabrata, 392
Candida guilliermondii, 392
Candida spp., 380, 390–92
Candidiasis, 386
Capsid, 417–18, 595
Capsomere, 411, 413
Capsule stain, 279
Caramelization, 469
Carbol fuchsin, 277–78
Carbon dioxide, 132, 134, 217, 310
Carbon monoxide, 73, 548
Carbon tetrachloride, 194, 196
Carbon tetrachloride poisoning, 194, 196
Carcinogens, 596
Cardiolipin, 259
Cascade effect, 231
Case studies, 456
Casts, 517, 521–22
Casts in urine, 521–22
Catabolism, 596
Catalase, 317, 324, 327–29, 331–35, 344–46, 349–53, 355, 357–59
Catalase test, 317
Catalysis, 201
Catalyst, 596
Catecholamines, 209
Cathode, 29, 31–32, 60, 169, 200, 239
Cation, 596
Cell membrane, 104, 160, 170, 219, 355, 376, 411, 428, 440, 460, 539, 602
Cellulose, 34
Cellulose acetate, 32, 60, 179
Cell wall, 340–41, 345
Centers for Disease Control and Prevention, 297
Centrifugation, 286, 430, 463, 495
Ceruloplasmin, 223
Cestode, 396, 400
Chaga's disease, 254, 404
Chédiak-Higashi syndrome, 88
Chemical poisoning, 17, 92
Chemiluminescence, 212
Chemostat, 596
Chemotaxis, 232
Chickenpox, 83, 228

Chills, 385–86, 408, 481, 483
Chimera, 436
Chitin, 596
Chloramphenicol, 65, 390
Cholera, 348, 596
Cholesterol, 4, 132–33, 160–62, 168, 224, 518–19, 540–41, 549
Chromatography, 60
Chromogenic media, 290
Chromosomes, 426, 592, 594, 599, 602–3
Chronic granulomatous disease (CGD), 88
Chronic lymphocytic leukemia, 101, 537
Chronic renal failure, 218–19, 505
Circulatory (volume) overload, 480–81, 484–85
Circulatory overload, 485
Cirrhosis, 89–90
Citrate, 309–10, 331, 346–48, 353, 355, 469–70, 481, 485, 554, 557
Citrate phosphate dextrose (CPD), 469–70
Citrate toxicity, 481, 485
Citric acid cycle, 319
Citrobacter freundii, Cl. botulinum, 227
Citrobacter freundii, Cl. Botulinum, 227
Citrobacter freundii, Cl. difficile, 524
Citrobacter freundii, Cl. perfringens, 424
Citrobacter freundii, Cl. Perfringens, 424
Citrobacter freundii, Cl. tetani, 256
Citrobacter freundii, Cl. Welchii, 332
Classification, 139, 230, 415
Clinical laboratory scientist, 563, 572
Clinical microbiology, 4, 261
Clinical significance, 71–73, 75, 93–94, 101, 105, 110, 148, 152, 157, 161, 166, 176, 182, 194, 196, 199, 201, 203–5, 216–20, 441–51, 507, 510, 513, 518–22, 577–81, 584–86, 588
Clostridium spp., 318, 331
Clotting, 96, 100, 471
Clue cells, 357
Coagulation factors, 98
Cocci, 325, 344
Coccidioides immitis, 378, 381, 385, 391, 560
Coccobacilli, 275
Codon, 593
Coenocytic, 376, 380, 596
Coenzymes, 186–87
Cofactors, 98
Cold antibodies, 437
Colloids, 175, 476, 522
Colon, 156, 335, 357, 435, 524
Colony-forming unit, 300
Colorimeter, 20, 26
Compatibility, 431, 495
Complement, 4, 232–34, 241, 243, 253–55, 549–50, 571, 597
Complement-fixation, 243, 254–55, 597
Complement-fixation test, 255, 597

D

E. coli, 274, 276, 290–91, 298, 300, 343, 346, 515, 531

E. histolytica, 530

E

Ear, 295

Eczema, 72

Edema, 175, 485

EDTA, 46, 48–49, 51, 74, 76–77, 115, 132–33, 153, 166, 168, 177, 194, 202, 214, 408, 470, 554, 561, 579–80

Elective surgery, 471

Electrolytes, 4, 213, 215

Electron acceptor, 146, 167, 317, 319, 599, 603

Electron microscope, 22

Electrophoresis, 60, 179, 538, 545, 598

Elek test, 251, 333

Elephantiasis, 396–97

ELISA, 103–4, 171, 193, 212, 245–47, 404, 419, 477, 538, 550, 558–59, 598

Elongation, 366

Elution, 459, 488, 552, 598

EMB agar, 557

Embolism, 598

Emergency, 465

Emphysema, 211, 214

Employment outlook, 14

Endemic, 423

Endocarditis, 284, 329–30, 345, 359, 514, 522

Endogenous, 156, 226

Endospore stain, 278

Energy rich compound, 596

Enriched media, 289

Enteric fever, 83, 243–45, 351

Enterobacter aerogenes, 307–11, 313, 315, 317, 322

Enterobius vermicularis, 399, 528

Enterococcus faecalis, 285, 318, 320, 326, 329

Enterococcus faecium, 326, 329

Enterococcus spp., 285

Enveloped viruses, 234, 411

Enzyme Commission number (EC number), 187, 193

Enzyme-linked immunosorbent assay, 212, 245, 247, 558–59, 598

Enzyme Nomenclature and Classification, 187

Enzymes, 4, 186–87, 191–92, 204, 246

Eosin, 291, 534, 556

Eosinophilia, 399

Epidermophyton floccosum, 378, 383, 387

Epithelial cells, 357, 405, 533

Epitope, 598

Epstein-Barr virus, 418, 558

Erysipelothrix rhusiopathiae, 334

Erythroblast, 41–42, 92, 109, 436, 441, 466, 487, 541, 579

Erythrocytes, 3, 81, 89, 93, 199, 215

Freund's adjuvant, 236
Fructose, *A. fumigatus*, 388
Fungi imperfecti, 597
Fusarium spp., 391

G

G6PD, 63, 131, 145, 467
Gallbladder, 295, 575
Gamete, 599
Gamma globulin, 466
Gamma-glutamyl transferase, 204
Gamma hemolysis, 599
Gas chromatography, 20, 35, 37, 163, 168, 546
Gastric, 556
Gastrin, 210
Gaucher's disease, 110, 161, 172, 203, 549
Gelatin, 259, 314–15, 348
Gel system, 491
Genes, 305, 349, 366, 413, 421, 427, 429, 438, 443, 450, 595, 603–4
Genetics, 547
Genome, 332
Genomics, 364
Genotypes
   Geo. Candidum, 378
   Geo. capitatum, 373
Geographical distribution, 51, 442–51
Gestational diabetes, 137, 143
Giardia lamblia, 286, 526
Giemsa's stain, 82, 408–9
Glanzmann's thrombasthenia, 103, 107
Glomerular filtration rate, 153, 215, 221, 584
Glucagon, 138, 543
Gluconeogenesis, 139, 223, 543
Glucose, 3, 63, 91–92, 133, 137, 139, 142, 144–47, 193, 205, 308, 313, 315, 317, 320, 327, 333, 343–46,
   348, 357, 508–9, 543–44, 561
Glucose tolerance test, 544
Glucuronyl transferase, 181
Glutamate, 195
Glycerol kinase, 165, 167
Glycine, 436, 566
Glycogen, 139, 223, 543
Glycolysis, 144, 543
Glycoproteins, 175, 237, 429, 592
Glycosuria, 137, 143, 509
Gout, 545–46
Graft-versus-host disease, 481
Gram-negative, 268, 273–76, 281–82, 290, 297, 300, 302, 305, 310, 313, 317, 324, 332, 340–46, 348–50,
   353, 357–59, 363, 366, 422, 435
Gram-negative bacteria, 268, 281, 297, 300, 302, 317, 324, 340–43, 345, 435
Gram-positive, 272–77, 282, 289, 300, 305, 324–26, 330–32, 334, 336, 340–41, 357, 363, 366, 422

H

Kjeldahl method, 178
Klebsiella pneumoniae, 276, 279, 302, 309, 313, 317, 322, 347, 375
Klebsiella spp., 305, 307, 343
Koch's postulates, L. monocytogenes, 275

L

P

Pyruvate, 194–95, 197, 307–9

RPR test
  S. aureus, 274, 290, 327
  S. epidermidis, 422

S

Sabouraud's agar, 390–91, 424
Saccharomyces cerevisiae, 378
Safranin, 273–74, 278, 341
Salicylate, 585
Saline preparation, 525
Saliva, 429
Sallm. Typhimurium, 322
Salmonella spp., 290, 292, 307, 309, 343, 351, 531
Salm. paratyphi, Salm. Typhi, 244, 309, 351
Samples, 182, 202, 250
Saponification, 161, 166
SARS CoV-2, 416, 419–21
Scabies, 72
Schick test, 256
Schistosoma haematobium, 528
Schistosoma japonicum, 528
Schistosoma mansoni, 528
Secondary stain, 278
Secretors, 429, 499
Semen, 5, 532
Sensitivity, 36–37, 100, 103, 127, 179, 183–84, 200, 254, 302, 325, 366, 386, 421, 495, 498
Sensitization, 431, 440, 487, 499
Sepsis, 87
Septicemia, 604
Serological reactions, 226
Serotonin, 73, 210
Serratia marcescens, 309–11, 315–16, 348, 557
Serum, 3–4, 49, 55, 65, 131, 148, 152, 156–57, 160, 165, 177, 179, 181–83, 194, 198–99, 201, 218, 227, 255, 552, 581
Sexual reproduction, 377
Sheep, 255, 259, 562
Shigella dysenteriae sonnei, 351
Shigella spp., 288, 290, 292, 309, 322, 343, 375, 531
Sialic acid, 602
Sickle cell disease (SCD), 90, 93, 443, 449, 456, 472, 476, 537–38, 540
Sickle cell trait, 540
SIM medium, 307
Skin, 18, 72, 138, 241, 275, 295
Skin scrapings, 338
Smallpox, 228
Sodium, 46, 48, 60, 72, 76, 135, 177, 215, 223–24, 267, 291–92, 309, 320–21, 424, 469, 504, 530, 544–45, 561, 570
Solvents, 29, 160
Specific gravity, 50, 507
Specificity, 186, 241, 254, 421, 495

Typhoid, 71, 267, 559, 571

U

Ulcerative colitis, 84, 203
Ultraviolet light, 155, 186
Unicellular, 271, 330, 358, 376–77, 402, 594
Ureaplasma urealyticum, 310, 356
Urease, 149, 193, 310, 327, 333, 335, 339, 342, 347, 351–53, 355, 359, 556
Urethra, 269, 287, 298–99, 520
Uricase, 157–58, 193, 544
Urinary deposits, 518
Urinary tract infections (UTIs), 298, 302, 330, 346–48, 352, 515, 521
Urinometer, 507
Urobilinogen, 182, 508, 510–12
Urticaria, 484

V

Vaccines, 228, 264
Vaginal discharge, 386
Vaginitis, 392, 521
Valine, 59, 174
Van den Bergh reaction, 223
Varicella-zoster virus, 418, 558
Vasopressin, 207
VDRL, 251, 258, 358, 571
Vectors, 395
Venereal diseases, 251, 258
Venipuncture, 605
Venous blood, 47–48, 66, 72, 76, 94, 255, 486
Vibrio, 275, 288, 292, 319, 348–49, 531, 596
Vibrio cholerae, 288, 292, 319, 348, 596
Vibrio parahaemolyticus, 349
Vibrio spp., 292, 348–49, 531
Virion, 410–12, 419
Viruses, 5, 21, 227, 288, 410, 412, 414–15, 423, 605
Viscosity, 25, 50
Vitamin B12, 65
Vitamin K, 107, 547
Vitamins, 548
Voges-Proskauer test, 307–8
Vomiting, 530
von Willebrand factor, 555, 597

W

Waldenstrom's macroglobulinemia, 92, 436
Warm autoantibodies, 437, 459
Wassermann test, 254
Water, 20, 27, 72, 310, 318, 380, 504

Printed in the United States
by Baker & Taylor Publisher Services